More praise for *Pills That Work, Pills*

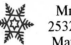
"Extremely practical . . . Refreshing and insightful analysis of one of the most important things a doctor does for his or her patient—prescribe medications for common, and sometimes life-threatening, ailments. . . . This remarkable book should be required reading for all health care consumers in this country, especially those who desire more personal involvement in, control over, and responsibility for their own medical care and that of their children."

—NORMAN CHRISTOPHER, M.D., FAAP
Associate Professor of Pediatrics and
Emergency Medicine
Northeast Ohio Universities

"Dr. Bosker raises the true flag for health care. . . . *Pills That Work, Pills That Don't* is a book that needs to be read, and Dr. Bosker's is a voice that needs to be heard. . . . Dr. Bosker returns to the physician's patient-centered roots. As the 'sleeping giant' of the health care profession slowly awakens, Dr. Bosker's book will help light the way."

—GEORGE R. SCHWARTZ, M.D.
Editor-in-Chief
Principles and Practice of Emergency Medicine

"In this excellent treatise on pills and their pitfalls, Dr. Bosker provides valuable and needed information. . . . Individuals who take advantage of this book can anticipate a better quality—and, hopefully, duration—of life by using the best medications available, and equally important, by avoiding the potentially serious and life-threatening problems associated with ineffective medications and drug-drug interactions. This groundbreaking book is recommended for all health care consumers who wish to assume greater control of and responsibility for their own health, personal pharmacology, and future well-being. Don't leave your pharmacy or doctor's office without it."

—ALBERT C. WEIHL, M.D., FACEP
Assistant Professor of Medicine and Surgery
Yale University School of Medicine

"Wow, what a book! . . . Consumers need ammunition . . . and this book gives new meaning to 'less is more.' . . . It is an invaluable tool all homes should have."

—Harry Henwood, Pharmacy Manager

"This excellent reference gives consumers the skills needed to work responsibly and communicate effectively with their doctors."

—*New Orleans Times-Picayune*

"Bosker's combination exposé and self-help guide is readable and even rousing. . . . An informed and responsible book."

—*Booklist*

PiLLS THAT WORK

−

PiLLS THAT DON'T

•

DEMANDING—AND GETTING—THE BEST AND SAFEST MEDICATIONS FOR YOU AND YOUR FAMILY

GIDEON BOSKER, M.D.

Fawcett Columbine
The Ballantine Publishing Group • New York

A Fawcett Columbine Book
Published by The Ballantine Publishing Group

Copyright © 1997 by Gideon Bosker

All rights reserved under International and Pan-American Copyright Conventions. Published in the United States by The Ballantine Publishing Group, a division of Random House, Inc., New York, and distributed in Canada by Random House of Canada Limited, Toronto.

http://www.randomhouse.com

Library of Congress Catalog Card Number: 98-96386

ISBN: 0-449-91273-6

This edition published by arrangement with Harmony Books, a division of Crown Publishers, Inc.

Cover design by Ruth Ross
Design by Nancy Singer

Manufactured in the United States of America

First Fawcett Columbine Edition: November 1998

10 9 8 7 6 5 4 3 2 1

To all my patients
who, over the years,
have taught me the difference
between pills that work, and
pills that don't

Contents

Acknowledgments

This book represents a gratifying collaboration among many talented and unusual individuals who, from my perspective, have been devoted not only to producing a book of the highest editorial quality, but were genuinely committed to publishing a volume that would make life better, safer, and healthier for those who read it. Working with people who are not only refined and rigorous in their editorial and publishing acumen, but who also maintain the highest professional standards, has made the completion of this project a challenge and a pleasure. However, working with such individuals, when they also share a commitment to improve quality of health and life for others through the written word, has catapulted this project into even more meaningful territory.

In this regard, I would first like to thank my editor, Leslie Meredith, whose guidance, insight, and command of the editorial, informational, and organizational issues that govern a book of this scope were essential. She provided the intellectual infrastucture necessary to produce a work that would serve an ambidextrous function; a book that would both articulate problems and pitfalls in the health care industry, and that would also provide practical, empowering solutions to these problems for its readers. Part-consultant, part-editor, part-taskmaster—and always on target—Ms. Meredith has the special gift of making a writer demand more of himself and his own work, and in the process, ensures that the reader also gets much more than they would have otherwise, had her turbocharged editorial wand not been hyperactive throughout the entire natural history of the project.

Deep respect and gratitude are also extended to Andrew Stuart, assistant editor. Always perspicacious, a consummate diplomat, and appropriately cajoling when conditions required it, Mr. Stuart played the difficult role of vigilant train master and conceptual confidant. I wish to acknowledge his many excellent suggestions for how features in this manuscript might be presented, his critical analysis of the book's important elements, and his discerning judgment throughout the book's development.

Special acknowledgment is also due to Mark Mayell. An accomplished writer, journalist, editor—and an especially sophisticated analyst of the contemporary medical and medication scene—Mr. Mayell helped provide an organizational scheme for the manuscript during its initial stages. I would like to thank Mr. Mayell for his critical reading of the manuscript in its early form and for his substantial rewrites and revisions of key sections in this book. Mr. Mayell's editorial input into this project during a critical step in its evolution was invaluable and deserves high praise.

Janet Biehl is also due special appreciation for copyediting the book, fact-checking drug names, and providing stylistic consistency. I am especially grateful for her insightful commentary as to how this information would best be presented for a general audience. I would also like to thank production editors Liana Parry and Chris Fortunato for their excellent assistance in this effort.

Many other people at Harmony Books and in the Crown Publishing Group supplied their creative talents, guidance, and professional expertise to ensure that this book would register on the health, self-empowerment radar screen, and therefore, would make a positive difference in as many people's lives as possible.

First and foremost, I would like to extend my respect and appreciation to Chip Gibson, publisher and vice president at the Crown Publishing Group. At a time when so many publishers take a distant seat from the day-to-day editorial, sales, and positioning issues that arise during a book's journey to the printer, Mr. Gibson commandeered this project with intelligence and grace throughout all its critical stages, providing illuminating commentary and midcourse corrections when required. Mr. Gibson has the unique talents of

providing encouragement and steadiness when required, but also the creativity to explore innovative venues for bringing a book to the widest possible audience.

I have special respect for and sincerely acknowledge the efforts, interest, and talents of Tina Constable and Brian Belfiglio of the Crown publicity department. I appreciate the time they took to give this book a careful reading, as well as their thought-provoking analysis of how this information should best be communicated to health care organizations and the media, so that the largest audience possible could benefit from the book's information. Ms. Constable's and Mr. Belfiglio's deep interest in and profound understanding of the book's subject matter and intended purpose have stimulated me to refine my approach to how consumers should be informed about issues surrounding medication use.

Many friends and family members provided support, humor, and insightful commentary throughout the project. I would especially like to thank my mother, Dorothy Bosker, Lena Lencek, Bianca Lencek-Bosker, Karen Brooks, Paul and Susan Stander, Joanne Day, Gene MacDonald, David Wilson, and the library staff at Good Samaritan Hospital, Portland, Oregon.

Finally, I would like to thank Richard Pine of Arthur Pine Associates. Although, as a literary agent, Mr. Pine does not have an MD after his name, he might as well have. It is a special and unusual pleasure to have collaborated with someone who not only is a stickler about editorial quality and originality, but who also shares a commitment to use the written word for the purpose of bringing information that can be used to improve quality-of-life to the general public. His commanding knowledge and unusual insights into contemporary issues governing the consumer health movement—and into the medical landscape, in general—explain why Mr. Pine was a cornerstone and valuable collaborator on this project from its inception.

Author's Note

The information in this book is intended to be used for educational purposes only. The reader is cautioned not to make any assumptions about, or make any alterations, additions, or deletions to, their medication intake based on information in this book. All the principles, concepts, and information contained herein should be applied only in collaboration with, and under the close, attentive, supervision of, a physician. All medications—including those that are mentioned or discussed in this book, as well as those that are not—should be taken, evaluated, monitored, and adjusted only under a doctor's close supervision. Medications should not be started without a prescription from your doctor. Moreover, no medication should be discontinued, have its dosage changed, have its dosing frequency altered, or be replaced with another medication, unless specifically instructed by a physician. This book is not intended to guide drug therapy in any specific individual or to serve as a guide for making drug choices, except under the care of a licensed physician. Recommendations regarding specific medications represent the author's opinion, are made for illustrative purposes only, and do not imply the superiority or inferiority of one medication over another.

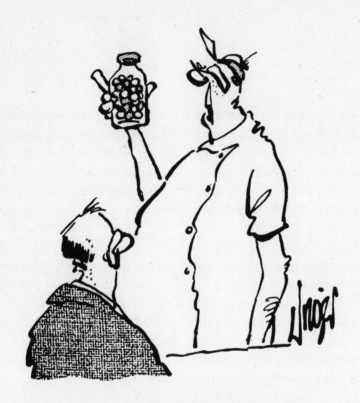

"I'm not sure what these are, but
take them for a couple of weeks
and let me know how you feel."

Introduction

EMPOWERING HEALTH CARE CONSUMERS

This book is about nothing less than a life-or-death, feel-well-or-feel-like-hell issue. The fact is, there are pills that you need and pills that you don't. There are pills that kill and pills that save; pills that cause adverse effects and pills that prevent disease. There are pills that work and pills that don't.

Unfortunately, making these distinctions is difficult even for the most talented physician. In the world of clinical medicine, however, experience is frequently the best guide. And after more than fifteen years of evaluating and treating patients who were suffering from the consequences of excessive, inappropriate, or suboptimal prescription drugs, I feel there is a need for this "fewer pills, better health" book that empowers consumers and families, in collaboration with their physicians, to improve the quality of medications prescribed on their behalf.

Pills That Work, Pills That Don't is the culmination of my lifelong goal to make medication use in the United States a safer and more effective enterprise. It combines unbiased, authoritative information about prescription drugs with an action plan for eliminating and replacing unnecessary, ineffective, and unsafe prescription medications. It helps get people off bad pills and on good ones. It distinguishes between tragic bullets and magic bullets. It encourages lifestyle changes that reduce the need for drug therapy. Finally, it makes physicians and institutions accountable for unsafe and irrational drug-prescribing practices, while encouraging patients and their families to take more responsibility for monitoring the progress of their therapy.

There has never been a greater need for involving patients and their families in medication decisions. The total number of prescription drugs, as well as the overall quantities taken by health care consumers, has skyrocketed in recent years. Better living through pharmacology has become a way of life—and with good reason: When used wisely, drugs are fundamental to maintaining good health. Few will disagree that appropriately prescribed medications can help keep people alive. Drugs can cure potentially fatal diseases. They make it possible for people like you and me to lead more productive, active, and pain-free lives. Stated simply, drugs are some of the most ingenious bio-molecular solutions ever devised to keep the Grim Reaper at bay.

That's the good news. Along with pill power, however, come pill problems. The bad news is that inappropriate, excessive, and sub-optimal drug prescribing is a silent killer. As essential as drug therapy is to the maintenance of good health, medications also have the capacity to make you feel bad or even sick. Many factors—some hidden and others clearly visible—have brought about the alarming in-crease in medication-related problems being reported in both medical journals and the lay press. The wide range of available medications complicates choices for physicians and, there-fore, increases the risks of excessive prescrib-ing, interactions, and side effects.

It is a problem that touches all of us—young and old, sick and well, rich and poor. In fact, in the current health care environment it constitutes a hidden epidemic—no age group, gender, or demographic profile is spared the pitfalls associated with prescription medica-tion use. Children develop serious infections because their antibiotics are ineffective against common bacterial pathogens; young adults become dependent on anxiety-reducing drugs such as Xanax; and the elderly suffer from the gastrointestinal complications of the non-steroidal anti-inflammatory drugs (NSAIDs) used to treat arthritis. Each of us knows some-one who has been the victim of a drug-related mishap. Accordingly, every family and every health care consumer must have access to de-finitive information—such as is provided here—that will empower them to evaluate the quality and safety of prescription medications prescribed on their behalf, and to guide their physicians toward optimum choices.

No other medical issue affects so many of us on such a regular basis or has such far-reaching implications for longevity and health. You may not be able to influence all the factors that cause inappropriate, unsafe, and suboptimal drug prescribing, but you can communicate and collaborate clearly with your prescribing practitioner. You can also be well informed in your approach to the health care plan or system that selects medications for your use.

Doctors, pharmacists, consumer advo-cacy groups, and public policy makers con-cur that a patient-driven program aimed at improving drug therapy could make a dra-matic impact on the health of millions of Americans. Armed with targeted, *Consumer Reports*-like recommendations about drugs in current use, and a proven action plan for medication reduction, people from all walks of life can become "physician assistants" in drug prescribing.

They will be able to direct physicians and other prescribers toward approaches that minimize medications to maximize re-sults; toward prescribing habits that im-prove health and increase longevity while maintaining quality of life; and toward a new, alternative mission statement for drug prescribing that encompasses all of the fac-tors involved in medication use: cost, user-friendliness, side effects, performance levels, durability, dose considerations, and preven-tive health maintenance.

THE PATIENT REVOLUTION

The information and health-improvement strategies contained in this book are the result of years of research, clinical experience, consultations, and interactions with health care professionals—including doctors, pharmacists, and nurses—who have devoted their lives to making medication use safer, simpler, and more effective. I have also reviewed and analyzed more than three thousand clinical trials published in the medical literature.

The reforms I advocate in this book have already helped thousands of patients maximize the safety and effectiveness of their medication use. Many of the concepts and specific drug choices I recommend in *Pills That Work, Pills That Don't* have been presented in more technical fashion in a book I wrote for professional health care providers called *Pharmatecture: Minimizing Medications to Maximize Results*. It was published in 1996 by Facts and Comparisons, one of the world's largest and most respected publishers of drug information. Their reference books and newsletters, updates, and drug evaluations, with more than 80,000 pharmacist and physician subscribers, are considered the primary pharmacotherapeutic resources for thousands of doctors of pharmacy (Pharm. D.'s), pharmacy directors, and physicians working in academic institutions, community hospitals, managed care networks, and health maintenance organization (HMO) pharmacy departments across the country.

Pharmatecture presents a hands-on approach to optimizing the selection of outpatient medications. One of the nation's leading doctors of pharmacy, Michael Reed of New York, has said that this book "should be required reading for anyone before putting a pen to prescription pad. . . . In fact, I would make this book required reading for all prescribers if it were within my power." Another Pharm. D., Stephen Ernest, has written, "*Pharmatecture* is the answer pharmacists and physicians have been looking for. Whether clinicians are practicing in a managed care environment or institutional setting, [this] book is the first comprehensive, broad-based pharmaceutical/drug therapy reference designed to meet the needs of prescribing practitioners, while, at the same time, focusing on comprehensive patient care . . . this book will produce superior clinical outcomes for the prescribing physician and pharmacist, regardless of their practice setting."

In the past few years I've described the concepts outlined in *Pharmatecture* in face-to-face appearances before 50,000 physicians at more than a thousand hospitals and clinics across the country. Professional, academic, and institutional support for these principles has been overwhelming. This systematic, "less is more" program for optimizing drug regimens has begun to penetrate deeply into both the physician and the pharmacy communities and has been widely adopted at hundreds of hospitals and clinics across the United States.

The *Pharmatecture* program was the beginning—and represents only one component of—a revolution in drug therapy. The second phase of this revolution is to bring all the benefits of this program *directly to health care consumers.* With so many new therapeutic agents tumbling into the physician's armamentarium, it's time for patients to take the lead in refining and upgrading prescribing patterns. Informed patients will hold physicians accountable for their drug choices. With the help of *Pills That Work, Pills That Don't,* they will be able to identify more effective and less toxic drug choices that are better tailored for their health needs. Armed with this information, and working in collaboration with their physicians, Americans will achieve better therapeutic results with fewer pills and side effects.

I am convinced that this consumer-driven revolution is the perfect—and at present the only—viable antidote to physician and institutional deficiencies in drug prescribing. A patient-activated medication-management plan can produce dramatic health improvements for people with problems ranging from premature skin aging and allergies to depression and heart disease. First and foremost, this book helps individuals distinguish between better drugs and worse drugs for the common ailments that affect 90 percent of the population. It helps people discriminate between medications that have been proven to prolong life by preventing disease and those that provide only symptomatic relief or temporary remissions.

Although consumers have to be part of the treatment process, much drug-related information is technical and appears to be beyond the comprehension of most nonphysicians. How does a patient like you safeguard the quality of your or your family's medication regimen? Without question, the recent publication of consumer-oriented pill information books that list medications and their essential properties—indications, side effects, contraindications, and interactions—are an important step in providing such information. A number of these books have been popularly received by the general public, but they all lack authoritative guidance or a ranking system that can help you distinguish between better pills and inferior pills, between pills that work well and pills that don't. They also all lack the unique 12-Week Action Plan in *Pills That Work, Pills That Don't* that provides a step-by-step approach for getting off pills that you don't need or that pose unnecessary risks.

A PLANNED PHARMACOLOGICAL ECONOMY

For all practical purposes, the health care industry in America today has made drug selection a mysterious, inconsistent, and erratic process, governed for the most part by bottom-line concerns linked to the sordid cash nexus. Profit-wise, pill-foolish decisions now dominate the inner sanctum of managed care organizations and HMOs, which have the power to decide which pills you will be able to take and which ones you won't. Call it a "planned pharmacological economy"—put simply, the market forces that would normally supply the best medications to the most demanding customers have completely broken down. The implications are staggering. Consumers have become increasingly powerless over their pharmacological destiny. Millions of people, like you, who pay premium dollars for health insurance are denied access to top-of-the-line pills. Complicating these problems is the fact that no reliable source provides the essential information required to make educated decisions about drugs.

What this means is that your freedom to choose the best and safest medications for you and your family is in serious jeopardy. Many of the critical decisions affecting medications you and your family need now occur behind closed doors, without your input and frequently without the input of even your doctor. In fact, many of these decisions are made by administrators who are driven by bottom-line money concerns affecting the profitability of health plans, rather than by the value issues—safety, efficacy, convenience, side effects, and versatility—surrounding a particular medication. Other considerations that have absolutely nothing to do with the quality of medications include discounts that health plans and HMOs get from pharmaceutical companies or drug wholesalers, and the personal and professional relationships between pharmacy directors or medical researchers and pharmaceutical companies.

What we do know is that you, as a health care consumer, are imperiled. You are an outsider and have been forced to play by the rules of a two-tiered health care system that is divided into medication "haves" and "have-nots." Lacking authoritative, unbiased sources of drug information, you may not even know to which group you belong.

Although the pharmaceutical landscape is full of wonderful medications that prevent disease and relieve symptoms rapidly, you may never have the opportunity to use the best available options. The fact is, some people have access to better medications than others. Much of this is determined by the health care plan to which they belong. Some have more restrictive medication policies than others. For example, one health plan may permit its physicians to prescribe Imitrex (for migraine), Norvasc (for high blood pressure), Prevacid (for ulcers), or Zithromax (for infections) without fear of penalty or reprisal, whereas others may discourage initial use of these top-of-line, "best-in-class" medications.

In large managed care organizations, pharmacists, doctors, and administrators hold regular "pharmacy and therapeutics" meetings to discuss drug policies, options, and procedures. Although the decisions they make have a profound impact on your health, your access to optimal medications, and your quality of life, the process is concealed from public scrutiny. It may even be hidden from view of most of the physicians who participate in the health plan. Once these people have decided which drugs will be available to your physician, you have little, if any, opportunity to overturn the decision.

Consider the following analogy. You go to a stockbroker whose research team analyzes, specializes in, and issues a certain group of stocks or mutual funds. The brokerage firm "makes market" in these stocks—it has a financial interest in and profits from seeing that its clients buy shares of them and in having them perform well. To enhance the sales of these equities, the brokerage encourages its sales brokers—in fact, it provides them with monetary and bonus incentives—to recommend that you purchase them. Meanwhile, you have learned from reliable sources that other stocks, in which your firm does not make market, are performing much better than those recommended by your broker. With enough pressure, you could encourage your broker to purchase whatever stocks you request, but your broker will profit more handsomely by recommending the stocks "affiliated" with his or her brokerage firm. Stated simply, your stockbroker has a powerful incentive to steer you toward those equities that have favored status within his or her particular company. If these stocks are high performers, you will benefit, but if they aren't, you will suffer due to these restrictive policies.

The same is true for the way medications are prescribed, especially if you belong to an HMO or managed care plan. In this case, the restrictive drug policies are imposed at the formulary level. A *formulary* is a list of medications that have been approved by a health plan for routine use by its physicians. If favorable pricing practices or strong affiliations with certain pharmaceutical companies motivate a health plan to include a specific group of medications on its formulary, these are the drugs that the health plan will encourage for initial use.

Of course, if your health plan has the vision to select the best medications, you are in luck. But if your health plan has selected drugs primarily on the basis of cost, to a great extent you will be denied access to optimal medications, at least on the first go-around. Your doctor usually won't tell you what other options are available because the health plan has encouraged him or her to prescribe, at least initially, only drugs listed in its formulary. These may not always be the best pills on the market. One of the purposes of this book is to teach you how to demand—and get—the best pills available for you and your family.

To a great extent, this is a secret society of pill selectors and pill prescribers. When your doctor writes a prescription for you, he is making a "pharmacological" referral. The question is, is he or she "referring" you to a better drug or a worse drug? To a drug that's more expensive or less expensive? More often than not, you are completely out of the loop. Imagine if you went to a real estate broker who showed you only houses that were listed by his or her particular firm. That would be outrageous. That's why real estate brokers use multiple-listing services, which present the full range of real estate properties that are available in a particular area.

Unfortunately, when it comes to drug selection, especially within the context of managed care plans and HMOs, there usually is no multiple-listing service for all available medications. Rather, the physician is restricted to choosing from a narrow range of options. You need a way out of this dilemma. One of the most important purposes of this book is to take you behind the scenes so that you can make informed decisions about medications. The MedRANK Checklists in Part II of this book will help you distinguish between optimal medications and less favorable alternatives.

PENETRATING THE DRUG SECRECY BARRIER: HOW DO YOU FIND OUT WHICH DRUGS ARE BEST?

In the current climate of pharmacological secrecy and closed-door policy making, it is not easy for the average health care consumer to identify which medications are best. The fact is, you are denied most of the critical information that you would normally need to make an informed decision. As a result, negotiating your personal pharmacological needs is a difficult process. When it comes to prescription drugs, for the most part you are operating in the dark. This presents an unusual paradox. Although consumers are deluged with information about many day-to-day products and services that do not have life-or-death, sickness-or-health consequences, they are poorly informed about their personal drug intake and its profound impact on their well-being.

In virtually every aspect of our lives, we try to make informed decisions based on quality, value, safety, and convenience. Why shouldn't quality-based issues govern decisions about medications as well? The point is, they should. We are an upgrade-obsessed culture. Whenever possible, we want our cars, hotel rooms, and software upgraded. Why shouldn't our drugs be upgraded too? The problem is, getting information about medications is much more difficult than it is for other products. You can't rely on customary channels of information or your "street smarts" when it comes to pills. Even from a purely logistical perspective, it is difficult if not impossible to gather a critical mass of information about most medications. You can't get a statistically valid sampling from your friends or neighbors, as you can from asking them how they like their Jeep Cherokee or whether they are happy with their Windows software or what quality of fish is available at the local supermarket. Because these kinds of products are in wide use, you can usually collect enough information to make an informed decision.

But you can't test-drive a drug. Generally speaking, it takes a long time—sometimes several weeks—before you know whether you are going to like a medication and whether it is going to produce the result you need. Proactive approaches to drug selection are limited because there's no one to ask and not enough people to provide a reasonable body of opinion. The fact is, you simply don't have enough friends who are taking the calcium channel blocker Norvasc, or who are using Imitrex to treat migraine headaches, or who have taken the antiviral drug Valtrex, to gain enough information to decide whether these are good pills or bad pills. You simply don't have enough friends to tell you whether a particular medication is convenient, whether it's user-friendly, or whether it works. Yes, you can ask your doctor, but many barriers at the physician and institutional level may prevent you from getting the real scoop there as well.

Herein lies the pharmacological rub. To a great extent, when it comes to deciding whether a medication is high quality or low quality, you are in the dark. Unlike automobiles, clothes, and real estate, you can't judge a pill by its cover. All pills and tablets, for the most part, look very similar, yet any two pills will usually cause vastly different benefits and pitfalls. The quality, risks, and effectiveness of various pills are essentially hidden from view. The medication rating system, i.e., the MedRANK Checklists, provided in Part II of this book, offer a sensible option for steering you and your physician in the right direction. They provide unbiased and authoritative rankings of medications. If you study them carefully, you can demand—and get—the best and safest prescription medications for you and your family.

DO YOU DESERVE THE BEST PRESCRIPTION MEDICATIONS?

You might ask yourself, "Do I deserve the best?" The answer is, of course you do! When it comes to sickness and health, you and your family deserve nothing less than the best. It is absolutely outrageous that your health plan would not make all optimal medications available to you and your family for a particular problem or medical condition. Let's say you pay $1,800 a year for health insurance. Some people require health care on a regular basis, but many others need to see their primary care physician only once or twice a year. What this means, from a purely dollars-and-cents point of view, is that many people are paying the equivalent of $900 for a biannual office visit. In other words, if you have to see your physician only a couple of times a year, those office visits carry a real premium.

Now, let's say you pay a visit to that physician for a common problem, such as a bacterial sinus infection. How would you feel if your physician prescribed a $12 antibiotic for your problem, rather than a $35 antibiotic, simply because the health plan provides strong incentives to him or her to prescribe the cheaper medication first? You would be outraged, as I would be. And what if you also learned that the cheaper medication required ten days of drug therapy rather than five days for the better drug, had a 20 percent chance of producing nausea or vomiting as opposed to 3 percent for the better drug, and was not the most effective medication for that condition? Does this kind of policy make sense? Is it appropriate for your health plan to save $25 on a course of antibiotic therapy when you are paying $1,800 a year for health insurance? Absolutely not!

It seems to me that the health plan should be more than willing to spend the additional $25 for the antibiotic that is dosed on a more convenient basis, has a lower risk of side effects, has a lower risk of interactions with other drugs, and is likely to be a more effective cure the first time around. Stated simply, it is inconceivable that a health plan would try to save $25 by putting your convenience and health on the line. But that is exactly what they do.

To overcome these institutional barriers and pitfalls and to help identify the best medications for a particular disease, you can consult the MedRANK Checklists. Armed with this information, you can then gently suggest to your physician that these are the medications you would like him or her to consider first for your medical problem.

LEGAL ISSUES COME TO THE FORE

Fortunately, the federal government has adopted new policies that limit the kinds of incentives that HMOs can pay to doctors as rewards for controlling costs. These new rules will likely set a standard for the entire managed care industry. They are part of an effort to address the fears of patients that, as they are drawn into HMOs and other managed care plans, financial factors will increasingly influence doctors' clinical decisions. In particular, there has been concern that doctors will deny patients needed services so that they can keep their costs in line with the annual budget generated by the health plan.

The New England Journal of Medicine summarized these concerns in an editorial in its September 1996 issue: "The quality of health care is now seriously threatened by our rapid shift to managed care as the way to contain costs," it said. "Managed care plans involve an inherent conflict of interest. On the one hand, they pledge to take care of their enrollees, but on the other, their financial success depends on doing as little for them as possible."

Most of the incentives and restrictions addressed by the federal regulations are those that apply to patterns of referral to specialists and to high-technology care. But these concerns are just as important for the world of drug prescribing. If a physician is given incentives to use a low-cost medication first, he or she is essentially "referring" you to a lower-cost drug option. From a legal and conceptual point of view, such cost-based "pharmacological referrals" should also be addressed by federal legislation. Restrictive drug-prescribing policies, from a conceptual and legal point of view, are simply limitations in treatment options. Although doctors say that the "gag clauses" that discourage them from discussing expensive treatment options apply primarily to specialized care, the fact is that they are equally relevant to drug prescribing. New rules governing drug prescribing in managed care organizations are desperately needed.

HOW TO USE THIS BOOK

Pills That Work, Pills That Don't is organized into three parts. Part I, "Why You May Not Be Getting the Best and Safest Prescription Drugs," contains three chapters. The first two summarize the benefits and dangers, respectively, of prescription drugs, and the third outlines the principal changes necessary to reform prescription drug practice.

Part II, "The MedRANK Checklists: A Rating System for Prescription Medications," is the bulk of the book, and consists of rankings of hundreds of prescription medications. The chapters are organized around specific medical conditions such as heart disease, allergies, and childhood ailments. The drugs are ranked as follows:

- **Optimal** (Highly Recommended/Best of Class)
- **Recommended** (Acceptable with Reservations)
- **Discouraged for Initial Use** (But May Be Required in Selected People)
- **Avoid If Possible** (Not Recommended)

The fact-filled analyses and the many "pearls" of drug-related information in these rankings can help you determine whether you are having drug-related problems and how to identify medications better matched to your needs, including prevention-oriented drug therapy. You will also learn what questions to ask your physician so as to direct him or her toward streamlined regimens consisting of safe medications that will enhance the quality of your life. It should be stressed that the advantages and disadvantages of medications often vary by drug class. In some cases they may be determined by the risk of drug interactions, in others by compliance patterns, side effects, or efficacy.

Part III, "The 12-Week Action Plan: Getting the Best and Safest Prescription Drugs," describes proven strategies for eliminating, consolidating, or replacing unnecessary, inappropriate, or unsafe prescription drugs. This Action Plan is the critical bridge on the road from medication *information* to *application*, a difficult and frequently treacherous path even for physicians. It has been a long time coming and is desperately needed. The Action Plan is a proven medication-reduction and -refinement program based on a dialogue between patient and doctor. It will inform and empower you to become a full-fledged collaborator with your physician. Using the Action Plan as an interface, you and your practitioner can work together to build a more durable, user-friendly medication program. You can use specific MedRANK Checklists to steer your doctor toward optimal drugs. The goal is for patients and physicians to work together to produce lean, mean drug regimens

that do more with less: that produce maximal results with the best drugs currently available, while minimizing the number of medications required to get the job done.

CONCLUSION

The analysis of the problem in Part I, the drug-by-drug recommendations in Part II, and the 12-Week Action Plan in Part III are all based on four basic principles:

1. Drugs are not created equal. Some are better than others, and all too often patients don't end up taking the optimal ones.
2. Many prescription medications that people are currently taking can be eliminated or reduced in dosage without adversely affecting their health or clinical condition. There are myriad opportunities for minimizing medications to maximize results. In addition, many medications that are useful for preventing disease are underused.
3. If consumers are armed with good information, they can approach their physicians with targeted inquiries and specific recommendations that can guide them toward medications that are more user-friendly, produce fewer side effects, are less toxic, and yield better outcomes. Over the long term, this process will reduce health care costs for these patients.

4. Lifestyle changes can reduce dependence on drug therapy and permit patients to manage their health status with nonpharmacological alternatives.

Although the analogy is perhaps a bit simplistic, *Pills That Work, Pills That Don't* is in one sense a "diet book for pills." The objective is to reduce not calorie intake but the intake of prescription drugs. Instead of shifting from high-calorie foods to low-calorie ones, consumers are presented with hundreds of options for switching from high-risk drug classes (such as tricyclic antidepressants and theophylline compounds) to low-risk drug classes (such as selective serotonin-reuptake inhibitors and inhaled beta-agonists). And instead of feeling better because they have lost weight, they will have an improved sense of well-being because they have shed the side effects and toxicity that accompany so many prescription medications.

The key to this approach is to make people aware of how they feel on their medications, provide them with state-of-the-art information—and specific recommendations—about commonly used drugs, and teach them how to ask their prescribing physicians the right questions. "Doctor, do I need a medication? Should I take this drug or that one? What are the advantages and disadvantages, the risks and benefits, of each? How should I take it? Should we add a drug to my current regimen? Do I need all the medications I am taking, or are there some that we can gradually discontinue? Do I need to tolerate the side effects of this drug, or is there another medication that is just as effective but has fewer side effects? Am I taking the best drug in its class, or simply the cheapest, because my managed care organization is trying to save money? When should I begin to question the length of time I've been on this drug?"

These are the kinds of questions this book answers in a clear, concise manner. But not only does it present a road map to optimum drug therapy, it also emphasizes lifestyle changes, such as dietary modifications, smoking cessation, exercise programs, and environmental controls, that make possible nonpharmacological approaches to health maintenance. The end result for you will be improved health, a longer life, fewer pills—and substantial cost savings.

PART I

—

WHY YOU MAY NOT
BE GETTING
THE BEST AND SAFEST
PRESCRIPTION DRUGS

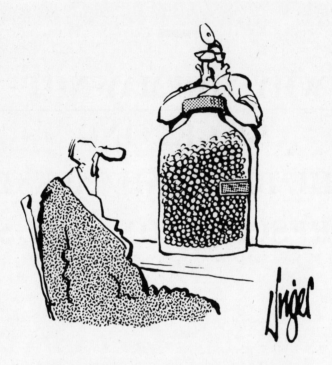

"I hope you're not one of those people
who have trouble swallowing pills."

CHAPTER 1

▬

PILLS THAT WORK . . .

When I first saw Jennifer S., her clothes were disheveled, her hair and skin were unhealthy looking, and her eyes seemed flat and lifeless. After talking with her, it became clear that she suffered from a number of problems. A college grad in her late twenties, she had just moved to the area to take a new job. The demands of work, plus the fact that she was having a hard time making new friends, were taking a toll on her. Normally outgoing and somewhat high strung, she was feeling increasingly listless and stressed out. In fact, her symptoms were significant enough to satisfy the criteria for a diagnosis of depression. Jennifer was also falling into poor dietary and lifestyle habits (eating junk food, not getting enough exercise) and was having trouble kicking a persistent vaginal infection.

After taking a medical history and examining her, I tried to help her address various issues in her life. I also gave her prescriptions for two drugs. I suggested the antidepressant Zoloft as a temporary crutch for her emotional

difficulties. Like its better-known cousin Prozac, Zoloft can often have a positive effect on mood and emotion. Unlike Prozac, Zoloft seems less often to be associated with over-stimulation as a side effect, so I thought it would probably be more appropriate for a high-strung person like Jennifer.

In the past Jennifer had found it difficult to comply with the necessity to take a prescription drug three times per day for an entire week to treat a vaginal infection. Fortunately, I was able to offer her an alternative medication—Diflucan, a broad-spectrum antifungal agent—that was much easier to use and just as effective. I knew that a single 150 mg dose of Diflucan, taken in my office, was probably all that she would need to clear up her vaginal condition.

Over the course of the next few months, Jennifer's physical and emotional condition improved remarkably. Some of the changes had nothing to do with the antidepressant—she was seeing a mental health counselor, and she joined a local health club, for example—but the medication definitely helped. The vaginal infection quickly disappeared and had not come back. More important, her outward appearance brightened up, her eyes regained their natural sparkle, and her confidence and zest for life seemed to return. Each time I saw her, we reevaluated her condition and adjusted the medication schedule, gradually tapering her dosage of Zoloft. After twelve months, she seemed healthy and well adjusted and no longer required the medication at all.

In these days of recurrent horror stories about prescription drugs, it is worth reminding ourselves that many medications can be beneficial and even life-saving. When drugs are used wisely and cautiously, they have the capacity to make people well, improve or relieve disabling symptoms, enhance their quality of life, and even prolong their survival. At least in the industrialized world, prescription medications are so widely available and so readily used that we have come to take their remarkable properties for granted. Yet anyone who lived more than a century ago and who had the misfortune to suffer from any of a number of intractable and frequently fatal conditions would have regarded as miraculous the drugs we have at our disposal today. Consider the following:

- **Penicillin:** The first modern antibiotic, penicillin, was identified only in 1928 by Scottish bacteriologist Alexander Fleming. Its acceptance and use were delayed until the last two years of World War II, when Allied doctors used it to save the lives of thousands of wounded soldiers. Since coming onto the consumer market after the war, penicillin has prevented the premature deaths of countless people who would have otherwise died from various systemic bacterial infections, including syphilis, pneumonia, osteomyelitis, and endocarditis.

- **Vaccinations:** Until effective vaccination campaigns against smallpox were developed in the 1950s, this virulent infectious disease had claimed the lives of millions of people for at least three thousand years. When smallpox struck a population that had not been exposed to it, it approached genocidal potency—upward of 90 percent of those infected succumbed to its effects. Though a cure was never discovered, the success of drugs to prevent smallpox led the World Health Organization (WHO) in 1980 to declare the disease eradicated worldwide.

- **Insulin:** First recognized in the early 1920s, it has allowed millions of diabetics to live full and active lives that would otherwise have been cut short by the adverse effects of diabetes on metabolism, circulation, vision, and other bodily systems.

- **Depression:** Since the late 1950s, medical researchers have been able to design drugs that raise or lower levels of certain brain chemicals that affect mood and emotion. These new classes of antidepressants—especially the selective serotonin-reuptake inhibitors (SSRIs), including

Prozac and its cousins, available only since the late 1980s—have benefited millions of people who would otherwise suffer from depression or experience the intolerable side effects of drugs previously used to treat the condition.

Of course, this list of medical successes does not even touch upon the myriad other modern drugs whose effects have been useful if somewhat less dramatic or one-sidedly positive. It is quite possible that chemotherapeutic agents to treat cancer, the "cocktail" of new drugs to help fight HIV infection, innovative cholesterol-lowering agents, and many other drugs will someday be recognized along with penicillin and insulin in the drug hall of fame.

Pharmaceutical companies are spending huge amounts of money to research, develop, test, and market new drugs each year. Admittedly, they stand to make hundreds of millions in profits if a new drug succeeds. Yet health care consumers are bigger winners when a medication comes along that eradicates a previously incurable condition, that alleviates the symptoms of a painful ailment, that prevents a costly hospitalization or invasive procedure, or perhaps most important, that prevents the spread of a deadly communicable disease.

AN OUNCE OF PREVENTION

Despite the dramatic health improvements that come from disease-prevention strategies (such as smoking cessation, weight loss, exercise, nutritional modifications, blood pressure control, and reduction of excessive alcohol intake), preventive medicine is still the battered stepchild of modern medicine. This is especially true when it comes to drug therapy. Many doctors and public health officials agree that the most overlooked group of potentially beneficial drugs are those that can be taken to *prevent* disease. Because of inadequate physician education, poor dissemination of clinical trial results, and time pressures exerted by cost-driven health care systems, millions of people are falling through the cracks and being denied the benefits of prevention-oriented medications. These drugs include:

- **Aspirin:** Studies have established that low daily doses (such as 80 mg) can help prevent heart disease.
- **Estrogen:** This hormone has been shown to reduce the risk of heart attack by 47 percent in postmenopausal women who have one or more risk factors for heart disease. Although estrogen's ability to prevent heart disease is well recognized by the medical community, many women in this age group have never had their physician fully explain its pros and cons. In fact, estrogen, much like aspirin, can be considered a "cardiovascular drug for a lifetime." You can take it at a constant dose for an unlimited duration, it does not require any add-on drugs to achieve its therapeutic effects, and it prevents heart disease and its attendant complications.
- **Cholesterol-lowering drugs:** We now

know that patients who have had a previous heart attack can reduce their risk of future heart attacks if they receive early treatment with a cholesterol-lowering drug such as Lipitor, Pravachol, or Zocor, even if their blood cholesterol level is *normal*.

- **Beta-blockers:** These versatile drugs are named for their ability to block certain receptors in the heart and lungs. They can prevent further damage to the heart muscle after a heart attack. Consequently, if you or a family member has had a heart attack, it would be appropriate to ask your physician whether you should be considered for this kind of prevention-oriented therapy.

Additional medications that have prevention-oriented properties include Cytotec (misoprostol, a drug that can help to prevent gastric ulcers), certain antidepressants (worldwide, only tuberculosis claims more lives than suicide among women aged fifteen to forty-four, according to WHO figures), and some blood thinners. Vaccinations to immunize against pneumonia as well as other common infectious diseases, including diphtheria, tetanus, polio, measles, mumps, and rubella, are essential preventive tools. Influenza and hepatitis B can also be prevented with the help of immunizations.

Physicians' failure to help their patients take advantage of these medications has reached alarming proportions. For example, although the prevalence of hypertension (high blood pressure) and elevated blood cholesterol are approximately the same (30 to 34 percent of adults), studies show that 85 to 90 percent of hypertensive patients get treatment, whereas only about 45 percent of patients with elevated cholesterol receive appropriate treatment. The consequences of failing to prescribe prevention-oriented medications can be devastating: depression goes untreated, heart attacks are not prevented, and more expensive and toxic drugs frequently are pressed into service to mop up prevention failures.

In other cases, new diagnostic tests and heightened awareness of disease symptoms can make it possible for people to take advantage of early, proactive drug intervention. Alzheimer's disease is an important case in point. Cognex and Aricept are the only medications currently approved by the FDA for improving mental function and memory in patients with mild to moderate Alzheimer's disease. Unfortunately, these drugs are maximally effective in the very early stages of this illness, which highlights the importance of early detection.

WOMEN: PHARMACOLOGICAL OUTCASTS

Women: misdiagnosed, undertreated, and poorly served. Of the 2.8 billion prescriptions written each year, about 1.7 billion are for suboptimal, inappropriate, or unsafe medications used in women and children who, as pharmacological outcasts, come up short and have to swallow a "bitter pill." There are many reasons for why women and pills don't mix as well as they could.

- **Misleading Prescription Medication Advertising to Women Health Care Consumers**. Direct-to-consumer (DTC) advertising for prescription medications, 85 percent of which is directed at the female health care consumer, has now been approved for expanded use and greater deregulation by the FDA. But much of this information is slanted in favor of the promoted medication, and conspicuously lacking in mention of side effects and downsides, including sexual dysfunction, risk of breast cancer, and life-threatening infections. What is the consumer to do? Worst of all, it is impossible for women to do "comparative shopping" and, as a result, they frequently accept the advertisement as gospel.

  Physicians are frequently under-informed, health plans restrict medications that can be used and, consequently, the female health care consumer is in a Catch 22 and doesn't know where to turn for guidance. The MedRANK sections in this book provide a desperately needed road map through this treacherous pharmaceutical landscape that, so often, is characterized by slanted, confusing, conflicting, and restricted information.

- **Infertility and Ectopic Pregnancies Rising Dramatically in Women as a Result of Inferior Medication Options Used in Managed Care Health Plans.** Despite increasing awareness of the dangers and long-term consequences of sexually transmissible diseases, medication therapy for these diseases in women has lagged in effectiveness and common sense. Chlamydia is the most common infectious cause for infertility and ectopic pregnancy. Unfortunately, studies show that the best medication to address the out-of-control chlamydia epidemic is grossly underused by the majority of health plans servicing 80 million women. In fact, many health plans do not even recommend the CDC-endorsed, "one-dose-cure-here-now" treatment (Zithromax) for chlamydia.

  Instead, they urge their doctors to use doxycycline, a cheap medication that requires 14 doses over 7 days—a treatment course many people never finish. Chlamydia is a $4 billion epidemic that is associated with infertility, tubal pregnancies, and chronic pain. It is an insidious, public health menace—that continues to grow because penny-wise, epidemic-foolish health plans refuse to see the wisdom of getting the job done with more reliable, fertility-protecting, single dose treatments.

- **Women Are Dying Before Their Time: Increased Risk of Death in Women from Use of Clot-Dissolving Medications.** In a sad twist, women are being exposed to health- and life-threatening side effects of medications that have been shown to be relatively safe in men, but are extremely dangerous to use in female patients with similar problems. In a study reported in the *Journal of The American Medical Association* by investigators from England and the University of Washington, women treated with Genentech's $430 million clot-busting Alteplase (tPA) were almost twice as likely as men to die within thirty days of their heart attack. They also had a significantly higher risk for nonfatal complications associated with this drug, including shock, heart failure, and serious bleeding.

This study has some very sinister implications. As pharmaceutical company–sponsored media and advertising campaigns ensure that physicians and consumers become increasingly enchanted with the "lifesaving" properties of powerful clot-busting drugs, the potentially devastating effects these agents can have in women have been ignored or poorly publicized. In a recent analysis of this article and its implications for women, Louis Lasagna, MD, Dean of The School of Medicine, Tufts University, writes: "It is disturbing if women who receive thrombolytic [clot-busting] therapy are at greater risk for both fatal and nonfatal complications. Can we change this for the better in any way?"

- **Deafness, Recurrent Infections, and Ear Tube Surgeries in Children on the Rise from Use of Inferior Antibiotics in Managed Care Health Plans.** Every mother has been there. . . . "This is the third ear infection Matthew has had in ten weeks, doctor," complains the discouraged mother. "What's wrong with these antibiotics? They don't seem to be working. There's got to be something that will take care of the problem, once and for all." Millions of cranky, frustrated, and sleep-deprived mothers just like this one are right when they suspect there is an antibiotic that can spare their child's suffering, prevent recurrent infections and hearing loss, reduce the need for surgical insertion of ear tubes, and get the job done the first time around. Unfortunately, their doctors—frequently under pressure to contain costs by their health plan—are financially motivated to prescribe less-than-optimal antibiotics the first time around.

Studies in a leading medical journal show that amoxicillin, the most widely used antibiotic to treat ear infections in children, is *not* effective against almost one-third of bacterial species producing this condition. With increasing antibiotic resistance to the bacteria that cause ear infections and pneumonia in children, these cost-driven therapeutic "experiments" produce unsatisfactory—and sometimes dangerous—results.

- **Bitter Pills, Sweeter Profits, Sicker Women**. Because employers and their employee health care consumers shift from one health plan to another on an average of once every 3.4 years, decisions about which medications women should and should not have access to are usually driven by short-term profit considerations, rather than by the capacity of medications to provide long-term prevention against life-threatening diseases. Under these ground rules, women are denied advantages of better antidepressants, estrogen replacement therapy, and safer anti-anxiety medications.

• **Pills of Omission: Women Are Dying Before Their Time.** Millions of Americans, especially women, are not prescribed lifesaving, prevention-oriented medications by their health plans and, therefore, are dying before their time. They are being denied counseling, advice, and consultation regarding prevention-oriented medications— estrogen, aspirin, beta-blockers, blood thinner, clot-dissolvers, cholesterol-lowering drugs, vitamins D and E, calcium supplementation, antidepressants, and many others.

The "failure to medicate, failure to educate" syndrome has become a growing problem in women's health care. For example, men are routinely counseled to begin taking aspirin at forty to fifty years of age in order to prevent heart disease and cancer. Women, however, rarely receive this advice despite the fact that studies show that females who consume four to six aspirins per week have a lower risk of developing cancer of the colon or rectum, above and beyond the protective effects against heart disease. In a recent *New England Journal of Medicine* study titled "Aspirin and Colorectal Cancer in Women," researchers from the Harvard School of Public Health report that women who took aspirin regularly over ten years showed a small drop in cancer risk, whereas women who took aspirin for twenty years were 38 percent less likely to develop cancers of the colon or rectum than aspirin nonusers!

• **Prescription Habits of Male Physicians May Be Harmful to a Woman's Health.** Many features of the "misdiagnosed, undertreated" syndrome that is endemic among women can be explained by gender differences among physicians treating this population. In this regard, a recent study by a Harvard School of Public Health group reported in the *Journal of Internal Medicine* confirms that women under the care of female physicians were 11.4 times more likely to be prescribed estrogen replacement therapy than those under the care of a male physician!

In practical terms, this means that the overwhelming majority of women receiving care of male doctors are being denied the life-prolonging, health-enhancing properties of estrogen replacement. Overall, only 3 percent to 15 percent of eligible women receive this treatment. Equally distressing was the finding that women with female physicians were significantly more likely to have received Papanicolaou (Pap) smears to screen for cervical cancer, breast examinations, and testing for blood in the stool. Do these and similar studies suggest that having a male physician may be a risk factor for premature death in women? Perhaps they do.

- **Sexual Function in Women Ignored When Prescribing Medications.** Because they use inexpensive, generic drugs, health plans are wreaking havoc on the sex lives of women. Using a questionnaire-based approach, a recent report outlined factors that influence physicians when they select drugs to treat high blood pressure or depression. The study revealed that 89 percent of physicians consider impairment of sexual function, adverse effects on orgasm, and compromised libido when choosing a blood pressure medication or antidepressant for men. But only 16 percent of doctors surveyed said they considered these basic life-quality issues when selecting antihypertensive medications or antidepressants for their female patients.

  The lust-compromising consequences of such cavalier approaches to drug selection in an estimated 21 million women with high blood pressure have now been clarified. Recent studies now point to the importance of considering the type and class of medication—as well as dietary habits and weight status—when choosing blood pressure–lowering drugs for women. The news for women, especially those with mild weight problems, is not good. Put simply, the two most widely used blood pressure–lowering medications—diuretics and beta-blockers—produce significant sexual impairment in women with hypertension.

  Fortunately, there is a sex-saving twinkle for women at the end of the pharmacological rainbow. Reporting in the *Archives of Internal Medicine* and using an evaluation instrument called the "Sexual Physical Complaint Scale," a group of investigators found that among mildly overweight female patients receiving a diuretic (water pill) for their blood pressure, 24 percent had marked worsening of sexual problems. Sexual problems, however, could be reduced significantly if these women followed a diet that achieved a 10 to 12 pound weight reduction.

- **Pills That Harm: Women Come Up Short at Managed Care Plans and HMOs.** Each year, more people in the United States die (140,000) or are injured (870,000) from prescription medication misadventures or misuse than from car accidents and airplane crashes combined. A disproportionate number of these casualties are *women*, who from 1977 to 1993 were officially barred from early drug trials overseen by the FDA, and now, studies show, must make more trips to the doctor, hospital, and emergency department because of medication restrictions imposed by their managed care health plans.

- **The Medication Information Gap Widens for Women's Health Needs.** Burdened by productivity, peer review, and performance pressures imposed by health care plans, doctors who prescribe medications day in and day out are undereducated about the effectiveness and safety of medications in women. In the case of heart disease, women are treatment outcasts from the get-go, because they oftentimes are not included—or are grossly under-represented—in seminal disease-prevention, life-prolongation studies. Consider, for example, that women comprised only 10 percent of the patients studied in the landmark Prospective Pravachol Pooling (PPP) project, a mega-trial designed to evaluate the effectiveness of medications used to prevent heart disease! This skewing toward male patients is outrageous, because women are afflicted with and die from heart disease as often as do men, only later in life.

THE PHARMACEUTICAL IMPERATIVE

Ironically, even as drug therapies succeed in preventing disease, curing illness, or reducing misery, new conditions are being recognized that require treatment with medications; and studies are uncovering more and more reasons for using currently existing prescription drugs. Furthermore, improved—and much more sensitive—screening and diagnostic tests, encouraged by national disease-awareness and screening campaigns, are detecting an increasing number of young adults with asthma, high blood pressure, bronchitis, blood cholesterol elevations, depression, and other disorders, all of which can benefit from opti-

mal long-term drug therapy. What all this means is that an increasing number of young and middle-aged people are joining the ranks of the "pharmacological establishment." Even parents of young children are now faced with difficult decisions about antibiotic use for ear infections, medications for asthma and allergies, and drug treatment for childhood behavioral disorders.

As recently as a few decades ago, only a limited number of prescription medications were available for the most common medical conditions. If you were dissatisfied with a drug, your options were probably restricted to either tolerating its side effects or not treating the condition at all. Fortunately, things have changed, and you have many more options today. A number of drug classes contain a dozen or more individual drugs from which your physician can choose, as the following table shows:

CURRENT MEDICATION OPTIONS

Drug Class or Therapeutic Group	Approximate Number of Medications Available
Nonsteroidal anti-inflammatory drugs (NSAIDs)	17
Insulin preparations	23
Thiazides and related diuretics	12
Angina medications	6
Anti-arrhythmia medications	25
Calcium channel blockers	9

Drug Class or Therapeutic Group	Approximate Number of Medications Available
Beta-blockers	12
ACE inhibitors	8
Bronchodilators	11
SSRI antidepressants	4
Seizure medications	14
Parkinson's disease medications	5
Oral antibiotics	26
Birth control pills	12
Cholesterol-lowering drugs	7
Sedatives	15

As welcome as this explosion in choices is, it presents consumers and physicians with a new dilemma: How can you sort through so many options to find the medication that is best suited for your health condition? How can you recognize the positive traits of the best medications?

"PILLS IN THE GRASS"—DANGERS LURK IN CURRENTLY AVAILABLE MEDICATIONS

After recent withdrawal from market of two potentially dangerous, high-profile prescription medications (weight loss pills) prescribed to millions of people, there is renewed concern about FDA safety nets and reporting procedures for potentially unsafe drugs. The real question is, "Just how many more pills are there *still* out there that probably should be taken off the market either because (a) they are po-

tentially dangerous, or (b) because they are in such wide use, but are so ineffective or marginally effective as to be harmful to health?"

Other drugs, clearly not dangerous enough to be pulled from the market because of harmful effects, but which in many cases may be inferior or ineffective enough to prompt careful reconsideration of their day-to-day usefulness and the harm they cause by *failing* to cure, to provide maximal effectiveness, or to treat serious conditions, include the following:

Amoxicillin (antibiotic)
Ceclor (antibiotic)
Suprax (antibiotic)
Cafergot (migraine drug)
Stadol (migraine drug)
Hismanal (allergy drug)
Posicor (new blood pressure pill)
Elavil (antidepressant)
Tagamet (ulcer medication)
Lescol (fluvastatin)
Mevacor (cholesterol-lowering medication)
Lopid (lipid-lowering drug)
Cognex (Alzheimer's drug)

The point is that when a drug is pulled from the market, we're just seeing the tip of the iceberg—those drugs that are really, really dangerous. Now, what about all the "awful" or "terrible" or "worthless" or "tricky" or "unpredictable" or "interacting" drugs—pills that are gray and can't be touched by the FDA—that don't fall in the Grim Reaper category, but are being used by millions of people day in and day out. These drugs, which will be discussed in this book, are even *more* important to bring to your attention, because they're still *circulating* for human use. There are lots of drugs that may not be quite nasty enough to yank, but are substandard enough to be avoided at all costs, and consumers need to know about them. This "dangerous, but not deadly" group will never be pulled from the market, yet will still go on wreaking havoc through their ineffectiveness and other problems. People are lulled into thinking they are getting effective treatment for their condition but, in fact, they are not.

THE QUALITIES OF PILLS THAT WORK

It's unfortunate, but many physicians do not have the drug-prescribing issue in clear focus. Consumers know this intuitively, and yet they are at a loss as to how to take the matter into their own hands. What they need are clearer guidelines to determine just what constitutes a pill that works and a pill that doesn't. In the next chapter we'll consider some of the most common pitfalls of drug prescribing, but first let's outline the qualities of pills that work.

Perhaps first and foremost, pills that work are safe and effective. This is a baseline criterion that many doctors never get beyond. Prescribing a drug simply because it is safe and effective is like buying an automobile because it has seat belts. Yes, seat belts are good and necessary, but all cars have seat belts—they're standard equipment. It's more relevant to know whether the car also has driver- and passenger-side air bags, antilock brakes, all-wheel drive, side-impact collision panels, and the like. Dodge Neons have seat belts and Volvos have seat belts, but that doesn't mean both cars are equally safe.

In the same sense, virtually all drugs that sneak through the Food and Drug Administration's radar are, in the broad sense, safe and effective. This is good, but the best drugs do more than satisfy these minimal criteria. In other words, it's not sufficient for a drug just to be safe and effective. It has to have other characteristics as well. Equally important criteria, which many physicians sometimes fail to consider in drug selection, include:

- Its side effects and impact on overall quality of life
- Its cost and convenience of dosing
- Number of conditions it can treat
- Its effectiveness over the long term
- Its risk for causing harmful drug-drug and drug-disease interactions

The fact is, drugs within any given class are not created equal. Among the 14,000 or so FDA-approved drugs currently available, some are clearly safer than others, and some are clearly more effective. For example, the antihistamine Hismanal (astemizole), has a much higher risk of causing abnormal heart rhythms (some of which can lead to death) than the antihistamines Claritin (loratidine) and Zyrtec (cetirizine). In other words, although all four medications, in the broad sense, carry the FDA safety and effectiveness "seal of approval," Claritin and Zyrtec have a clear safety edge. Thus, optimal medications—pills that work—have something extra over pills that work less well. They typically have a much cleaner drug-interaction profile, cause fewer side effects, offer convenient and simple dosing, and provide unparalleled effectiveness.

Clearly, physicians need to dig deeper and explore issues beyond a drug's safety and efficacy. They need to evaluate its extras. And with your help, and the information in this book, your physician will be encouraged to consider the value-added aspects of drug therapy.

Let's take a closer look at each of the criteria for pills that work.

☺ *Pills that work cause fewer side effects and have neutral or beneficial effects on your overall quality of life.*

Side effects and quality-of-life issues should always be main concerns. If you suspect that your medication is producing troublesome side effects, ask your physician to review your current drug intake. In many cases, the association between your symptoms and a specific drug will be obvious. If so, an appropriate substitution can be made. Without such a review, the opportunities for introducing a better, more user-friendly medication are limited.

It only stands to reason that if people take a medication to treat a chronic problem but have to endure troublesome side effects, then something is wrong. For example, if high blood pressure pills or an anti-allergy medication make people too sleepy to watch an entire episode of *Masterpiece Theater*, then the disadvantages of the drug probably do not outweigh its benefits.

Clinical studies demonstrate that the majority of drugs used to treat the most common illnesses—including high blood pressure, depression, heart disease, and arthritis—have the potential to produce a wide range of adverse side effects, including subtle impairments in sleep, mental function, sexual performance, and emotional stability. Increasingly, how patients *feel* while taking a particular medication, to what extent it improves their quality of life, and its negative side effects have become just as important as its ability to get the job done.

Unless your physician searches out such side effects, these kinds of problems may never be recognized. And you and your family members will be the ones who suffer most.

☺ *Cost and convenience.*

Because a variety of drug options exist for most medical problems, you should talk to your doctor about the issues of greatest concern to you. For example, if cost is an important consideration, clearly communicate this concern to your doctor. Significant price variations can be found among medications in any therapeutic class, and you should not be embarrassed to inquire about less expensive alternatives. (Cost is a tricky issue that also gets into considerations of cost to the consumer versus cost to society [due to insurance copayments and the like] and the relative values of generic versus trademarked drugs. We'll look into these aspects of the cost issue in Chapter 3.)

On the other hand, if convenience is more important to you, you may want to tell your doctor that you prefer a prescription for the drug with the easiest and simplest dose schedule, regardless of its cost. I have a saying: "Once-a-day keeps the doctor away." I've found that, generally speaking, pills that work best are once-daily medications, and pills that don't are medications that have to be taken three times or more per day. When it comes to the world of prescription medications, more is frequently less: less effective, less comfortable, and less convenient. Many medications, including penicillin, indomethacin, erythromycin, doxycycline, amoxicillin, propranolol, cholestyramine, and diphenhydramine, which were once considered state-of-the-art treatments, have been superseded by better drugs that are dosed less frequently (and associated with fewer side effects).

Interestingly, many patients express concern about whether they can really reduce the number of times each day a medication has to be taken—they *perceive* that drugs taken more frequently are better equipped to treat their condition. In fact, just the opposite is true! Drugs that have to be dosed more frequently put people at higher risk for poor compliance, unnecessary therapy, and medication-related problems.

Antibiotics are a good case in point. Most antibiotics have to be given for several days to cure many common infections. In some cases, one or two weeks of daily doses are necessary. Recent innovations in drug therapy, however, have produced antibiotics that have to be given only once. Others require only three or five days for a complete treatment course. Some of these "tissue is the issue" antibiotics stay at the site of the infection for several days after you have finished taking them. In other words, they are still fighting the infection even though you are no longer actually taking pills.

If you are like most people, you will prefer the convenience of a drug with a shorter course. Studies show that fewer than 10 percent of patients on antibiotics are even taking their medication on the tenth day of a ten-day course. In other words, many people bail out well before the drug has done its job. But once-daily medications can provide around-the-clock coverage with more simple dosing. This is true not only for chronic diseases, such as high blood pressure, heart disease, arthritis, depression, allergies, and diabetes, but for short-term conditions such as infection and musculoskeletal injuries. In fact, once-daily medications used to treat high blood pressure, arthritis, ulcers, infections, depression, and pain-producing diseases frequently are even more effective than older drugs requiring more frequent administration.

One-dose and short-duration therapies are currently available for many *infectious* conditions, including chlamydia, vaginal candidiasis, nonspecific bacterial vaginosis, gonorrhea, urinary tract infection, nail infections, head lice, sinusitis, childhood ear infections, pneumonia, bronchitis, and skin infections. Some drugs are clearly better choices than others, too. For example, among the twenty-seven antibiotics widely used to treat bacterial infections causing community-acquired pneumonia or bronchitis, only three drugs (azithromycin/Zithromax; levofloxacin/Levaquin; and clarithromycin/Biaxin) cover *all* the bacteria that predictably cause these infections. (See the MedRANK checklists in Chapter 13 to determine which antibiotic and antifungal regimens are best suited for your pattern of recurrent infections.)

☺ *Pills that work are versatile, in the sense that a single drug can treat more than one condition simultaneously and thus reduce the need for taking multiple medications. These are also called "smart drugs."*

One of the most important objectives of this book is to identify for consumers versatile, "high-productivity" medications. Or, so-called "smart drugs." Your physician must become familiar with those drugs that are able to treat *more than one* condition or symptom. Examples include anti-allergy drugs that treat indoor allergies, seasonal allergies, and hives (cetirizine/Zyrtec); antidepressants that treat depression and improve insomnia (sertraline/Zoloft; paroxetine/Paxil); blood-pressure-lowering medications that treat hypertension, lower cholesterol levels, and improve prostate function (doxazosin/Cardura); and hormonal replacement therapy (Premarin) that prevents bone wasting, alleviates menopause-related symptoms, may prevent onset of Alzheimer's disease, and decreases the risk of heart disease and stroke.

Clearly, versatile—or so-called "smart"—drugs are preferable to medications that have the capacity for treating only one condition or symptom. As a general rule, if you suffer from a number of medical problems and are being treated with many different medications—each targeted at only one disease or symptom—you will benefit from "smart" medications that can treat multiple conditions. You should consider the following examples:

- If you have diabetes and are taking one drug to treat high blood pressure and yet another drug to treat congestive heart failure, it may be more appropriate to consolidate your drug regimen with a single agent such as an ACE inhibitor (Vasotec, Zestril), which can treat all three conditions at once. (*ACE* stands for angiotensin converting enzyme; *angiotensin* is a protein that narrows tiny blood vessels and thus increases blood pressure. Thus, ACE inhibitors dilate [relax] blood vessels and aid in the treatment of hypertension.)

- If you are taking one medication to treat high blood pressure and another medication for angina-related chest pain, it usually makes much more sense to use a single calcium channel blocker such as Norvasc. Calcium channel blockers and beta-blockers can provide symptomatic relief for the chest pain as well as to help control blood pressure.

- If you are a man over the age of 60 and have high blood pressure and urinary flow problems caused by an enlarged prostate, you will benefit from a peripheral alpha-blocker such as Cardura or Hytrin, which are indicated for the treatment of hypertension *and* prostate problems. (Alpha-blockers prevent certain nerve cell receptors from binding with neurotransmitters that would otherwise tend to increase blood pressure.)

- If you are taking a diuretic for treatment of high blood pressure plus an oral potassium supplement, your physician can simplify your regimen considerably by prescribing what's called a potassium-sparing diuretic (Maxzide, Aldactazide). This would require you to take only a single pill per day, without the need for what is usually a poorly palatable oral potassium supplement.

The lack of attention to versatile drugs runs deep among doctors and is a problem infecting many medical subspecialties, including gynecology. Even though physicians still treat hundreds of thousands of women suffering from *Candida* (fungal) vaginitis with a seven-day course of intra-vaginal Monistat suppositories, the one-pill, cure-here-now medication mentioned at the beginning of the chapter (Diflucan/fluconazole) is just as effective yet less expensive and has to be given orally only *once.*

☺ Pills that work are durable, in the sense that their effectiveness lasts indefinitely, over the long haul.

All too often, physicians inappropriately select a drug that works for only a short period of time. Within weeks he or she is forced to prescribe an add-on medication—a "pharmacological tow truck"—to maintain the desired therapeutic result. This predisposes the patient to the risks of polypharmacy, or treatment with multiple medications. In contrast, pills that work have been proven to maintain their effectiveness predictably—when used alone—*over the long haul.* It only makes sense to use those medications first that keep ticking year after year without the need for reinforcements.

☺ Pills that work cause fewer than average adverse interactions with other drugs you may be taking.

In 1996, physicians wrote 2.8 billion prescriptions, or about eight prescriptions for every man, woman, and child in the United States. This widespread medication use was accompanied by a corresponding epidemic of adverse reactions. Most recent studies estimate that from 10 to 15 percent of all hospitalized patients experience an adverse reaction to a drug at some point during their stay, and that up to 25 percent of all hospital admissions in the elderly are associated with or caused by a drug-related incident. All this emphasizes the importance of identifying medications known to have a lower risk for drug interactions.

Within some classes of drugs—including antibiotics, beta-blockers, calcium channel blockers, and anti-ulcer medications—certain medications are known to place patients at high risk for drug interactions, whereas other drugs in the same class are less likely to do so. For example, among the calcium channel blockers, verapamil (Calan) is associated with a fairly extensive list of drug-drug interactions, whereas felodipine (Plendil) and amlodipine (Norvasc) are associated with very few drug-drug interactions. Among commonly used antidepressants, fluoxetine (Prozac) is more likely to produce drug interactions than is sertraline (Zoloft). The ulcer drug cimetidine (Tagamet) is more problematic than famotidine (Pepcid). The MedRANK Checklists in Part II cover hundreds of similar examples.

Whenever possible, you should ask your

physician to put you on a medication that is the *least likely* to be incompatible with other drugs.

....

THE PHARMACOLOGICAL FUTURE

The future will no doubt bring more and better drugs. Previously difficult-to-treat conditions, including possibly AIDS, will respond to innovative drugs. More effective vaccination programs may help measles go the way of smallpox. Advances in cancer treatment are promising, and antidepressant formulas seem to advance every year. Again, however, the two-edged sword appears. With new and more numerous drugs comes an increased risk of drug-related problems, the scope of which I'll detail in the next chapter.

CHAPTER 2

━━

. . . PILLS THAT DON'T

Jonathan M. limped into my examining room not long ago and slumped into a chair. Referred by his internist for "headaches, high blood pressure, back and chest pain, and other complaints of unknown origin," it soon became clear that I was one of a half-dozen physicians Jonathan was seeing.

Not surprisingly, what these other doctors had told Jonathan sometimes conflicted, and in the aggregate it was all extremely confusing to him. His battery of doctors (I wouldn't call them a team, because they seemed to operate almost totally independently of each other) had also prescribed almost a dozen drugs, many of which Jonathan had been taking for nearly three years. Complying with his regimen meant he had to be taking some twenty-four pills per day. He was taking a diuretic for the blood pressure, a painkiller for the headaches and another for the backache, a short-acting, generic calcium channel blocker for the chest pain, and many other questionably useful drugs. He was also taking medica-

tions for nausea, sleeping problems, and lack of energy, problems that in all likelihood were resulting from other medications he was taking.

If Jonathan was a physical mess, his medication schedule was a bigger mess. It took a number of months to narrow his diagnosis to two underlying conditions: high blood pressure and migraine headaches. Using the 12-Week Action Plan (described in Part III), we were able to sort out what drugs Jonathan really needed and could benefit from, and what was unnecessary or simply redundant. We soon reduced his medications to only *two* drugs: Norvasc, a calcium channel blocker that has the advantage of treating *both* high blood pressure and chest pain; and Imitrex, a highly efficient migraine medication that he could take on an as-needed basis. Eventually, he showed positive signs of regaining his overall health on a more rational medication program.

Unfortunately, Jonathan's medication problems are closer to the rule than the excep-

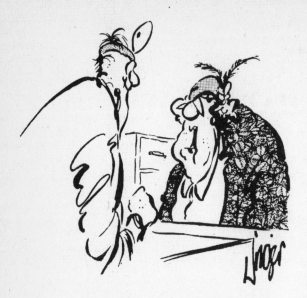

"I feel a lot better since I ran out of those pills you gave me."

tion. Many people today are taking too many drugs, too frequently, and for too long. During this time of "pharmacological imperative," the number of prescription ingredients in an average drug regimen has swelled dangerously out of control. In the United States, two out of every three physician visits result in a drug prescription. It has been estimated that a patient seeing a physician in the United States for a specific complaint receives about four times more medication than a person with a similar complaint in a European country.

PILLS: TOO MUCH OF A GOOD THING

One thing is for sure: The risks of drug-related problems will grow as time goes on. Recent information suggests that we are currently in the middle of an epidemic of excessive and suboptimal drug prescribing. Consider the following:

- An estimated 150 million physician visits per year, at a cost of about $7.5 billion, are due to drug-induced problems.
- Approximately 140,000 Americans die each year from failure to consume their drugs properly.
- Approximately one-fourth of all nursing home admissions result from the inability of patients to manage their medication use appropriately on their own.
- As many as 28 percent of all hospital admissions (more than 8 million per year), at a cost of more than $45 billion, appear to be due to or associated with drug-related problems.
- At least 770,000 and possibly as many as 2 million hospital patients in the United States are injured each year from medication errors, resulting in extra hospital costs estimated at $4.2 billion.
- The direct annual cost of managing the complications of inappropriate drug therapy exceeds the annual cost of all diabetes care ($45 billion in 1994). Add to that the indirect costs (such as lost productivity and wages) of inappropriate drug intake, and the total bill associated with failures in drug management approaches the cost of managing all cardiovascular diseases ($117 to $154 billion in 1994).
- Noncompliance with prescription medications produces a loss of more than 20 million work days each year.

- Up to 60 percent of physicians prescribe antibiotics to treat the common cold, a viral condition not affected by antibiotics.

The bottom line is, millions and millions of people—children, tweeners, boomers, and the chronologically gifted—are suffering on a daily basis from havoc wreaked by inappropriate or excessive drug prescribing. In the current drug-prescribing climate, no age group, no sex, and no demographic profile is spared the pitfalls of medication use. In fact, virtually every American is familiar with a drug therapy misadventure, whether it has been their own or that of a friend, child, or parent.

A NEW PHILOSOPHY

Along with increased prescription drug use in all segments of society comes the potential for distressing side effects, quality-of-life impairment, and unnecessary financial hardship. With the dramatic expansion of drug classes and pharmacological interventions, physicians and their patients are being forced to reexamine conventional drug use. In the final analysis, state-of-the-art prescribing requires close *collaboration* between patient and physician. Drugs should be introduced not only to correct abnormal test results but, more important, *to service the real-world health goals*, quality-of-life objectives, and expectations of people who must take drugs to stay well.

Every family must be empowered to guide their physicians toward better prescription medications tailored to their needs.

Physicians are being increasingly challenged to promote safe, appropriate, effective, and economical drug use. They should strive to foster precision in drug therapy and identify and resolve drug-related problems and misadventures. Accomplishing these goals requires patients' help.

Not surprisingly, perceptions about the relative risks and benefits of conventional drug therapy are changing. Although patients and physicians may think of coronary angiograms and surgical interventions as "invasive procedures," the fact is that writing a prescription for a short-term medication such as an antibiotic or a long-term medication for high blood pressure has the potential for being one of the *most invasive*—and dangerous—acts in which your physician can participate. Committing a patient to a medication for five or ten years is a profound step that exposes him or her to possible side effects and, perhaps, a burdensome financial commitment. These risks must be balanced against the possible health benefits of the drug. Prescribing a drug, therefore, carries with it all the attendant responsibilities of long-term monitoring and periodic reviews to confirm the safety of and necessity for continuing medication therapy.

This doesn't mean that all—or even the majority of—medications are harmful. But it does mean that many drugs have the potential to make you feel bad, while others can cause drug interactions, lead to financial hardship, or impair quality of life.

What can be done to remedy this sad situation? First, we must consider the three most prominent actors in the drug play: you, the health care consumer; your doctor, the health care provider; and the larger institutions that govern and control the drug industry, including regulatory agencies like the FDA, insurance companies, and, especially, HMOs and managed care organizations. Each of these actors must begin to recognize the pitfalls they face and thus begin to share some of the responsibility when things go wrong.

....

THE PILL IS GONE: WHAT HEALTH CARE CONSUMERS DO WRONG

Health care consumers need to become more active partners in their medication programs. Here are some common errors they need to avoid making.

☺ Many health care consumers fail to take their medications at the right times and in the proper doses.

Physicians refer to following medication directions as *compliance*, a word that has some unfortunate connotations of passivity on the part of the patient, but that is the term we'll use nevertheless. There are many potential pitfalls relating to noncompliance. Studies show that about 30 to 50 percent of the 2.8 billion prescriptions dispensed in the United States each year are not taken properly by the patient. For medications prescribed for high blood pressure, the compliance rate after a period of three years is no better than 32 percent. In addition, up to 20 percent of patients never even get their prescriptions filled in the first place—the most serious example of noncompliance.

Patients fail to comply for various reasons. One of the most common reasons is dissatisfaction with the drug itself: The patient perceives that its "noise level" (such as distressing side effects, inconvenient dosing, and exorbitant cost) is *greater* than the noise level of the disease (such as severity of symptoms, discomfort, and fear of serious illness). He or she may take sanctuary in the relative "silence" of the illness rather than tolerate the noise level of the medication. Put simply, such patients do not comply with their drug regimen, and in the long run they suffer the consequences of inadequate therapy.

In general, if you have a relatively "silent" condition—one that doesn't produce a lot of obvious symptoms, such as high blood pressure, an elevated cholesterol level, or diabetes—you may be inclined to place less value on the probability of *future* health benefits from drug therapy and to place more value on its *present* inconvenience and side effects. This predisposes you to comply erratically with your drug regimen. I am reminded of the patient who, during an office visit with an associate of mine, once commented, "I feel a lot better since I ran out of those pills you gave me."

In the long run, patients who are noncompliant, for whatever reason, will suffer the consequences of inadequate therapy: diseases that are poorly controlled, progressive or disabling symptoms, or decreased longevity. But unless the benefits of a drug outweigh its disadvantages, at least as perceived by the person taking them, noncompliance will undermine a successful outcome for the patient.

☺ *Medical checks and balances are lost when health care consumers go to multiple doctors and don't inform each about what the other has prescribed.*

The road to polydrug use is often paved with good intentions. But when a number of different subspecialists are contributing to your medication "stew," your drug list will need a thorough going-over. In some cases subspecialists such as cardiologists, urologists, and gynecologists may focus narrowly on just one of your medical problems. Subspecialists may also be familiar with only one or two therapeutic classes of medications. Consequently, drug regimens designed by multiple sources put you at higher risk for drug interactions and for long-term therapy with medications that may no longer be indicated. The old saying "Too many cooks spoil the broth" certainly applies to the world of drug prescribing.

Studies show that if you make six or more visits to your physician each year, or if more than one practitioner is prescribing drugs for you, then you are at higher risk for medication misadventures. You will probably want to review your medications on a regular basis and compare your drug list against those recommended in the Action Plan Checklists in Part III. When you evaluate your prescription medications, you should make note not only of the drugs themselves but also their prescribers, who may be physicians, nurse practitioners, physician assistants, or pharmacists. If you discover that your prescriptions have been written by more than one person, your primary health care provider should screen your drug regimen for possible duplications and incompatibilities. Whenever possible, you should urge your primary physician to be the *only* source for your prescription medications.

Another solution to this problem is to encourage your prescribing providers to communicate with each other. It is also important for you to communicate changes that one prescribing practitioner makes to all the other health care providers responsible for your medication program. Usually your primary care physician will be the person who is responsible for most of your drug therapy, and it is perfectly natural for this physician to call the others to consult about possible changes in your medication program. On occasion, it simply may not be possible for your primary provider to coordinate all of your prescriptions. If this is the case, you will generally be better off if the other doctors write prescriptions *only* in their area of specialty. This will reduce the likelihood that multiple or duplicate medications are prescribed for the same medical problem.

Sometimes, patients take over-the-counter (OTC) drugs and fail to inform their doctors. This, too, can be a problem since adverse interactions are possible between OTC and prescription medications. If there is a potential conflict between two medications, one or both drugs should be changed. Some commonly used OTC medications that are associated with a high risk for potential drug-drug interactions include aspirin, antihistamines, and cold remedies.

☺ *Health care consumers fail to fully inform their doctors about side effects and other medication problems.*

Is it the drug that's making you feel blah? Or is it your job? A personal problem? More often than not, drug-related impairments cruise beneath the radar of clinical detection. An open and honest exchange between you and your physician will make his or her job easier and, in general, will produce the best results. In many ways, you know your body and mind better than your physician does. You can turn this to your advantage because, after all, you are charged with the responsibility of monitoring only a single patient—*yourself*. Compared with your time-pressed doctor, you will also be better able to assess your response or that of your family members to newly prescribed drugs. For example, a physician may fail to link the onset of a new symptom—whether it be a rash, headache, diarrhea, or fatigue—with the recent introduction of a drug into your regimen. When this kind of association falls through the cracks, you must provide the tip-off for your physician.

☺ *Subtle side effects are the most difficult to evaluate.*

With so many drugs available in the current pharmaceutical arsenal, many physicians, and even pharmacists, are simply not aware of the full range of subtle side effects associated with common medications. Those who are aware of them frequently fail to take a history that is detailed enough to uncover insidious, quietly festering side effects.

Even the more obvious symptoms may be difficult for a doctor to connect with a drug. For example, blood pressure medications have the potential for producing cough (ACE inhibitors), sexual dysfunction and altered sleep patterns (beta-blockers), or leg swelling (nifedipine). Antidepressant medications can cause agitation (Prozac), muscle tremors (Prozac, Effexor), high blood pressure (Effexor), diarrhea (Zoloft), and impotence (Serzone). If you, as the patient, can be made aware of these possibilities and can take the time to practice the art of *medication self-evaluation*, you will be better positioned to recognize side effects, discuss medication options with your physician, and press your doctor to prescribe drugs with better, more patient-friendly profiles. (To help you identify these problems, complete the Action Plan Side Effect Checklist on page 375, as part of your 12-Week Action Plan.) Drug-associated side effects are not unavoidable. In fact, in most cases, they are avoidable. It's just a matter of selecting a drug that is appropriate for you.

☺ *Health care consumers cling irrationally to long-standing drug regimens.*

You need to be open to change. Many patients have a tendency to identify *too strongly* with their drugs. They become fearful that any change will disrupt their lives, even when side effects or other problems are already evident. You must open-mindedly consider any modifications proposed by your practitioner. These may involve new medications with reduced side effects and greater user-friendliness. By the same token, don't be reluctant to question your physician or pharmacist about the necessity for continuing a medication that you are currently taking. Not uncommonly, medications started years ago can have their dosage adjusted downward or discontinued altogether.

....
TOXIC DOC SYNDROME: WHAT DOCTORS DO WRONG

Unfortunately, many of the problems associated with drug therapy begin in the physician's office. Some are due to inadequate information, others are due to poor communication between patient and doctor, and others are caused by intrinsic problems with the drugs themselves. Again, I want to emphasize that as well intentioned and educated as your doctor may be, most busy practitioners simply cannot keep track of all the side effects, the unique advantages of new drugs, antibiotic resistance patterns, the risks of drug interactions, and all the implications of recent clinical studies. Before we consider solutions, let's take a look at the scope of the problem and see just how bad it is. What do doctors often do wrong?

☺ Doctors overprescribe.

That is, they prescribe too many drugs in too high quantities. If you are taking more than eight pills per day or more than three different prescription medications, your doctor may be overprescribing.

Not too long ago, the problems associated with multiple medications affected primarily the elderly. But today the use of multiple medications has become much more common in the young and middle-aged adult populations as well. With screening campaigns for heart disease, the rise of sexually transmitted diseases, and improved diagnostic methods for common conditions such as asthma, Alzheimer's disease, high blood pressure, and depression, medication use among middle-aged adults has surged dramatically. Millions of young and middle-aged individuals are taking antidepressants for premenstrual dysphoria, panic attacks, and obsessive-compulsive disorders; heart pills to lower blood pressure and cholesterol levels; hormonal drugs for life changes; and antibiotics for recurrent infections.

As a result, increasing numbers of people are at risk for adverse drug interactions. The risk of drug interactions increases by tenfold when the number of medications in the regimen jumps from only three to four. Drug interactions may be harmful or even life-threatening. For example, many drugs (including Seldane, Tagamet, erythromycin, Biaxin, theophylline, and Coumadin) that function well *in isolation* of other agents can cause serious problems *when combined* with other medications. (See the Action Plan Checklist of Selected Medications with Significant Risk of Drug-Drug Interactions on page 372 to assess your own risk for drug interactions.)

☺ Physicians may delegate to others their responsibility to fashion an optimum drug regimen.

In many health care settings, drugs are prescribed by nurses or physician assistants. Although these professionals may be well trained in primary care, they are usually even less equipped than doctors to make subtle distinctions regarding drug selection. Clearly, in order to protect themselves, consumers require more control over the drug-prescribing process than they currently possess.

☺ Because of institutional pressures physicians may fail to spend sufficient time to customize the drug regimen for the patient.

If your physician is typical, he or she has a prescribing pattern that can be summarized as "not defined, not refined." Because of current pressures on health care providers to see as many patients as possible as quickly as they can and thereby maintain "physician productivity," the majority of doctors do not always have enough patient contact time to explore all the subtleties or ramifications of their drug choices. In many cases, they end up relying on scanty information gleaned from face-to-face office visits that last an average of only three to four minutes. On occasion, a practitioner may be too busy to review medication-related information in your chart. Spending insufficient time taking your case history will place you at a higher risk for excessive and inappropriate medication choices.

Doctors also get into a rut of using only those medications that are available through their health plan formulary and furthermore often prescribe something merely because they perceive that's what the patient wants. What's more, few physicians are familiar with alternative approaches—herbal remedies, vitamin therapy, acupuncture, short-duration drug therapy—which may be suitable for many patients. No wonder drug prescribing is oftentimes random, reckless, and rudimentary.

☺ Make your physician be a splitter rather than a lumper.

One of your overarching goals as a patient is to help convert your physician from being a "lumper" to being a "splitter." Lumpers prescribe drugs without considering the special needs, risks, or goals of the *individual* patient. They also tend to prescribe drugs according to the *broad* class of medications to which they belong, rather than evaluating the subtle but important differences among the drugs within a *specific* category. Physicians who are splitters, on the other hand, carefully weigh the subtle advantages and disadvantages of many different drugs and the impact they will have on the patient's condition. Needless to say, when it comes to prescribing drugs, splitting is better than lumping. A good example can be found among the ulcer medications: Tagamet and Zantac both belong to the same drug class, but Zantac is preferable because it is less likely to cause drug interactions.

☺ Physicians may use drugs as a quick fix.

Making optimal, patient-friendly drug choices requires having the time and freedom to perform full examinations and come to precise diagnoses. Unfortunately, either because of time constraints or because they don't always have the full range of diagnostic options at their disposal, many practitioners take the path of least resistance. It's not that physicians have bad intentions—it's just that in today's world they are overwhelmed with too many patients, too many restrictions, too much paperwork, and too much conflicting information. Many are overworked and burnt out.

Because patients can't always count on their physicians to make customized drug decisions, patients are faced with the challenge of detecting unsafe and faulty prescribing patterns themselves, and communicating potential problems to their physician in the hope that corrective action will be taken.

☺ Many physicians are undereducated.

Doctors are simply unable to keep up with all the new drug information. The staggering explosion in our pharmacopoeia has created an information deficit and education gap among physicians that is so profound, it threatens the quality of contemporary drug therapy. By the time a physician completes a three-year residency program, five years have elapsed since his or her course in clinical pharmacology. During this interval, approximately 130 new drugs will have become available. Add to this the ongoing political pressure on the FDA to expedite the approval process for a wide range of drugs used to treat cancer, HIV infection, Alzheimer's disease, and many other conditions. The result is that many physicians have received no formal education for many of the drugs they prescribe.

The seriousness of this drug information blackout was highlighted recently by the Health and Public Policy Committee of the American College of Physicians, which warned in a white paper, "After completion of formal medical school and house officer training, there is no exposure to intelligent, informative, and unbiased assessments of drug therapy." The committee went on to comment that the "entire educational process" is largely random, incomplete, and subject to distortion.

☺ Many physicians take a trial-and-error approach to medication therapy.

Sadly, this expeditious "I'm prescribing as fast as I can!" approach to drug prescribing is all too common. In many cost-conscious health care settings, physicians are prevented from using sophisticated diagnostic tests to pin down a specific diagnosis. As a result, they sometimes start patients on drugs without a confirmed diagnosis. After a trial course of the drug therapy (during which the patient may suffer side effects as well as "financial toxicity"), they see whether the patient has improved. This "shoot from the hip," trial-and-error approach is becoming increasingly common and poses considerable health risks for patients. As a doctor in one *Herman* cartoon so aptly put it, "I'm not sure what these pills are, but take them for a couple of weeks, and let me know how you feel."

Fortunately, there are solutions to the problem of prescribing on the fly. Prescribing drugs *reflexively* must give way to prescribing drugs *selectively*. Informed patients can help physicians be more selective about their drug choices.

☺ Doctors may prescribe drugs for unapproved purposes.

Most of the time, physicians prescribe medications only for uses that have been approved by the FDA. On occasion, however, you may find yourself taking a drug that is not officially approved by the FDA for use in your condition. This is known as off-label or unlabeled prescribing. When you are using a drug for off-label purposes, you should ask your doctor for a clear assessment of its risks and benefits, and an explanation of why the drug hasn't been approved for your condition.

☺ *Doctors may fail to look for delayed, medication-related complications.*

One of the most common questions people ask is, "If I feel fine taking my pills now, does that mean I don't have to worry about side effects?" The answer is no, absolutely not. Medication problems may take minutes, hours, days, or months to surface. In fact, many drugs are time bombs. You won't experience complications until you've been on the drug for a while. For example, many drugs—tacrine (Cognex) for Alzheimer's disease, diclofenac (Voltaren) for pain, methotrexate for arthritis, oral ketoconazole (Nizoral) for fungal infections—that can lead to liver problems may take months before lab tests show abnormalities. With other drugs, however, allergic reactions, skin rashes, diarrhea, or gastrointestinal problems become apparent within hours of administration. (This is especially true of some antibiotics.)

In still other instances, problems declare themselves only after another drug has been added to the program. For example, you may take Advil, Motrin, Aleve, or some other over-the-counter pain reliever for a prolonged period and not experience any problems. Then one day your doctor puts you on a blood-pressure-lowering drug such as an ACE inhibitor (perhaps Vasotec, Capoten, or Monopril), and with no warning you develop kidney problems, or your blood potassium rises to a level that could cause an irregular heart rhythm.

Medications used to treat older individuals for heart problems or high blood pressure are of special concern. Let's say you or a family member have been prescribed a calcium channel blocker such as Calan or Cardizem for high blood pressure. Everything seems to be going fine until your physician decides to add a beta-blocker to help keep your blood pressure down. Suddenly you develop a very slow heart rate, incapacitating weakness, and dizziness, causing you to be rushed to the hospital. In this case, the combination of the calcium channel blocker plus the beta-blocker caused your heart rate and blood pressure to drop to a level that was insufficient to sustain an adequate blood flow to your brain.

A recent study confirmed that almost 25 percent of people 65 or older were taking medications considered inappropriate for their age or health status. Unfortunately, senior citizens may not notice any problems until something unexpected or dramatic happens. They may not realize they have been taking a pharmacological time bomb until they fall and break their hip because the drug they were taking made them sleepy; until a life-threatening bleeding episode in their gastrointestinal tract develops from the anti-inflammatory drug they were taking; or until they develop congestive heart failure because of the calcium channel blocker or beta-blocker they were taking in excessive doses.

The only safe approach is to *anticipate* problems with your medication intake. You must be *proactive* about evaluating your own drug regimen. You must try to get on drugs at the *outset* that have little or no chance of producing complications or interactions.

Problems related to medication intake may surface quietly and gradually, or suddenly and without any warning. This is certainly the case for medications such as non-steroidal anti-inflammatory drugs, blood thinners, and anti-arrhythmic medications. (See the Action Plan Checklist for Medication Time Bombs on page 370 for a list of medications that may pose significant problems over time.)

☺ Doctors may fail to reduce drug dosages over time.

For many common conditions such as high blood pressure, physicians may fail to attempt what is called "step-down" therapy. A drug-reduction technique advocated by the Joint National Commission Consensus Report on Hypertension, step-down therapy involves reducing a medication dose gradually over a period of days or weeks under the supervision of a doctor. It is estimated that about 20 percent of patients currently on a single blood pressure medication can be weaned off the drug and still have their blood pressure well controlled. Despite these impressive success rates, only a small percentage of the 40 million Americans with high blood pressure are ever considered for a step-down program.

☺ Doctors may fail to stop some drugs that should not be used at all or continued over the long term.

This "failure to eliminate" is one of many ways in which drug-prescribing patterns have spun dangerously out of control. A number of routinely prescribed medications tend to be used beyond their normally accepted duration limits. You may have been started on a drug several months or even many years ago, and though you may have been refilling prescriptions for the drug during this entire period, the medication may no longer be needed or appropriate for the original condition.

Other medications are frequently prescribed without adequate indications to justify their long-term use. These include Persantine for stroke; long-term Tagamet for ulcers; anti-arrhythmic drugs for irregular heart rhythms; digoxin for patients with suspected heart disease; antipsychotic medications for behavior control in skilled-care facilities for the aged; and Cognex for advanced symptoms of Alzheimer's disease.

Still other drugs that should be considered for possible elimination include medications that have been (inappropriately) maintained long beyond their window of therapeutic opportunity. Special attention should be focused on anti-ulcer medications, antibiotics, blood pressure medications, and anti-asthma drugs. On occasion, medications may become obsolete (such as short-acting verapamil for high blood pressure) because newer, safer drugs (in this case, amlodipine) that are more effective and have fewer side effects have become available.

Millions of Americans are taking medications that they simply do not need or that are outdated. For example, not everyone on antidepressant medications requires long-term therapy. Many people with *minor* stress- or situation-related depression who have been started on drugs such as Prozac, Zoloft, and Paxil, after 9 to 12 months of treatment should be given an opportunity to discontinue their therapy under careful supervision. Excessive use of blood-pressure-lowering medications is also rampant. Routinely, medications are being added to patients' drug regimens without considering opportunities for *eliminating* the drug that may not be working and *replacing* it with one that does.

In all these cases, you can spare yourself further years of unnecessary drug therapy (and wasted money) merely by calling your physician's attention to the medication.

Prolonged drug therapy for ulcer disease is an excellent case in point. Over nine million Americans have been put on chronic therapy with the rather costly H2-blocker anti-ulcer medications. Although many of these people may still require long-term-maintenance therapy with these medications, it is now generally accepted that the majority of gastric ulcers not caused by NSAIDs are the result of infection with a bacterium called *Heliobacter pylori*. This organism can be eradicated and peptic ulcers healed with as little as two weeks of intensive antibiotic therapy, in combination with other medications that inhibit secretion of gastric acid.

In practical terms, this means that many individuals are being maintained unnecessarily on long-term anti-ulcer drugs, simply because they have not received the proper treatment to eradicate the infectious agent responsible for the disease. You may be one of these individuals. Accordingly, if you or a family member are currently taking an H2-blocker for the treatment of ulcer disease, you should consult with your physician to determine if you are an appropriate candidate for the alternative short-term treatment directed against *H. pylori*.

 Doctors may unwittingly treat drug side effects with more drugs.

At times, physicians may unwittingly prescribe medications to treat symptoms that are being caused not by an underlying medical condition, but by the *side effects* of a drug the patient is already taking. This is just one factor contributing to the slippery slope leading to polypharmacy (the use of multiple medications). I once took care of a woman who came to me with a brown sack bulging with medications. She sat down in my office and explained: "Dr. Bosker, I take the blue pills to counteract the effects of the pink ones, and I take the pink ones to reduce the side effects of the green ones, and the green ones I take for the yellow pills, and the yellow pills help me tolerate the red capsules—and I forget why they put me on the red ones in the first place!"

Considering the recent explosion in the uses of drug therapy—combined with a corresponding expansion in our pharmaceutical arsenal—it is not surprising that polypharmacy and therapeutic mishaps have become a way of life and a concern for many individuals and their families.

TRAGIC BULLETS: WHAT HEALTH CARE PLANS, HMOs, AND OTHER INSTITUTIONAL ACTORS DO WRONG

If enough pressure is exerted by a sufficient number of informed consumers, it is possible that health plans, insurance companies, government agencies, managed care organizations, and other institutions will be forced to remedy some of the problems they contribute to medication use. Some of these problems are more serious than others, but all deserve our attention.

☺ Managed care organizations and HMOs may push generic drugs for bottom-line reasons.

Generic medications—widely endorsed, prescribed, and promulgated by health plans serving more than 75 million Americans—are at the center of a fierce debate in the medical world. Because the controversy is not entirely black and white, the relative advantages and disadvantages of generic drugs must be appreciated in order for you and your doctor to make improvements in your drug regimen.

First, a little background. Generic drugs, as you probably know, are very attractively priced medications that, for all practical purposes, contain the same active chemical ingredients as the brand-name drugs after which they are modeled. From a legal and proprietary standpoint, however, generic preparations cannot be manufactured until the patent for the brand-name medication has expired. Patents on medications usually last for up to fourteen years. As a rule, the majority of prescription medications that are currently available as generic preparations are pharmaceutical products that were first introduced for public consumption about ten years ago or longer.

Many insurance plans and managed care organizations have strongly endorsed a "generic first" approach to prescription medications, primarily as a cost-cutting maneuver to maximize profits. Alarmingly, many group care plans give physicians powerful incentives to prescribe generic drugs. In fact, a doctor's profit-sharing payout or year-end bonus may actually increase if he or she adheres strictly to the plan's limited stable of inexpensive generic medications.

The conflict of interest in such "prescribing for profit" practices is obvious: The health plan and the doctor (and even the shareholders) profit on the bottom line, but the patients suffer because they are denied better medications. No wonder that some physicians, in jest, have commented that HMO stands for "hokey medication organization." The so-called "gag rules" that attempt to prohibit physicians from talking about alternative (usually more expensive) medication therapies have now been found to be unconstitutional, so you will want to ask your physician whether he or she feels your medication options have been compromised by restrictive plan policies.

☺ Generic drugs usually mean lower quality at lower cost.

For the most part, the argument over generic medications boils down to price versus quality. Excessive reliance on generic medications is a form of "drug rot." Almost without exception, generic drugs are dirt cheap. But they simply don't provide as many conveniences, quality-of-life enhancements, safety benefits, and therapeutic advantages as brand-name medications. As we have seen, most prescription drugs that are available generically were first introduced for public consumption at least ten years ago and sometimes even twenty-five years ago! Most generic medications, even if they are chemically *identical* to the brand-name drugs they are replacing, are less *technologically* advanced than current brand-name drugs still under patent protection. In the world of pharmaceuticals, less technologically advanced usually means having less convenient dosing, more side effects, a higher risk of drug interactions, or less likelihood of producing real-world results.

Like vintage automobiles, generic medications are "older models" that constitute a type of "pharmacological obsolescence." Older cars may have their charms, and most can still get you to the mall and back, but from an engineering perspective they are not up to the standards of what's rolling off the assembly lines today. Car makers would never dream of making "generic" versions of their older models, yet pharmaceutical manufacturers make a fortune selling generic medications *representing an outdated state of product development!* No wonder your health will usually be better served by newer drugs—assuming you can afford them—that are not yet available as generic preparations.

One patient put it very succinctly: "Whenever my previous doctor gave me a prescription for a generic drug, I expected the instructions on the bottle to read something like, 'Take one teaspoon, three hundred times a day.'"

Nevertheless, proponents of generic medications argue that you can get the same pharmacological ingredients from them that you can from much more expensive brand-name equivalents. Although true, this kind of analysis misses the point entirely. From my perspective, as well as the perspective of many physicians and pharmacists, it is less a matter of whether generic drugs are as good as their brand-name equivalents than whether generic medications are as good as more *current* agents for which generic equivalents *are not yet available.*

That's why I sometimes refer to generic drugs as "moldy oldies." The fact that generic propranolol is probably just as effective as the brand-name product Inderal, or that generic verapamil is just as effective as the brand-name drug Calan, skirts the issue. Both the brand-name *and* the generic versions of these medications are suboptimal today. From your perspective as a patient, the critical issue is whether older brand-name drugs—purchased as generic formulations—have as much pharmacological value as newer drugs that are still on patent and that, therefore, have no generic version available. Nine times out of ten, they don't. It's that simple.

Consequently, you should be very concerned if your drug regimen contains an overwhelming preponderance of generic medications. Why? Because the *exclusive* use of generic medications—whether it be to treat high blood pressure, infections, or arthritis—suggests that a health plan or insurance company may be leaning on its physicians to prescribe with *purely cost* rather than quality and value considerations in mind. If this is the case, you will want to discuss the situation with your physician.

If you are being prescribed generic medications, do you have any recourse? Will your physician be permitted to switch you to better, brand-name drugs? The answer, almost without exception, is yes. Although most health plans encourage physicians to use an inexpensive generic medication *first*, almost all of them have brand-name drugs in reserve for special situations. If, for one reason or another, you express dissatisfaction with the side effects, dosing features, or effectiveness of a generic medication, *your physician will have the option of upgrading you to a brand-name medication.* Your level of concern, how well informed you are, and your ability to identify specific generic drugs for replacement are your "upgrade coupons." You must, however, make yourself heard, and the Action Plan (described in detail in Part III) is the ideal platform for communicating this kind of information.

Without question, some generic preparations (aspirin; atenolol/Tenormin; trimethoprim/sulfa-Septra) can be useful and cost effective in selected patients. A recent study showed that levothyroxine, a generic drug, was as effective as Synthroid, a brand-name medication, for treating people with thyroid problems. But these are exceptions to the rule. In general, the premium you or your health plan may have to pay for brand-name drugs is usually worth the price. After all, it is your health, nothing less. Generically available drugs such as amitriptyline, cimetidine, verapamil, and erythromycin simply do not have the same real world, clinical value as the brand-name drugs Zoloft, Pepcid, Norvasc, or Zithromax, respectively. The problem with generic drugs is not that they are generic, but that they are not the most value-oriented drugs within their respective class.

For these reasons, they cannot be considered equivalent substitutes for more advanced brand-name preparations still under patent. For example, the brand-name antidepressant Zoloft, unlike the generic antidepressant amitriptyline, is better tolerated, does not produce as much sleepiness, and does not increase the risk of falling in older patients. The blood pressure medication Norvasc, unlike generic verapamil, is approved for the treatment of both high blood pressure and angina, can be used safely in patients with congestive heart failure, and does not run the risk of slowing heart rates. Compared to generic cimetidine, Pepcid is less likely to produce harmful drug interactions. And unlike generic erythromycin, the brand-name antibiotic Zithromax is less likely to cause drug interactions, has to be taken only once a day for five days, and has better coverage for routine lung infections. (See the Action Plan Checklist for Generic Medications on page 373 to identify generic medications that, in most cases, ought to be replaced with better, brand-name drugs from a similar or related drug class.)

Many professional organizations, such as the American Academy of Family Practice, support the use of brand-name drugs, especially when it comes to treating life-threatening cardiovascular and neurological disorders. Antiseizure medications, digoxin, and drugs used to treat rhythm disturbances of the heart have been highlighted as drug classes for which brand-name medications are preferable.

In summary, compared with generic drugs, many newer brand-name drugs, which are not yet available in generic form, are characterized by improved drug-delivery systems, more favorable side-effect profiles, and more convenient dosing forms. And although brand-name drugs are much more costly on a pill-to-pill basis, they are usually worth the extra cost. Because they are safer, more versatile, more effective, and better at promoting compliance, over the long run they have the potential to reduce the total amount of money you spend on your health needs.

Naturally, if purchasing *all* brand-name drugs is simply not within your budget, be assured that a well-balanced mix of generic and nongeneric drugs represents a compromise that will work to your benefit. As part of your drug regimen reform, you and your physician can decide what combination of generic and brand-name drugs is best suited for your needs. In any event, if you are being treated primarily with generic drugs, you will benefit considerably from a program designed to replace these suboptimal medications.

MALPRACTICE IN THE PRESS: DIRECT TO CONSUMER ADVERTISING

After more than fifteen years of diagnosing and treating patients suffering from the consequences and potential hazards of unsafe and less-than-optimal prescription and over-the-counter medications, I felt there was an urgent need for a "fewer pills, better health" book that would empower consumers and their families to get the most out of medications and supplements, so they could add *high-quality, pain-free* years to their lives.

The need for a "less is more, safety first" program for medication use has never been greater. You and I have both read—and have been very troubled by—the recurring headlines we read in our daily newspapers and the health reports we see almost every day on prime-time TV:

- "Weight Loss Drugs Linked To Fatal Heart Problems: Pills pulled from market!"
- "Medication errors responsible for 100,000 unnecessary deaths each year"
- "Natural antidepressant remedy found safer, cheaper, and better tolerated than prescription medications used for mood problems"
- "FDA Yanks Allergy Pill That Can Cause Fatal Heart Rhythms"
- "Ineffective Antibiotics Cause Increased Use of Ear Tubes in Children: Better Prescribing Patterns Urged"
- "Pharmacists Fail To Recognize Deadly Drug Interactions"
- "Women: Misdiagnosed and Underserved For Life-Threatening Illnesses—Better Use of Medications Urged by Government Panel"
- "Thousands of Americans Dying Before Their Time Because of Failure to Get Preventive Medications"
- "New Miracle Drug Promises Relief For Arthritis Pain Sufferers"

As these articles suggest—and as you well know, these problems with prescription medicines are only getting worse—we are in the midst of an *epidemic* of inappropriate, suboptimal, and excessive drug prescribing that is affecting the health and well-being of *every* American family.

Much of the problem has to do with direct-to-consumer advertising. How can you protect yourself against misleading claims about advertised medications? The information in the MedRANK Section in Part II of this book will help you navigate through the landscape. Why? Because you will find not only drug descriptions, but you can look up the disease and see whether the drug being advertised is appropriate or not, and even better, you can see where the advertised drug falls as far as optimal, recommended, or avoid, thereby providing a check and balance.

☺ *Pharmaceutical company advertising and marketing may play too prominent a role in the prescription process.*

Oftentimes the pendulum swings the other way, toward unnecessarily expensive new drugs for situations in which a less expensive medication works just as well. For example, thousands of men with prostate problems are prescribed a costly medication called Proscar, even though a less expensive alternative such as Cardura or Hytrin may produce equivalent or, in many cases, more dramatic improvement in urinary symptoms (see Chapter 18). A similar trend has been observed with antibiotics. For bronchitis, physicians frequently prescribe Biaxin rather than Zithromax. Even though both drugs are effective, the former costs about $60 for a course of therapy whereas the latter costs about $40.

When physicians unnecessarily write prescriptions for expensive drugs that offer no significant advantages, it is often because they are influenced by sales pressures and promotional activities of the $88 billion-per-year pharmaceutical industry. I once overheard a physician comment to his patient: "I'm going to prescribe something that works like aspirin but costs much, much more." Clearly, consumers need a mechanism for overcoming this barrier to optimal drug therapy.

☺ *Managed care organizations and HMOs may restrict the drugs that prescribing practitioners can initially use for their patients.*

Because of drug formulary restrictions (limits on the medications that are accepted for use) in many cost-conscious managed care plans and HMOs, physicians are urged—some would say coerced—to use *inferior* drugs, at least as *initial* therapy. These would include, among others:

- Calcium channel blockers such as felodipine (Plendil) for patients with high blood pressure, which is known to produce a higher incidence of leg swelling than other calcium channel blockers, such as amlodipine (Norvasc)
- Diuretics to help control high blood pressure, which often cause unnecessary side effects and are considered by many experts to be the Ford Pinto of blood pressure medications
- Antibiotics such as amoxicillin and cefaclor to treat ear infections caused by bacteria that have a high likelihood of being resistant to these drugs
- Antihistamines that, compared with newer drugs, have a higher risk of side effects such as sedation
- The cholesterol-lowering medication fluvastatin (Lescol) for lowering cholesterol levels, even though atorvastatin (Lipitor) is more potent and therefore better able to achieve target goals of the National Cholesterol Education Program (NCEP)

In managed care settings, which now service the majority of all health-insured Americans, initial drug options typically are limited to those identified as "cost effective" by the health plan. In fact, physicians are encouraged to make such distinctions even among *brand-name* drugs. In the worst case, these plans slavishly advocate the least expensive agents even when they are "technologically" inferior, produce more side effects, and are therapeutically less effective than newer medications.

☺ Drug research and testing have treated women and the elderly as "pharmacological outcasts."

Certain groups of people are at higher risk for suboptimal drug therapy. For many years, studies evaluating medications were conducted primarily on males. Women were simply out of the loop. To some extent, this reflected the fact that men had a higher risk for heart disease and certain kinds of cancer. But the result was that the effectiveness of many medications was measured primarily according to how they performed in the male population. For example, only 10 percent of women with heart disease are treated aggressively enough with cholesterol-lowering drugs. The precise advantages and disadvantages of many commonly used drugs, such as those used to treat high blood pressure and heart disease, were not evaluated with the same intensity in women, who are frequently underserved and underprotected when it comes to drug therapy.

The same can be said for the elderly population. Although clinical trials for medication must now include a significant percentage of elderly patients, many medications currently on the market were tested in younger individuals who were not taking multiple medications. Because older patients are more likely to take many different drugs for their medical conditions, the risk of drug interactions is significantly greater in this group. The MedRANK Checklists in Part II attempt to account for the unique advantages and disadvantages of various medications in these groups of "pharmacological outcasts."

☺ Managed care health plans and HMOs frequently permit substitution of one drug for another at the pharmacy level.

This is sometimes called "blind" or "transparent" substitution. What is this widespread practice? Let's say you have been doing well taking a medication that belongs to a certain drug class. But you change health plans. Now, when you go to fill your prescription for that drug under the auspices of the new plan, the pharmacist is preauthorized to substitute what is perceived to be a "therapeutically equivalent," less expensive—and not infrequently, generic—drug for the one you have been taking for years with good results. Frequently, such drug substitutions present no problems. But in some cases, the new drug reflects important differences (involving convenience factors, user-friendliness, efficacy, or side effects) that can undermine the effectiveness and comfort level of your medication regimen.

You should not permit such brand interchanges. For example, you should not allow your pharmacist to change from one brand of digoxin to another, one calcium channel blocker to another, one antibiotic to another, or one antiseizure medication to another, without first consulting your doctor to see whether that interchange is safe.

☺ *Managed care organizations and HMOs may be overly dictatorial in determining which drugs their physicians may prescribe.*

Many managed care plans dictate to physicians their initial and secondary drug selections, in the form of drug utilization "report cards" and so-called "critical pathways." These reports, usually generated by the health plan's pharmacy department, rank medications of a given class according to their acquisition price and/or their desirability as an initial drug-of-choice for common medical conditions.

For example, a health plan pharmacy panel may issue the following antibiotic recommendations to its physician providers: "As your first choice, prescribe erythromycin for treatment of a bacterial lung infection. If this drug fails because your patient is intolerant of the gastrointestinal side effects caused by this medication, or if the patient fails therapy because he or she has an infection caused by *H. influenzae*, then upon reevaluation you may prescribe a newer macrolide such as Zithromax, which has a lower incidence of side effects and better coverage."

The annotations on the report card tell the story. The more costly medications—which frequently but not always will have advantages—are followed by several dollar signs ($$$$),

whereas less costly drugs are followed by only a single dollar sign ($), indicating their attractiveness. It goes without saying that physicians, who are held accountable for the profitability of their health plans—and whose own personal profit-sharing plans are usually linked to the HMO's overall financial performance—are encouraged to forgo the high-ticket medications in favor of the lower-priced options. As we've seen, in many cases this may mean generic medications that have fallen out of favor for one reason or another.

What does this mean for you? For all practical purposes, so that the health plan may save $20 on your pill bill, its directives have turned you into a "therapeutic experiment." Why? Because, to take the case just described, about 20 percent of patients show some degree of intolerance to erythromycin. Furthermore, up to 25 percent of pulmonary infections in adults—especially in people who smoke, have asthma, or suffer from lung problems—are caused by *H. influenzae*, bacteria against which erythromycin is completely ineffective. Zithromax would have been a more effective, user-friendly option from the outset.

The point is obvious: This system encourages doctors, at least in the first go-round, to use the least expensive—and not necessarily the most effective—medication, reserving the "top dog" drug only in the event of failure. Remember, in most health plans the amount you pay for a prescription is usually a *fixed* co-payment, so *you* usually don't save any money by having your doctor prescribe a less expensive medication. In the best case, you get an acceptable medication, and your plan profits handsomely by steering your practitioner, with the help of the drug report card, toward a less expensive drug. In the worst case, you get an inexpensive medication with an inferior side-effect profile, decreased effectiveness, and a more challenging dosing schedule. If treatment with this first drug fails, you may have to come back for a second try with a more expensive medication. The health plan has covered its bases, but at the expense of a return visit for you, inconvenience, time lost from work, and sometimes delayed resolution of your health problem.

You undoubtedly have read about these "pill-wise, penny-wise, patient-foolish" problems. Managing cost rather than managing care, in fact, has become a public policy issue in prescription writing. It should not come as a shock to learn that money is an important ingredient in the drug-prescribing equation. Perhaps the problem is best summarized by a cartoon in which a doctor explains to his patient, "This is time-released medication; it doesn't go off until your check clears."

Not surprisingly, patients are not the only people who are concerned about these trends. Physicians practicing in managed care settings are feeling increasingly "pillstrung and peeved." They are voicing increasing *opposition* to restrictions placed on them by health plans that discourage or prohibit prescribing current, more effective, and safer medications. By voicing *your* concerns about the quality and range of the drug options available for your health needs, you and your physician can work together to open up your health plan's drug arsenal and make better medications available to you and your family.

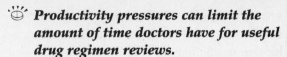 ***Productivity pressures can limit the amount of time doctors have for useful drug regimen reviews.***

Patients may not have the chance to benefit from better medications because their restricted access to physicians limits opportunities for their doctors to perform diligent, timely, and detailed reviews of their drug regimen. Patient education also is compromised. Without these reviews, the opportunities for introducing better, more advanced medications are limited.

Drug costs may impose significant barriers to medication compliance.

The financial strain associated with long-term drug therapy is highlighted in a cartoon in which a patient, prescription in hand, asks the pharmacist, "Are there any side effects to these pills apart from bankruptcy?" The message is clear: Drugs can be expensive—so expensive that people are often deterred from complying with their regimens. You may be one of them, or you may have a family member for whom drug costs are the *primary* determinant of faithful adherence to a medication program. If this is the case, you must identify these factors during the 12-Week Action Plan.

The importance of cost in determining medication compliance is a fiercely debated issue. Clearly it is a factor, but its effect on noncompliance will vary from patient to patient, according to their financial status. When the barriers to drug intake are primarily economic, cost should take precedence in drug selection; but if cost factors are not your principal concern, you should attempt to get your practitioner to select medications that emphasize versatility, quality, convenience, quality-of-life maintenance, and disease prevention. In many cases, higher cost is accompanied by better quality and superior results.

☺ *The FDA drug-approval process is a bottleneck that may prevent optimal and timely introduction of medications.*

Recent legislation permitting pharmaceutical companies to partner with the FDA in performing statistical analyses of clinical trials has helped expedite the drug-approval process. But the process still has bottlenecks, and many medications do not make it through the system in expeditious fashion, thereby denying Americans their health-promoting benefits.

☺ *Pharmacies sometimes provide insufficient or confusing labeling of pill bottles.*

Certain precautions that your prescribing provider or your pharmacist can take will help keep you fully informed about what a drug does, how frequently it should be taken, and so forth. Your prescribing practitioner should request that the name and the purpose of each drug be placed on each prescription container. This is very important, because in order to know whether you might benefit from reducing the number of medications you are taking, you need to transcribe specific drug information into a drug chronicle. (See the Drug Chronicle Checklist on page 337.) Moreover, labeling pill bottles this way significantly reduces the chances for error, especially those kinds of errors that are made when you are receiving prescriptions from more than one physician, or when prescriptions are filled by more than one pharmacist or pharmacy.

Giving careful attention to labeling, of course, requires that your physician be willing to take the time to write the purpose of each drug on the prescription, and that the pharmacist be willing to talk to your doctor if the instructions are not clear. Your doctor will usually honor your request to have such information included. The labeling should be simple, direct, and written in a language that is easily understood, regardless of your age or educational level. Simple examples would include "ampicillin—antibiotic for infection," or "hydrochlorothiazide—water pill for high blood pressure," or "digoxin—heart pill."

Every time you get a prescription filled, check the label to make sure that it tells you simply and clearly:

- The generic and brand names of the drug
- The purpose of the medication
- How often, how much, and how many pills must be taken
- Food or other incompatibilities

DON'T DESPAIR

Certainly a long list of problems can conspire to prevent you from obtaining pills that work. Some of these problems are more easily addressed than others, but all are capable of being resolved over the long term. What is needed is patience, dedication, and perseverance. Using the strategies discussed in the next chapter, we can usher in a new pill philosophy that will promote better health for all.

CHAPTER 3

TOWARD A NEW AND BETTER "PILLOSOPHY"

What can you do to overcome problems associated with less-than-optimal drug therapy? Armed with specific *comparative and precautionary* information about the medications that you or a family member is taking, and working in close collaboration with your physician, you will be able to achieve better health, at lower risk, by modifying and upgrading your current medication regimen. Many factors influence the safety and efficacy of drug regimens; a better understanding of how they may either enhance or compromise the quality of your regimen is essential for improving it. Among the most important issues that should be considered are how to do the following:

- Review your drug regimen to identify better pills and inferior pills. (The MedRANK Checklists in Part II provide a road map to help you make these distinctions.)

- Communicate with your physician or prescriber.
- Improve compliance with your medication regimen.
- Distinguish pills that work from pills that don't.
- Learn to better observe the effects of your drugs on yourself.

After taking a closer look at these points, I'll also offer some insights into special considerations for medication use in children and the elderly.

REVIEW YOUR DRUG REGIMEN

Regardless of the specific drugs you or a family member may be taking, virtually all regimens could benefit from careful screening and evaluation. If any of your drugs have to be taken more often than *once* a day, it is probably worth consulting your pharmacist or physician to see whether your regimen can be streamlined for more convenient (once-daily) dosing. Also, risky drug combinations and any unnecessary medications should be eliminated from your regimen.

If a drug cannot be eliminated from your regimen, however, you still have options for increasing the safety and friendliness of your medication program. Perhaps the most important of the other opportunities for reducing drug costs and side effects is reduction of drug dose. Screening your regimen to identify medications that can be taken at much lower doses is one of the most important guiding principles of this book. It is staggering to think how many medications are used today at far lower doses than just a few years ago, while still maintaining the same degree of therapeutic effectiveness. Unfortunately, despite rigorous FDA mandates and regulations governing clinical trials, many new drugs are still introduced into popular use at doses that exceed what is necessary to produce excellent clinical results.

Do not accept drug-associated side effects as unavoidable. In fact, in most cases, they *are* avoidable. It's just a matter of selecting an alternative drug that is appropriate for you. What's more, don't be reluctant to question your physician or pharmacist about the necessity of continuing a medication that you are currently taking. If possible, resist the tendency to cling to long-standing drug regimens. Rather, consider any opportunities for drug modification that your physician proposes. These may involve new medications with reduced side effects and greater user-friendliness.

PILL TALK: LEARN TO COMMUNICATE WITH YOUR PHYSICIAN

To maximize the health benefits of drug therapy, make sure you have a forthright exchange of information with your physician—in both directions. First, you as the patient must be provided with accurate information about your medical condition and the medications prescribed for you. Moreover, you must

FRANK & ERNEST ® by Bob Thaves

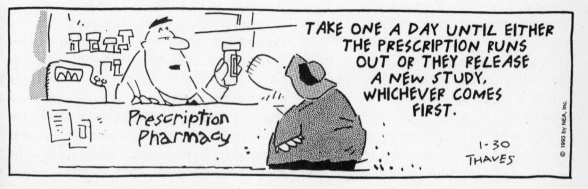

TAKE ONE A DAY UNTIL EITHER THE PRESCRIPTION RUNS OUT OR THEY RELEASE A NEW STUDY, WHICHEVER COMES FIRST.

Prescription Pharmacy

1-30 THAVES

© 1993 by NEA, Inc.

understand why your prescribing health care provider has made certain recommendations.

In turn, your physician must know your concerns about medication intake. Are you worried about cost? Convenience? Side effects? Quality-of-life changes? If you have any such concerns, communicate them at the time your medication is prescribed. If some of your questions surface after you have been taking your medication, let your physician know about them as soon as possible. Your knowledge of your medical condition and the drugs you are taking will influence your compliance. A considerable amount of noncompliance is caused by misunderstandings or poor communication between patient and provider. Common errors in medication instruction that you should be aware of include:

- Medications prescribed without adequate discussion
- Lack of information about how long you should take a medication
- Incomplete written instructions

The importance of asking your physician for adequate information cannot be overemphasized. One study showed that among patients who misunderstood their drug regimen poorly, only 17 percent complied with their prescriber's instructions. In contrast, more than 50 percent of patients with accurate information cooperated with their therapeutic program.

Remember, medications do not work optimally by themselves. For best results, you need to work with them. In other words, you

may need to adjust dietary, drinking, or lifestyle habits to maximize their effectiveness. Your physician should provide you with information about the medications that you are currently taking. The National Council on Patient Information and Education has established guidelines to help patients obtain essential facts that pertain to prescription medications. These guidelines include a number of issues you should clarify with your physician before taking any medication:

- What is the name of the drug, and what is it supposed to do?
- How and when do I take this drug—and for how long will I need to take it?
- What foods, drinks, other medications, or activities should I avoid while taking this drug?
- Are any side effects associated with this medication, and what should I do if they occur?
- Is there any written information about this drug? If so, where is it available?

Your physician or pharmacist should take the time to present you with a wide range of information, including helpful hints on how to take your drug, safety warnings, and significant side effects. You should receive instructions on how to take it with regard to meals. You should be instructed when to avoid alcohol, and what to do if you have missed a medication dose. Specific reasons for notifying your physician should be outlined. Information on problems associated with sudden discontinuation of the medication and brand interchange should be communicated in a clear and concise fashion. When laboratory tests are required to monitor your drug therapy, these requirements should be made clear at the outset. Naturally, if you have any additional questions concerning the use, indications, precautions, or side effects of a medication, ask your pharmacist or physician prior to beginning it.

☺ Self-advocacy is your best communication tool.

You are your own best advocate when it comes to detecting potential benefits, concerns, and inadequacies associated with your medication intake. Although your knowledge of the technical or pharmacological aspects of your drugs may be somewhat limited at first, the information in this book will provide the basis for effective communication about them with your physician. After reviewing and studying the recommendations in the Med-RANK Checklists in Part II, you will be better able to judge whether your drugs are working, how they make you feel, and whether you are taking the *best* ones available for your condition.

Safeguarding your personal pharmacology requires both information and communication. Some of the information will have to come from your physician or pharmacist, and some will come from the MedRANK Checklists. In any event, improving your medication intake will require keeping the channels of communication open between you and your doctor. This is especially true if you have a chronic condition requiring long-term medication, if you are taking more than two differ-

ent prescription medications, or if you are older than 60. Your objective is to distinguish between pills that harm and pills that cure, between wasteful drugs and wonder drugs, between drugs that cause disease and those that prevent it.

☺ Talking drugs: Collaborate, then medicate.

Engaging your physician in a discussion or review of your current medications does not mean that you are being confrontational. You shouldn't feel defensive, or feel as if you are undermining the authority of your physicians. Most physicians—and, especially, pharmacists—will welcome your participation in such discussions. The fact is, you know how your body and mind are feeling better than your physician does. You can turn this to your advantage because, after all, you are charged with caring for only a single patient—yourself—whereas your prescribing practitioner may be overwhelmed from having to keep track of hundreds of patients, with little more than scanty information gleaned from short encounters. A candid exchange between you and your prescriber about your drug regimen will make his or her job easier and, in general, will produce the best results for you.

As I emphasized earlier, many prescribers simply don't have the time to analyze a patient's medication regimen in the kind of excruciating detail they would like. Consequently, your practitioner can use your help, especially if the information you provide is accurate and your motives are well intentioned. In this day and age, informed consumers learn about advantages and indications for newly introduced drugs not only in books such as this one but in the lay press and popular media, sometimes long before their physicians do. Admittedly, physicians are not always comfortable with being upstaged, but for the most part they have accepted the fact that patients are becoming increasingly knowledgeable about matters relating to their drug therapy.

☺ *Don't become your own doctor.*

Although communication is key, it is important that you reassure your prescribing practitioner that your intention is not to prescribe medications for yourself, or to determine which drugs are best for you. Rather, you are interested in providing helpful information—and working in collaboration with your physician—so he or she can tailor drug choices to your specific needs.

....

IMPROVE COMPLIANCE

You may wonder why physicians and pharmacists so emphatically stress medication compliance—taking a medication at the dosage it was prescribed, at the appropriate intervals or time of day, and with or without meals, as instructed. One of the most important benefits of compliance is the opportunity to manage an illness with *fewer* rather than more medications. As ironic as it may seem, patients who *fail* to take their medications as prescribed actually *increase* the likelihood that they will become victims of polypharmacy.

For example, if you have to take a medication more often than twice a day, there is a good chance your therapy will fail. People simply aren't very good about taking drugs more than twice a day. If you are noncompliant and the medication does not have a chance to work, your laboratory results or physical signs (such as blood pressure, wheezing, or coughing) will tend to be abnormal. Unfortunately, abnormal laboratory values and physical signs are the primary reasons physicians prescribe medications. And herein lies the pharmacological problem.

☺ *When erratic medication intake produces unsatisfactory results, physicians usually try to correct the problem by throwing more medications at the patient.*

They do this in order to "get the numbers square on a piece of paper"—that is, to get the laboratory values corrected into the normal range. Naturally, if you inform your physician that you have failed to take the medications as prescribed, you may be able to avoid this problem. Your doctor may be wise enough to understand that what you need is a new drug to replace the one you haven't been taking, rather than a stern talk about compliance. But if your doctor thinks you *have* been taking the medication as prescribed, it can be the beginning of a vicious cycle in which more pills are prescribed to "put out the fire" of your supposed poor compliance. The end result may be inappropriate and unnecessary drug prescribing. The solution is to use and have confidence in medications that are dosed on a once-daily basis.

The phenomenon of medication noncompliance, in part, explains why millions of

Americans are prescribed second or even third courses of antibiotics to cure their infections, and why so many people with hypertension are taking several medications to keep it under control.

Improved compliance usually translates into better therapeutic results. It should be emphasized, however, that lower doses of medications don't always work in every patient. Some medications simply don't perform well at low doses in certain individuals, and you may be one of them. It may be necessary for your doctor to select a *replacement* medication that can be dosed at lower levels and still produce equivalent or better results, but with far fewer side effects.

☺ *Despite some exceptions, the advantages of decreased dosage have been observed in a number of commonly prescribed medications.*

Consider, for example, the once-popular anxiety-reducing medication Halcion. When this drug was first introduced, the manufacturer recommended using it at a dose of about 0.5 mg at night for sleep. After physicians and pharmacists gained sufficient real-world experience with this drug, however, it became clear that doses of that magnitude, especially in older patients, could produce undesirable side effects, including memory loss, confusion, and disorientation. Eventually, when dosage recommendations were lowered by about 75 percent to 0.125 mg, the safety of the drug and its side-effect profile improved dramatically. At this dose, Halcion maintained its effectiveness for sleep disorders and anxiety-related conditions but had a significantly re-duced risk of troubling side effects. Similarly, a number of other commonly used medications have also been shown to produce good results at lower doses than their manufacturers originally recommended. Although not an exhaustive list, these medications include estrogen, birth control pills, blood thinners, aspirin, AZT, ACE inhibitors, and antidepressants.

Other factors can also improve compliance. For example, studies show that compliance with your medication regimen will improve as your social networks improve, as you receive more education about your regimen, and as you obtain closer supervision over it. For elderly people who are taking complicated multiple-drug regimens, their drug intake will be enhanced if nurses make visits to their homes, if they are warned about the negative consequences of poor compliance, and if their drug intake is monitored. The best results are achieved if the pharmacist and physician provide clear information about a medication's risks and benefits. Doctors should emphasize information about adverse side effects and the efficacy of the treatment plan they are proposing. Ideally, they should provide written instructions.

EMBRACE "LESS IS MORE"

The importance of "starting low and going slow" cannot be overemphasized. When it comes to using drugs at excessive doses, we have learned our lessons the hard way. Over the years, it is estimated that thousands of hospitalizations and even many deaths could have been prevented if only researchers had conducted clinical trials using smaller doses of many common medications. Fortunately, however, the "less is more" approach now appears to be a permanent part of our therapeutic philosophy. It is even fair to say that some drugs are more effective at a reduced dosage because they are associated with fewer side effects and as a result patients are better able to comply with taking them.

☺ When more is less: Another red flag is the presence of medications that are being prescribed at levels that approach their highest recommended daily dose.

You can make a significant impact on the quality of your drug therapy, as well as on your sense of well-being, by asking your physician whether any of the medications you are taking have been prescribed at or near the highest recommended daily dose. When drugs *are* prescribed at their higher dose limits, the risk of side effects is increased, the cost is usually greater, and the therapeutic effects may be less than optimal. Although you, in fact, may require these high doses, some medications simply don't perform well in individual patients, of whom you may be one. It may be possible for your physician to select a replacement that can be dosed at lower levels and still produce equivalent or better results.

The wisdom of using lower doses has been confirmed for many commonly used medications, including thyroxine supplements and antibiotics. Three examples worthy of a closer look include estrogen, ulcer drugs such as Tagamet, Cytotec, and Zantac, and blood pressure–lowering medications.

☺ Optimal doses of estrogen.

Estrogen replacement therapy (ERT) reduces the risk of osteoporosis, heart disease, and perhaps even stroke in women who begin taking these hormone supplements shortly after the onset of menopause or following hysterectomy. These disease-prevention benefits—which may also include delay in the onset of symptoms of Alzheimer's disease—come in addition to estrogen's quality-of-life-enhancing properties, including clarity of mind, improved skin tone, vaginal lubrication, and reduction in hot flashes. On the downside (although the studies are conflicting on this issue), epidemiological data suggest that estrogen replacement therapy may increase slightly the risk of developing breast cancer in women over the long term. But other studies fail to confirm the link between ERT and breast cancer. Therefore, the decision to initiate hormone replacement should be made on a patient-by-patient basis.

The overall trend, however, should be to *encourage* estrogen use in postmenopausal women, since its advantages far outweigh its potential liabilities in the overwhelming majority of patients. And although there is clear evidence that ERT increases the risk of endometrial cancer, this problem, for the most part, can be prevented by the use of progestin hormones in combination with estrogen.

As far as the dose is concerned, you should be aware that there is an apparent increase in the risk for developing blood clots among women who are prescribed more than

1.25 mg per day. Consequently, doses in this range should be avoided. You should confirm with your physician that you are taking the lowest recommended dose of estrogen shown to prevent heart disease. In women who have had a hysterectomy, treatment with conjugated estrogen (Premarin) at a daily dose of 0.625 mg is appropriate. In women without hysterectomy, progestins should be added to estrogen to minimize the risk of endometrial cancer. The standard recommended, low-dose estrogen/progestin regimen consists of 0.625 mg conjugated estrogen plus continuous low-dose progesterone (2.5 mg per day of medroxyprogesterone) per day.

☺ *Pills for ulcers and indigestion.*

Drugs used to treat gastrointestinal problems, especially ulcers and "acid indigestion," can cause many unpleasant side effects at high doses. When taken at high doses, H2-blockers such as the popular ulcer drug Tagamet can cause confusion, breast tenderness and enlargement, and impotence in men. Consequently, if you are taking one of these medications—Tagamet, Zantac, Pepcid, or Cytotec—you should review your prescription with your doctor to be sure that you are taking the lowest effective daily dose. Curiously, in the case of Tagamet (which is now available over-the-counter without a prescription), reductions in daily dose have been quite dramatic. When Tagamet, the first H2-blocker approved for treatment of peptic ulcer disease, was introduced into the market, daily doses as high as 1,600 to 2,000 mg per day were routinely recommended. Unfortunately, these dosage lev-

els were associated with a significant risk of disabling side effects, especially confusion, which necessitated discontinuation in a large percentage of patients. Subsequent experience with Tagamet has shown that doses as low as 400 mg per day, or 25 percent of the initial recommended dose, are sufficient for ulcer healing and symptom relief.

Similar dose reductions apply to Cytotec, a popular drug used to *prevent* ulcers in older patients who are taking NSAIDs (including ibuprofen, Motrin, Aleve, and naproxen) for arthritis and related medical conditions. Originally this drug was used at doses of 200 mcg four times a day. At these levels, it produced diarrhea and stomach cramps in up to 50 percent of people who had to take it on a regular basis. As with the H2-blockers, dose reductions for Cytotec have been approved, and as expected, the medication is much better tolerated at these new dose levels. (See Chapter 12 for more information on drugs for ulcers and other gastrointestinal problems.)

☺ *Blood pressure–lowering drugs.*

Some of the most dramatic advantages of lowering dosage are observed with drugs used to treat high blood pressure. One of the most popular class of drugs used to treat hypertension, the ACE inhibitors were introduced at dosage levels that could cause kidney failure in a small but significant percentage of people for whom they were prescribed. For example, captopril (Capoten) was initially recommended at doses as high as 25 to 50 mg three times a day. Subsequent experience with this drug, however, revealed that blood pressure reduction could be accomplished with doses as low as 12.5 mg twice or three times daily. Consequently, if you or a family member are taking any medications, including Vasotec, Zestril, Capoten, or lisinopril, that belong to the ACE inhibitor class, you should see your physician to ensure that your dose reflects current recommendations.

The problem with thiazide diuretics is of even greater concern, since these drugs are routinely recommended by national expert committees and many cost-conscious health plans as medications of first choice for the treatment of high blood pressure. Put simply, these drugs that are used to get rid of water are used like water—and not without risk. Unfortunately, as inexpensive, well tolerated, and effective as thiazide diuretics may be at low doses, a lethal snake in the grass lurks, especially for people with severe heart disease who are prescribed very *high* doses of the drug. The problem appears to be aggravated in people who do not receive protection against the potassium losses these medications can cause. Recent studies suggest that dose reduction is especially important for thiazide diuretics. It is estimated that more than 40 million Americans are currently taking these drugs for high blood pressure and/or heart disease.

As recently as ten years ago, physicians were "carpet bombing" patients with excessive doses of diuretics. It was not uncommon for patients to be treated in the range of 100 to 150 mg per day. Although the drugs were clearly effective at this range, they were also notorious for producing a number of side effects, ranging from low potassium levels to sudden death. Presumably, the latter was caused by serious cardiac arrhythmias—irregular heart rhythms. In fact, recent studies using high-dose diuretic therapy—that is, hydrochlorothiazide doses of 50 mg or greater per day—in patients with heart disease and high blood pressure revealed an unexpected increase in sudden cardiac death. The increase in sudden death negated more than 50 percent of the benefits seen with improved blood pressure control. As the daily dose of thiazide diuretics increased from 25 mg to 50 mg to 100 mg, there was a corresponding increase in sudden death. Fortunately, the risk of sudden death could be reduced significantly if a potassium-sparing medication was added to the thiazide prescription.

If you are one of the millions of people in this country who is taking a thiazide diuretic, your 12-Week Action Plan must include a careful review of the dosing. Initial therapy with a thiazide should be at a low dose (12.5 mg to 25 mg per day). If higher doses are required (50 to 100 mg per day), you should ask your physician to add a potassium-sparing drug to your regimen. Even better, if you are taking high doses of these drugs for high blood pressure, you should probably encourage your physician to switch you to a different drug class altogether. (Additional recommendations for drug reduction and replacement in people with high blood pressure can be found in Chapter 6.)

In addition, making lifestyle changes (such as weight loss, regular physical activity, smoking cessation, or reduction of alcohol consumption) can reduce your dependence on prescription medications. Many commonly prescribed drugs are amenable to elimination or dose reduction as a result of positive lifestyle changes. These include medications used to treat blood pressure, heart disease, diabetes, bronchitis, asthma, allergies, chest pain, back pain, childhood infections, urinary tract infections, sexually transmissible disease, and many others.

BECOME A BETTER DRUG OBSERVER

If you "know thyself" and use the information in this book wisely, you can become an important participant in achieving better health. Moreover, you will also be in a better position to assess and evaluate your response to a prescribed drug.

Without question, any precise, detailed information you can provide to your physician will be considered valuable. If you suspect you are experiencing troublesome side effects, and these side effects discourage you from taking your medications exactly as prescribed, your doctor will want to know so that alternative medications can be considered. For example, you may be one of the millions of Americans currently taking a Prozac-like antidepressant. Like most such individuals, you may not be aware of the differences in side effects among the three widely used SSRIs. Some people will respond in a more or less exaggerated fashion to these medications, and consequently one agent may be a much better match for you than another. This emphasizes the importance of telling your physician about any uncomfortable symptoms, however subtle they may be, that you may have.

GETTING THE BUGS OUT: SPECIAL ISSUES FOR CHILDREN

Especially among children, parents must begin working with physicians to eliminate the routine use of medications associated with troublesome side effects, inferior treatment outcomes, or poor medication compliance. For example, amoxicillin suspension is an antibiotic routinely used for the treatment of ear infections in children—it is prescribed to more than 14 million patients each year. Yet its proven cure rate is one of the worst in the antibiotic business. Given this track record, why is it prescribed with such frequency? Because physicians are pressured by health plans to use this inferior, cheap ($8 per course of therapy) antibiotic first, before trying better, slightly more expensive agents that are known to get the job done the first time around. In the process, however, children suffer. Approximately one child in three has to be retreated. Even worse, the complications of treatment failures can include recurrent infections requiring surgical intervention, deafness, and the development of resistant bacteria.

Why doesn't this antibiotic work? One reason is that it has to be given for too many days and for too many doses. What's more, it can produce diarrhea, which deters parents from administering the entire course of therapy. In addition, over the years, certain strains of bacteria that cause middle ear infections (*Streptococcus pneumoniae, Hemophilus influenzae,* and *Moraxella catarrhalis*) have become resistant to amoxicillin. Moreover, amoxicillin is not "day-care proof": it has to be administered three times daily, which means that parents may have to depend on unreliable day-care centers to administer at least one dose. These critical palatability, "poopability," and predictability factors combine to produce a high rate of treatment failure. The patients lose. The only winners are the health plans, which increase their short-term profits—and of course, the bacteria, which survive the antimicrobial onslaught and go on to reproduce.

Are there other options besides amoxicillin? Of course there are. If physicians did weigh all the factors, they would routinely prescribe Zithromax Oral Suspension, a $28 antibiotic that covers all the bugs, has to be given only once a day for five days, and produces side effects so minimal that kids take the drug willingly and reliably.

Prescribing antibiotics for children involves critical "give and take" issues. That is, parents have to want to give the drug, and kids have to want to take it. Keep it simple. If you can take only one in the morning, why bother with a drug that requires one dose in the morning, one at lunch, and another after dinner?

••

GETTING GRANNY OFF PILLS: SPECIAL ISSUES FOR THE ELDERLY

We continue to learn from our elders. In fact, older Americans were the first to call our attention to the potentially devastating consequences of unnecessary prescription medications. The complications associated with excessive, inappropriate, and unsafe medication practices in nursing homes helped cata-

pult this issue into the public spotlight. Either directly or indirectly, the problems associated with excessive drug prescribing in the elderly population have touched virtually every American family in one way or another. Millions of people have visited or heard about elderly relatives—many of them with Alzheimer's disease—who deteriorated dramatically after being placed in skilled nursing facilities or foster homes. We now understand that many of these problems—sedation, disorientation, excessive sleepiness, confusion, and loss of vigor—are caused by the excessive use of antipsychotic medications (particularly tranquilizers such as Haldol, Thorazine, and Navane) that physicians prescribed to control behavioral disturbances in the elderly.

These problems are gradually being addressed by educational programs and medication-reduction plans in thousands of nursing facilities across the country. In the face of growing evidence that many sedating and tranquilizing medications could be discontinued in older individuals without adversely affecting their behavioral state, the government has stepped in with its own legislative action plan. The Nursing Home Reform Amendments of 1987 (Omnibus Reconciliation Act-87, or OBRA-87, Regulations) sought to narrowly restrict the use of these drugs in nursing home patients. Although their use is justified in many demented patients with uncontrollable agitation and behavioral disturbances, they can also produce a wide range of disabling symptoms, including chronic movement disorders, impaired alertness, social withdrawal, and increased risk of falls and hip fractures.

☺ *If you have a family member or close friend who is in a nursing facility on multiple medications, you can use the Action Plan Checklists in Part III to ensure that OBRA-87 regulations are being applied and also to identify specific drugs that ought to be considered for elimination.*

If you are informed about studies that confirm the safety of medication elimination and dose reduction in nursing home residents, you will be better positioned to persuade the physician caring for your relative or friend to initiate the Action Plan in this book. First, you should be aware that the OBRA regulations attempt to restrict antipsychotic medication use in dementia (Alzheimer's disease) only for those whose behaviors are considered dangerous to the patient or others, or that interfere with provision of adequate patient care.

Most likely you will have to educate your physician about OBRA regulations, since most practitioners are not familiar with the specific mandates they contain. First, emphasize to your doctor that these regulations require a trial of nondrug therapy to control behavior problems before introducing medications. In addition, in patients who have been stable for several months, they recommend a gradual reduction in antipsychotic medications. One important study conducted in nursing homes showed that a 36 percent decrease in the use of psychotropic drugs was accompanied by no increase in behavioral problems. Nursing homes that reduced the use of these powerful sedating drugs by 18 percent saw no increase in behavioral problems and less deterioration in short-term memory among the residents

who had their drugs discontinued. In another study conducted in twelve community nursing homes, a reduction in psychotropic drug use actually decreased psychiatric symptoms by 21 percent in patients who had their drugs eliminated.

☺ *The good news for the cognitively compromised elderly person is that less can be more, and in a greater number of cases than physicians ever expected.*

Study after study has shown that the availability of alternative behavioral techniques and better medications justifies withdrawal of antipsychotics and psychotropic medications in a selected group of patients. If you have a close friend or relative in a nursing facility who is suffering from dementia and is taking multiple mind-altering drugs (whether sedatives, hypnotics, or sleep medications), you are on solid ground in urging his or her physician to *consider* strongly a trial of drug tapering.

Unfortunately, it is difficult to predict in which older patients drug withdrawal is likely to succeed. But at least two factors strongly correlate with success. Medication withdrawal is more likely to be successful, first, in nursing home residents who are receiving *lower* doses of antipsychotic drugs, and second, in those who are using only a *single* psychotropic agent.

If one of these profiles fits your friend or relative in a nursing home, and this person seems adversely affected by sedating medications, you should make them aware of the 12-Week Action Plan in this book. This usually means working in collaboration with the physician and the nurses to ensure that OBRA-87 guidelines are being followed. With a carefully monitored program of drug elimination or dose reduction, you can help restore vigor, brightness, and a sense of engagement with life that would never have been possible under the mind-altering cloud of powerful medications. Nothing is more gratifying than helping to lift the veil of overmedication that deprives so many older patients of the pleasures of emotional engagement with relatives and loved ones.

If you or a family member is elderly and you are using this book to evaluate the medications being taken, you should keep in mind a number of other issues and potential pitfalls. Perhaps most important, elderly patients are at higher risk for experiencing drug-related side effects and potential medication errors than other groups of health care consumers. Unfortunately, older individuals have a tendency not to communicate the problems, side effects, or even financial concerns associated with their medications.

☺ *It is always helpful for elderly patients to ask their physician or pharmacist if any of the drugs they're taking are considered unsuitable or inappropriate for older individuals.*

Physicians should know the possible adverse effects that many drugs may cause in elderly individuals, but many do not. A careful review of the patient's current regimen is the best approach for uncovering potential problems.

A number of drugs are best avoided by senior citizens. These include sedative/hypnotic drugs (sleeping pills) such as Valium, Dalmane, Librium, and meprobamate. NSAIDs, especially Indocin, are best avoided unless absolutely necessary. Blood pressure–lowering drugs that have a tendency to cause sleepiness and sedation are best avoided, including Aldomet, reserpine, and propranolol. Unproven therapies for dementia (cyclandelate, isoxsuprine), tricyclic antidepressants (amitriptyline, doxepin), analgesics (propoxyphene/Darvon; pentazocine), muscle relaxants, and short-acting barbiturates (pentobarbital) will usually produce little benefit in the older patient. Evaluate each medication in your or your family member's regimen one by one, and ask your physician about any special considerations or precautions relating to the drug's use in the older individual. (See the Action Plan Checklist for Inappropriate Medications for the Elderly and the Action Plan Checklist for "Mental Manglers" on page 369 for additional medications that are unsuitable or require extreme caution in senior citizens.)

A recent landmark study published in *The Journal of the American Medical Association* reported an alarming incidence of prescriptions inappropriate for the elderly. Geriatric experts in the United States and Canada developed explicit criteria and showed that almost one-quarter of people aged 65 years or older—which corresponds to some 6.6 million Americans—received at least one of twenty contraindicated drugs. While 80 percent of the people receiving potentially harmful medications received only one such drug, about 20 percent received two or more. Among the drugs considered inappropriate in this population, the most commonly prescribed were dipyrimadole, propoxyphene (Darvon), amitriptyline (Elavil), chlorpropamide (Diabinese), diazepam (Valium), indomethacin, and chlordiazepoxide (Librium), each of which was taken by at least 600,000 individuals 65 or older. The study concluded that physicians prescribed potentially inappropriate medications for nearly a quarter of older people.

More good news for the older, cognitively compromised person who has been overmedicated: Various drug classes, including medications used to treat high blood pressure, heart disease, and gastrointestinal problems, can be withdrawn or have their dose reduced in up to 60 percent of older patients.

One landmark study evaluating the complications of withdrawing medications concluded that, although 62 percent of patients experienced problems when their medication was discontinued, the overwhelming majority (72 percent) of these problems were of a minor nature. Overall, the most important finding was that 60 percent of all discontinued medications were not reinstituted. In other words, these drugs were no longer needed to maintain patients in good health.

For example, among the people who had drugs eliminated in this study, the ulcer medication ranitidine (Zantac) had to be reinstituted in only 17 percent of patients, theophylline in 25 percent, and Haldol in only 20 percent. Dilantin had to be restarted in 30 percent of patients, digoxin in 40 percent, and the diuretic furosemide in 72 percent. These findings lend strong support to the drug-elimination goals of this book. They also confirm that drug-reduction programs have a high degree of success and pose very acceptable risks for those willing to undertake them.

—

PART II

THE MedRANK CHECKLISTS: A RATING SYSTEM FOR PRESCRIPTION MEDICATIONS

KNOWING AND DEMANDING THE BEST AND SAFEST PRESCRIPTION MEDICATIONS FOR YOU AND YOUR FAMILY

The MedRANK Life Prolongation and Enhancement Checklists

INTRODUCTION

Personal pharmacology is anything but a level playing field. When you are sick and need medications, there are better pills and worse pills. Part II consists of an easy-to-use, "pill-for-disease" ranking system that will give you all the tools and information you will need to make these important distinctions. Although several drugs may be approved to treat a particular symptom or disease, these medications are not necessarily equally safe or effective. In most cases, the significant differences among them deserve thoughtful consideration. A comparative evaluation that considers convenience, effectiveness, safety, versatility, quality of life, disease prevention, and life prolongation will help steer you and your doctor toward the best medications, and away from those of marginal or questionable quality.

Perhaps a car analogy can illustrate the point. The automobiles on display in a typical Ford showroom differ dramatically from one another, yet they are all Fords. A Ford Escort is not a Contour or a Taurus or a Lincoln Town Car. These automobiles—in particular, their safety features, road performance, styling, and user-friendliness—are as different as night and day. You will prefer one model over another because it is built better, drives better, and looks better than another car in the Ford "family." Differences among pills are much more difficult to identify—unfortunately, you can't test-drive several different ones in an afternoon—yet the dissimilarities are every bit as dramatic. For example, medications that belong to the class of blood pressure–lowering pills called calcium channel blockers are as diverse as the Ford models described above. Among the eleven available calcium channel blockers, some can impair contraction of the heart muscle and can cause life-threatening complications, whereas others do not. Some can interact with other medications and slow the heart rate to dangerous levels, whereas others do not. And yet all are calcium channel blockers. Equally important differences characterize antibiotics, drugs used to lower cholesterol levels, and antidepressants, as well as virtually every other class of drugs.

Differences among drugs can have a profound impact on health and well-being. The fact is that some medications have advantages over others. In some cases, these advantages are linked to safety, in others to prevention, in still others, to efficacy. From a quality perspective, some pills are considered to be "top of the line"—or "best of class"—medications, and others fall far short of the mark. If you intend to feel as well as you possibly can, if one of your goals is to prolong your life or the lives of your family members, then you should demand—and know how to get—high-performing medications. But to get the best and safest pills our health care industry has to offer, you must have a road map that will steer you and your prescribing providers to them.

PILLS OF WISDOM: THE ROAD TO BETTER MEDICATIONS AND OPTIMAL HEALTH

The information contained in Part II is intended to take you on the journey from inferior drugs to superior drugs. The information is organized by chapters, which correspond to the most common medical conditions. Each chapter contains sections called "Pills of Wisdom," which provide a broad overview of the treatment options available for that medical condition, an analysis of the risks and

benefits of using certain medications, and a brief discussion of recent innovations in drug therapy. Medications that represent leaps in effectiveness and/or user-friendliness are highlighted, and drugs that are associated with inferior results or safety problems are flagged.

This is where you will learn about the pearls and pitfalls associated with *specific* pills. When relevant, a thumbnail sketch of the most common symptoms associated with the condition is presented. Practical pill-related issues—effectiveness, cost, compliance, rapidity of cure—that favor some drugs and compromise others are highlighted, and specific recommendations are offered. You also will learn what diagnostic tests or screening procedures may be required before a particular medication can be prescribed. You will want to read this section carefully before making a final decision on the appropriateness of a particular medication for your problem.

THE MedRANK LIFE PROLONGATION AND ENHANCEMENT CHECKLISTS: IDENTIFYING THE BEST AND SAFEST PRESCRIPTION MEDICATIONS

The Pills of Wisdom sections in each chapter are followed by a MedRANK Checklist that is pegged to a specific medical condition. The MedRANK Checklists are a *Consumer Reports*–like ranking system that highlights medications that work well and those that don't. Simply turn to the chapter that discusses your disease or condition, and use these checklists to look up detailed information, pill rankings, and glean specific recommendations that will help you compare and analyze the medications that your doctor has prescribed.

It should be emphasized that the Med-RANK Checklists are meant to be a *consultative* guide only. *The ultimate decision as to which drug or drugs will best serve your needs should be made by—and in collaboration with—your physician.* Moreover, although the MedRANK Checklists provide detailed comparative information about side effects, compliance features, and effectiveness of medications, they do *not* indicate the relative suitability of a specific medication for *your* particular medical condition. Once again, this is a decision for your doctor to make.

All drug therapy must be *individualized.* Just because a drug is ranked more favorably than another doesn't mean you or your physician must blindly substitute this pill for a drug that has a lower ranking. As a rule, however, a drug that is ranked in a higher—let's say, "Optimal"—category will be preferable to a drug appearing in a lower—let's say, "Discouraged for Initial Use"—category. But it will not *always* be preferable. Drug selection should be customized for the individual patient. For people who have special needs or unique concerns, a drug with a lower ranking may be a better choice.

Still, this will be the exception rather than the rule. Usually, the pills appearing in the most favorable categories will represent the best and safest drug choices for the greatest number of people. The MedRANK Checklists have been generated based on results from hundreds of published clinical studies, consultations, and years of clinical experience. As a result, they reliably discriminate between better pills and worse pills, between pills that heal and pills that harm. If, after reviewing the information in a MedRANK Checklist, you suspect that one medication may be better suited for you than another, it is certainly reasonable to present this information to your doctor, so that he or she may consider making an adjustment. In addition, you will want to use this information as a starting point for the 12-Week Action Plan in Part III.

The decision to prescribe one drug rather than another ultimately rests with the physician who is responsible for weighing the benefits and disadvantages of one therapeutic class—as well as specific drugs within that class—against others. Most doctors are aware that some drugs within a class are more effective, user-friendly, or convenient than others, or are less likely to cause side effects or interactions, and they make their drug selections accordingly. Unfortunately, many prescriptions are not made with all these considerations in mind. That's why the MedRANK Checklists are essential. They provide a pharmacological "safety net" so you can demand and get the best and safest prescription drugs for your family's health care needs.

HOW ARE THE MedRANK CHECKLISTS ORGANIZED?

The medications listed in the MedRANK Checklists are ranked into four categories:

1. **Optimal** (Highly Recommended/Best of Class
2. **Recommended** (Acceptable with Reservations)
3. **Discouraged for Initial Use** (But May Be Required in Selected People)
4. **Avoid If Possible** (Not Recommended)

The medications are listed by both brand names and generic names, with the brand name appearing first. For each drug, its special advantages and disadvantages are discussed. Specific guidance is given, and answers are provided to important questions such as: How effective is this medication? Is it the best one available to treat this condition? If so, why? Is it convenient to take? Does it have a user-friendly side-effect profile? Does it treat more than one condition at a single time? How does it compare with other drugs ranked in the same category? How does it compare with drugs ranked in other categories?

WHAT FACTORS GO INTO THE DRUG RANKINGS?

A number of factors have been considered when ranking medications, including their safety, effectiveness, side-effect profile, daily dose frequency, risk of drug-drug or drug-disease interactions, and versatility. Drugs ranked in the "Optimal" category usually represent the safest and most effective medications available for that particular medical condition. In addition, Optimal medications tend to have simple (once-daily) dosing sched-ules, a lower risk of drug interactions, and a side-effect profile that is quality-of-life friendly.

Optimal medications are by no means perfect; nor are they universally suited for all patients. But compared with other drugs used to treat the same condition, they usually are the most effective and user-friendly choices available. As a rule, medications ranked Optimal represent top-of-the-line, best-in-class options for treating a specific condition. What about cost? For the most part, cost is not one of the factors considered in the rankings. But for medications that are either extremely expensive or very attractively priced, this factor will be highlighted.

Some of the MedRANK Checklists list no Optimal drug for the medical condition under consideration. For example, in the case of Alzheimer's disease, a number of medications have been approved to treat behavioral problems associated with this condition, but all have significant limitations—side effects and drug interactions—that preclude their categorization as Optimal. The same is true for medications used to treat obesity: Some are better than others, but none can be considered Optimal.

Medications ranked as "Recommended" are almost always acceptable for a particular condition. They are good, solid choices but are usually not the very best choice available. Because of dosing considerations, side effects, or drug interaction problems, Recommended pills may be less than optimal but perfectly acceptable. Generally speaking, Recommended medications can be used with a great degree of confidence by most patients. Many of the drugs that appear in this category are considered to be the standard for many common diseases.

Pills that appear in the "Discouraged for Initial Use" category usually are less favorable choices. As a rule, these medications usually have to be given more often than once a day, are known to produce side effects that can compromise quality of life, or are not as effective as the medications listed as Optimal or Recommended.

For selected individuals, however, it may be necessary to use medications that appear in the "Discouraged for Initial Use" category. For example, if you have had an allergic reaction to a Recommended or Optimal drug, you may have no choice but to use a Discouraged drug. In some cases, an Optimal or Recommended medication will prove to be *ineffective*, in which case it may be necessary to resort to a medication less favorably ranked. Oftentimes the medications that appear in the "Discouraged" category are last-resort medications that are pressed into service only if more favorable medications fail. Caution is frequently required when using drugs in this category, because they tend to have a higher risk of drug-drug interactions.

Without question, you should try to stay away from medications that appear in the "Avoid If Possible" category. Many of these drugs are third- or fourth-line choices, and for the most part they are no longer considered state-of the-art treatment for their respective conditions. Once again, on rare occasions, such as for particularly difficult or stubborn cases when reinforcement or add-on drugs are needed, it may be necessary to resort to a medication in this category.

Clearly, however, if you find yourself taking a medication in the "Avoid If Possible" category, you should probably consult with your physician or pharmacist to find out whether it can be changed.

Most drugs are used for a number of different conditions, and a medication may play a more important role in one disease than in another. You may find a drug listed as Optimal for some conditions but as Recommended or Discouraged for others. This usually means that the medication is particularly good for one condition but not as successful in another. For example, H2-blockers are considered Optimal for treating mild acid indigestion and heartburn, but they represent second-line choices for ulcers and gastroesophageal reflux disease (GERD). Similarly, the antibiotic Biaxin may be an Optimal drug for the treatment of *Heliobacter pylori* ulcer disease, but it falls to the "Recommended" category for "walking pneumonia." The point is, the rankings in the MedRANK Checklists take into account the specific value of a drug for a specific medical condition.

....

HOW TO USE THE MedRANK CHECKLISTS

The MedRANK Checklists are very easy to use. Simply look up the condition that concerns you, read the "Pills of Wisdom" section, and then study the drug rankings for that particular disease. If you find that your physician has prescribed a medication that is Recommended and you have never been given the option of taking an Optimal drug, you will want to find out why. Is it because your physician is not aware that there is a better drug? Is it because your physician feels the Recommended drug is every bit as good as the Optimal drug? Or is it because your health plan favors using the less-expensive Recommended drug first?

You should present these issues and highlight possible deficiencies to your physician during the 12-Week Action Plan, discussed in Part III. For example, if you are taking a pill that appears in the "Discouraged" or "Avoid If Possible" category, you will certainly want to call it to the attention of your physician or pharmacist. There will usually be much better options available.

You should bring these MedRANK Checklists to your physician's office and point out alternative pills that appear to be more advantageous than those you may currently be taking.

In general, you can use the MedRANK Checklists to help steer your prescribing practitioner toward better, safer, and more user-friendly medications. Individual medications or drug regimens ("cocktails") that have been have been shown to prolong life are also highlighted in the MedRANK Checklists. If, for some reason, you have not been prescribed a medication proven to prolong life or prevent a disease for which you are at risk, you should raise this issue as part of the 12-Week Action Plan.

Each MedRANK checklist contains an icon that indicates special features, warnings, or advantages associated with a particular drug. The following glossary explains each icon used in the book.

Glossary of Icons

Life Enhancement. MedRank Checklists annotated with this icon contain pills that improve quality of life, treat common illnesses, and restore health.

Life Prolongation. MedRank Checklists annotated with this sand clock "life prolongation" icon contain pills that have the potential to extend life.

Drug Interactions. This symbol identifies prescription and over-the-counter medications that can cause drug interactions, and therefore, should be used cautiously in combination with certain other medications.

Side Effect Warning. This symbol will help you identify medications that have a propensity for causing side effects that may be extremely harmful or impair quality of life.

Elderly Warning. This symbol identifies specific medications that either should be used only with great caution, or should be avoided entirely, in the elderly individual. If you are elderly and are taking a medication that appears on a list with this symbol, you should consult with your physician.

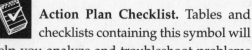

Action Plan Checklist. Tables and checklists containing this symbol will help you analyze and troubleshoot problems related to specific pills you are taking.

CHAPTER 4

PILLS 'R' US

The Best and Worst Medications for Children

"This is the third ear infection Matthew has had in ten weeks, doctor," complained one discouraged mother. "What's wrong with these antibiotics? They don't seem to be working. There's got to be something that will take care of the problem once and for all." Over the years I have seen hundreds of cranky, frustrated, and sleep-deprived mothers just like this one. And they were almost always right. Usually there was an antibiotic that would have spared their child's suffering and gotten rid of the ear infection the first time around. Unfortunately, their doctors—frequently under pressure to contain costs by their health plan—prescribed less-than-optimal antibiotics the first time around.

Not surprisingly, given the increasing antibiotic resistance to the bacteria that cause ear infections and pneumonia in children, these cost-driven therapeutic "experiments" produced unsatisfactory results. For the most part, the thought of giving young children, so precious and helpless, anything less than the best and safest medication is simply unacceptable. With a little guidance and common sense, you can help steer your child's physician in the right direction.

If there is one medication arena that requires a new "pillosophy," it's the use of antibiotics in children. Antibiotics should never be used unless they are necessary, but when they *are* required, you should insist on one that works. In the best of all worlds, you would like your doctor to prescribe an antibiotic that will cure your child's infection the *first time around*—the last thing you need is to keep bouncing back to your pediatrician because the antibiotic did not work. And yet this happens as the rule rather than the exception for many families. Recurrent ear infections, sinus problems, and allergies can make life miserable for you and your child.

The MedRANK Checklist "Antibiotics for Ear Infections in Children" in this chapter ranks medications for this common condition. The best and safest antibiotics are those that reduce the various *barriers* to clinical cure. The choice of an antibiotic should take into account all the *real-world* factors that determine success: the cost of the medication, its taste, and how well it works against the most common bacteria causing infections. When selecting an antibiotic, your child's doctor should also consider the time you have lost from work in order to care for your child, the cost of medications or other devices (diapers) to service the gastrointestinal side effects (diarrhea) of the medication, and the consequences of treatment failures or repeated episodes of infection. These can include hearing loss, linguistic difficulties, placement of ear tubes, and other problems.

☻ *Overcoming resistance.*

The journey from prescription pad to cure requires negotiating all forms of resistance. To optimize your child's chances of getting rid of an ear infection—or any other outpatient infection, for that matter—you and the physician will have to consider which medications are best able to overcome these barriers. Ensuring medication compliance in a young child is a delicate process that requires collaboration between parent and child. In the "give and take" of antibiotic therapy for children, the success of any medication will depend on whether you, as a parent, want to "give" the drug, and whether the child wants to "take" it. If your child resists the drug or encounters palatability or side-effect problems that hamper its ingestion, compliance will be compromised.

The first barrier to cure is *prescription resistance*, or the *cost* of the medication. Pre-

scriptions for drugs that are too expensive don't get filled as often as those that are more reasonably priced. Tell your doctor if you have any concerns about the price of the antibiotic prescribed for your child. In addition to cost, prescription resistance may also involve: (1) your doctor's persuasiveness in convincing *you* that the child needs the antibiotic; (2) word of mouth about the drug (is it perceived by others in the community as a tolerable or poorly tolerated medication?); (3) previous experiences you may have had with the medication; and (4) your perception of the seriousness of your child's condition. Get all the facts you need to ensure that you are sufficiently motivated to follow through with the prescription exactly as instructed.

You have your limits too, which I call *parent resistance*. Because children do not self-administer medications, children's compliance depends, to a great extent, upon the willingness and motivation of parents to *give* them the antibiotic. Yet at least one study has shown that poor medication compliance is the most common cause of antibiotic treatment failures. In other words, there is a limit to your patience. Drugs that require too many doses to be taken for too many days, and that produce too many side effects, will deter you from giving your child the full course of therapy. It's a fact—you're only human. The downside of such antibiotics is a poor result and treatment failure. For example, amoxicillin has been a gold standard for initial treatment of ear infections for many years, but because of its dosing schedule and ten-day treatment course, it may be associated with high parent resistance.

Similarly, medications that require refrigeration, that have to be administered by daycare or school personnel, or that require special timing requirements with respect to food intake, increase parent resistance and, therefore, may compromise proper, timely administration. Drugs with gastrointestinal side effects, especially diarrhea, create a cleanup factor that may discourage parents from completing the course of therapy.

Potential problems are also associated with day-care-mediated administration. Day-care workers are not as vigilant about giving children medications as their parents. Consequently, the only "day-care-proof" antibiotic is the one whose dosing schedule permits its entire course to be administered by parents *outside* the day-care environment. Generally speaking, once-daily medications (Zithromax, Vantin) are optimal in this regard, whereas medications dosed three times per day (Amoxil, Pediazole) may be associated with poor compliance. Although once-daily medications are associated with the best compliance, antibiotics dosed on a twice-daily basis are also acceptable in most circumstances.

Children have their limits too. What I call *patient resistance* are the barriers that prevent a patient from taking a medication. The principal factors determining patient resistance are a drug's palatability (its taste and the consistency of the suspension) and its gastrointestinal side effects (nausea, abdominal cramping, diarrhea). Or as I like to put it, the best antibiotics address the issues of "palatability and poopability," of "taste and waste." Poor palatability can adversely affect pediatric patient compliance. Parents who perceive that their child dislikes a medication may have trepidations about "forcing" it upon them. Alternatively, infants who find oral suspensions to be distasteful may spit up portions, a response that can produce a suboptimal intake unless the expelled dose is vigorously replenished by the parent.

Medications that have been associated with *poor* palatability, bitter taste, significant gastrointestinal side effects, or less-than-optimal consistency (granular taste, bitterness, and the like) include Biaxin, Vantin, erythromycin, Augmentin, and Cefzil. Liquid suspensions associated with a more *favorable* taste include Amoxil, Suprax, Lorabid, and Zithromax. The problems of patient resistance should never be underestimated.

The last barrier to success is *drug resistance,* or the effectiveness of the bacteria against the antibiotic. Naturally, it is your doctor's job to consider drug resistance when selecting an antibiotic. A medication that is inexpensive and well tolerated but fails to provide optimal activity at the business end—fighting the bacteria—will have a less-than-optimal cure rate. The best and safest antibiotics for children are characterized by low levels of prescription, parent, patient, and drug resistance.

☺ *Immunizations.*

The best approach to infection in children is prevention through immunization. (See the MedRANK Checklist "Vaccinations" on page 70.) Generally speaking, modern vaccines are safe and effective. Many recipients will experience only minor local side effects or none at all. The severity of side effects depends on many factors, including the dose and the individual patient. Possible side effects include tenderness, muscle stiffness at the ejection site, hives, and swelling.

Agents for active immunization consist of either killed or weakened live viruses or bacteria that are capable of producing antibodies in the host recipient. These bacteria and viruses do not cause disease. As a rule, active immunization with bacterial and viral vaccines and toxoids provides long-term protection (immunity) against a number of infections. Despite their safety, however, certain precautions should be noted with vaccines. For example, live or weakened virus vaccines should not be given to people with deficient immune systems. These include patients with leukemia, lymphoma, or other cancers, as well as individuals taking corticosteroids or receiving radiation. Children who have symptomatic AIDS should not be given live-virus and live-bacterial vaccines. After exposure to measles or chicken pox, however, these patients may receive passive immunization with immune globulin or varicella zoster immune globulin.

Live, attenuated virus vaccines are not generally given to pregnant women or those likely to become pregnant within three months of receiving the vaccine. But measles, mumps, rubella, and oral polio vaccines may be given safely to the children of pregnant women. When a vaccine has to be given to a woman during pregnancy, it is generally safest to wait until the second or third trimester, to minimize any possible fetal damage. At present, there has been no evidence of congenital rubella syndrome in infants born to mothers who received rubella vaccine during pregnancy. Generally speaking, there is no evidence of risk to the fetus from immunization of pregnant women using inactivated virus vaccines, bacterial vaccines, or toxoids. Tetanus and diphtheria toxoids should be given to inadequately immunized pregnant women because it affords protection against neonatal tetanus.

DTP vaccines provide active immunization against diphtheria, tetanus, and pertussis. There are strict guidelines for their timing and administration. Primary immunization with DT and DTP ideally begins at age two to three months, coinciding with the six-week postnatal checkup. This immunization is given on three occasions at four- to eight-week intervals, with a fourth injection administered six to twelve months after the third injection. Booster doses are given when the child is four to six years of age, preferably prior to entering kindergarten or elementary school.

Tetanus boosters need to be given only every ten years, when wounds are minor and presumed to be uncontaminated. For more serious wounds, a booster is appropriate if the patient has not received tetanus toxoid within the preceding five years.

Hemophilus influenzae type B, which is responsible for serious bacterial infections in children, was once the cause of most cases of bacterial meningitis between the ages of two and six. The peak incidence of infection occurs between six months and one year. The *Hemophilus* B vaccine provides long-term protection against infections caused by this bacterial organism. It is used for routine immunization of children of two months to five years of age. Because there are slight variations in the timing of various formulations, you should consult the immunization schedule in the MedRANK Checklist.

The oral polio vaccine (OPV) series is administered in three doses. It should be started at six to twelve weeks of age, usually in combination with the first DTP immunization at two months. The second OPV dose is generally given not less than six and preferably eight weeks later. Finally, the third dose is given eight to twelve months after the second. When entering elementary school, all children who have completed the primary series should receive a single follow-up dose of OPV, unless they received the third dose on or after their fourth birthday.

There has been a lot of publicity in the lay media about paralysis occurring following the use of live poliovirus vaccine. The Centers for Disease Control reported that during the years 1973 through 1984, approximately 274 million doses of OPV were distributed in the United States. During this same period, 105 vaccine-associated cases of paralysis were reported. Of these, 35 "vaccine-associated" and 50 "contact vaccine-associated" paralytic cases were reported. It appears that the risk of vaccine-associated paralysis is extremely small for those vaccinated, for susceptible family members, and for other close personal contacts. The measles, mumps, and rubella (MMR) virus vaccination is now recommended to improve control of measles. It includes a two-dose schedule. Generally speaking, MMR is given after fifteen months of age, followed by a second dose upon school entry.

ANTIBIOTICS FOR EAR INFECTIONS*
(Otitis Media, "Hot Ear," "Middle Ear Infection," "Red Eardrum")

 MedRANK Life Enhancement Checklist

☕ **Pills of Wisdom:** Convenience. Comfort. Effectiveness. Cure—the first time around, every time around. This is the mission statement for selecting the best antibiotics. The trick to treating ear infections in children successfully is to find a bacteria-killing medication (usually a liquid suspension) that, in the "give and take" of antibiotic administration, parents "like" to give and kids "like" to take. Unfortunately, even with more than fifteen antibiotics available for ear infections, satisfying both sides of this "give and take" is easier said than done. The antibiotic suspension must be easy for parents to administer—which means giving as few doses a day for as few days as is necessary to cure the infection—and easy for children to take. This usually means a suspension that tastes good and that doesn't cause gastrointestinal problems such as cramping and diarrhea. Put simply, the best antibiotic suspensions avoid "palatability and poopability" problems. Finally, you will want your doctor to choose an antibiotic that will get rid of all the likely

* Regardless of which antibiotic is prescribed for your child, be sure to give the entire course of therapy exactly as prescribed. Consult your physician if you have any concerns about dosing, missed doses, safety, or side effects.

bugs (bacteria) that are causing the infection. With so many strains of bacteria now developing resistance to older antibiotics, be sure your child is prescribed a medication that will be active against bacteria that are becoming resistant. In short, demand the best. Antibiotics such as Zithromax and Augmentin are top-of-the-line and offer the best coverage.

It must be stressed that many infections are caused by viruses, including 10 to 20 percent of all middle ear infections. These infections do not require antibiotics. In fact, in some European countries children with very mild ear infections—even those caused by bacteria—are not prescribed antibiotics immediately, and a high percentage of them get better on their own. But this is not the standard practice in the United States, where children with suspected bacterial infections of the middle ear are treated with antibiotics.

Be aware, however, that the overuse of antibiotics is not a good thing and can potentially produce more resistant strains of bacteria. If your physician advises against antibiotic treatment because a viral infection is suspected, he or she may very well be offering the best advice. But when an antibiotic is needed, there is no reason you shouldn't use the best. Our children deserve that much, and price differences of $25 between optimal and second-best options shouldn't stand in the way of convenience, comfort, and cure—the first time around.

OPTIMAL
(HIGHLY RECOMMENDED/ BEST OF CLASS)

Zithromax (azithromycin)

This is an effective antibiotic indicated for ear infections that answers the "give and take" for liquid suspensions. With only five doses (that's right, five swallows!) given for only five days, and a pleasant cherry taste, this antibiotic is a parent and child's dream come true. Parents want to give it, and kids want to take it. It covers all the appropriate bacteria, has an excellent safety profile, and has a very low risk for drug-drug interactions. This "less is more" antibiotic gets the job done with minimal inconvenience for parent or child.

An important and practical point of information: Although Zithromax is taken for only five days, it works "as if" your child were still actually taking it on the sixth through tenth days. That's because the antibiotic stays in the tissue at the site of infection for several days after the last dose has been taken, wiping out bacteria until the job is done. With all these features, this drug costs about as much as an oil change ($28), which makes it a good deal.

Augmentin (amoxicillin-clavulanate)

Now that this gold standard for the treatment of middle ear infections is available for twice-daily dosing (as opposed to the old three-doses-a-day variety) and is much less expensive than it once was, it deserves to be ranked Optimal. It still requires twenty doses over ten days, which isn't ideal, and 10 to 15 percent of kids will still get diarrhea. (Get those extra diaper packs ready!) This drug has also been shown to be effective in children who have persistent fluid behind their eardrums, or what's called chronic otitis media with effusion (OME).

RECOMMENDED
(ACCEPTABLE WITH RESERVATIONS)

Amoxil (amoxicillin)

I buck the trend with this antibiotic. Widely used, cheap, and tasty, amoxicillin has been, for quite some time, an institution—"big pink," the AT&T of antibiotics for ear infections. Despite its endorsements from many organizations and physician panels, however, amoxicillin is rapidly losing its effectiveness against many bacterial strains (*Streptococcus pneumoniae, Hemophilus influenzae*) known to cause middle ear infections. In addition, it is inconveniently dosed at three times daily (which can create problems for parents with kids in day care) and requires a full ten days of administration. The retreatment rate runs as high as 30 percent.

My position is: Why risk the window of bacterial vulnerability, and why inconvenience yourself and your child, when you don't have to? The "leaner and meaner" antibiotics listed in the "Optimal" category are my drugs of choice for a convenient, comfortable, and confident cure.

Bactrim, Septra (trimethoprim/sulfamethoxazole)

An inexpensive, twice-daily antibiotic that is widely used and quite effective. Resistant bacteria are being seen with increasing frequency.

Lorabid (loracarbef)

This very palatable, twice-daily, slightly pricey suspension gets the job done. It provides good coverage of the bugs.

Vantin (cefpodoxime)

Vantin is recommended because it has excellent coverage of the bugs and is conveniently dosed, once daily. Its important downside is its taste, which many kids simply detest.

DISCOURAGED FOR INITIAL USE (BUT MAY BE REQUIRED IN SELECTED PEOPLE)

Ceftin (cefuroxime)

This highly effective antibiotic has a less-than-pleasant taste and a less-than-pleasant price tag ($53) compared with other equally effective (Augmentin and Zithromax) options.

Cefzil (cefprozil)

Poor taste is a problem for the kids. It requires twice-daily administration. But it provides good coverage of the bugs.

Biaxin (clarithromycin)

The twice-daily dosing is less than ideal, but coverage of the organisms is excellent. Its principal problem is its suboptimal palatability, a problem it shares with Ceftin, Vantin, and Cefzil.

Pediazole (erythromycin/ sulfamethoxazole)

This old warhorse has excellent coverage, but with its four-times-daily dosing and unpleasant taste, it's not the most convenient or comfortable option available.

AVOID IF POSSIBLE (NOT RECOMMENDED)

Ceclor (cefaclor)

Ceclor was once very widely used for ear and sinus infections. Unfortunately, recent studies show it's losing some of its punch against bacterial strains involved in middle ear infections. Better, more convenient drugs are now preferred.

Suprax (cefixime)

This suspension has a pleasant taste and the convenience of once-daily dosing for ten days. That's the good news. The bad news is that more and more strains of *S. pneumoniae*, a common organism implicated in many middle ear infections, are becoming resistant to Suprax. As a result, other antibiotics with better coverage are preferred.

Cedax (ceftibuten)

The good news is that, like Suprax, this well-tolerated, once-daily antibiotic is approved for ear infections. The bad—and very curious—news is that this pricey drug (about $59 per course) will not kill a significant percentage (perhaps as much as 25 percent) of the bacterial strains *(S. pneumoniae)* that can cause middle ear infections in children. As a result, it should be avoided for initial use in this condition.

VACCINATIONS*

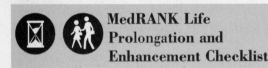

MedRANK Life Prolongation and Enhancement Checklist

Pills of Wisdom: Generally speaking, modern vaccines are safe and effective. Recommended immunization schedules have been developed by infectious disease experts, vaccines are approved by the FDA, and standards are issued by the Centers for Disease Control (CDC). The benefits of being vaccinated—a reduction in diseases that can lead to disability and death—far outweigh the extremely rare complications that have received such wide media attention. A resurgence of measles in 1989 and 1990, for example, produced 55,000 cases and 166 deaths. The main cause of this epidemic was the failure to vaccinate children at the recommended age of twelve to fifteen months.

Studies have uncovered serious deficiencies in compliance with immunization standards. As a result, one current pediatric immunization standard issued by the CDC is that parents be educated regarding immunization standards in "general terms."

Fortunately, most children will experience no or only minor local side effects with their immunization. The severity of side effects depends on many factors, including dose and the individual patient. Possible side effects include tenderness, muscle stiffness at the injection site, hives, and swelling. Agents for active immunization consist of either killed or weakened live viruses or bacteria that are capable of producing antibodies. These bacteria and viruses do not themselves cause disease. As a rule, active immunization with bacterial and viral vaccines and toxoids provides long-term protection (immunity) against a number of infections.

Despite the safety of vaccines, certain precautions should be noted. Live or weakened virus vaccines should not be given to people with immune deficiency—a reduced ability to produce antibodies and fight infection. They also should not be administered to people who have a decreased ability to mount

* Your local or state public health department maintains current vaccination recommendations. Please consult with them or your physician if you have any additional questions or concerns.

an immune response, including those with leukemia, lymphoma, or other cancer, as well as those taking corticosteroids or receiving radiation.

Measles, mumps, rubella, or oral polio vaccines may be given safely to the children of pregnant women. When a vaccine has to be given during pregnancy, it is generally safest to wait until the second or third trimester to minimize the possibility of fetal damage. At present, there is no evidence of congenital rubella syndrome in infants born to mothers who received rubella vaccine during pregnancy.

OPTIMAL IMMUNIZATION SCHEDULE

Diphtheria Toxoid

This vaccine is given at 2, 4, 6, and 15 (or 18) months of age; then again at 4 to 6 years. After this, a booster is given every ten years to maintain immunity. Usually given combined with tetanus and pertussis (DTP).

Tetanus Toxoid

This vaccine is given at 2, 4, 6, and 15 months (or 18) months of age; then again at 4 to 6 years. After this, a booster is given every ten years to maintain immunity. Usually given combined with diphtheria and pertussis (DTP).

Pertussis Vaccine

This vaccine protects children against whooping cough. It is given at 2, 4, 6, and 15 (or 18) months of age; then again at 4 to 6 years. After this, a booster is given every ten years to maintain immunity. Usually given combined with tetanus and diphtheria (DTP).

Hemophilus B Vaccine

This vaccine protects against serious bacterial infections caused by Hemophilus influenzae (type B only), which is responsible for causing meningitis, ear infections, pneumonia, and many other serious and even life-threatening conditions. The vaccine HibTITER (which is used for children between 2 months and 5 years of age) is given at 2, 4, 6, and 15 months.

Trivalent Oral Polio Vaccine (OPV)

This vaccine protects against paralysis caused by the poliovirus. Paralysis has been reported in people following the use of live poliovirus vaccine as well as in adults who were not previously vaccinated against polio but were in close contact with individuals who had recently been vaccinated. Overall between 1973 and 1984, about 105 cases of paralysis were reported as a result of 274 million doses distributed in the United States.

Oral polio vaccine is given at 2, 4, 6 (optional except in high-risk areas), and 15 (or 18) months, and then again between 4 and 6 years. The oral vaccine (OPV) is recommended by the CDC. However, inactivated poliovirus vaccine (IPV) is given to children (by injection) who have immune-deficiency problems or to those whose household members have this condition. Consult your physician for specific recommendations about indications for IPV.

Measles Vaccine

This vaccine protects against measles. It is generally given at 15 months and again between 4 and 6 years of age. It may be given in a combined measles, mumps, and rubella (MMR) live vaccine.

Rubella Vaccine

This vaccine protects against rubella. It is generally given at 15 months and again between 4 and 6 years of age. It may be given in a combined measles, mumps, and rubella (MMR) live vaccine.

Mumps Vaccine

This vaccine protects against mumps. It is generally given at 15 months and again between 4 and 6 years of age. It may be given in a combined measles, mumps, and rubella (MMR) live vaccine.

Varivax (varicella/chicken pox)

This relatively new vaccine is safe and reasonably effective in preventing chicken pox and shingles (a reactivation of the varicella zoster virus). A single injection is recommended for all healthy children between the ages of one and twelve years. Do not give aspirin for six weeks after the vaccination. It is not yet clear just how long the vaccine will be effective, or whether a booster dose later in adult life is required.

START LOW, GO SLOW, AND MONITOR THE SHOW
Pills for Attention Deficit/Hyperactivity Disorder

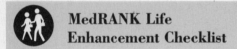

MedRANK Life Enhancement Checklist

Pills of Wisdom: The most important thing about treating children who have attention deficit/hyperactivity disorder (ADHD) or attention deficit disorder (ADD) is to be sure that the diagnosis of ADHD is properly established. Because the medications used to treat this condition are powerful—with a litany of undesirable side effects—it is essential that children not be started on them *unnecessarily*. If the drugs are started, it is absolutely essential to establish a baseline of the child's behavioral and educational activities. This is done both with subjective impressions and with an objective measurement tool called the Connors Hyperactivity Scale.

In broad brush strokes, the child with ADHD or ADD has an intrinsic inability to maintain attention, which leads to a state of overactivity or the disruption of his or her educational program. In general, girls are less likely to have hyperactivity, but they can have other symptoms of ADHD or ADD. There are very strict criteria for confirming that children merit this diagnosis. Unless they have at least six of the following symptoms, the need for drug therapy should be reconsidered.

Inattention Symptoms
1. Lack of attention to details or careless mistakes in schoolwork
2. Difficulty sustaining attention in tasks or play activities
3. Impression of not listening when spoken to directly
4. Failure to follow through on homework or other duties
5. Difficulty organizing tasks and activities
6. Avoiding tasks or activities that require sustained mental effort
7. Tendency to lose things

8. Excessive distractions by extraneous stimuli
9. Forgetfulness in daily activities

Hyperactivity Symptoms

1. Fidgeting with hands or feet or squirming in seats
2. Not remaining seated when expected
3. Running about or climbing excessively—restlessness perceived by older persons
4. Difficulty in engaging in leisure activities quietly
5. Often "on the go" or "driven by a motor"
6. Excessive talking

To be diagnosed with ADD or ADHD, a child must develop these symptoms before the age of seven. In addition, the symptoms must be present in at least two settings (at school and at home), and significant impairment in social, educational, or occupational functioning must be clearly evident. Finally, these symptoms cannot be the result of some other mental or developmental condition.

Once you, your child's teacher, and your pediatrician or family doctor are convinced that your child has ADHD or ADD, drug therapy is usually necessary. It should be combined with appropriate educational and psychosocial support. Paradoxically, the most successful medications are stimulants, which are associated with many side effects. Consequently, it is essential that your child be stabilized at the lowest possible dose of the medication required to reduce symptoms and permit the resumption of normal educational and social activities. Almost without exception, stimulants are not useful for anxious or depressed children, so if your child does not respond to one or more of them, you and your doctor may need to reconsider the diagnosis.

Not all children respond to the same medication, and some trial and error may be necessary. In fact, some children will respond to one medication but not another, and they may do so either at very low or at very high levels. To a great degree, the response will not be predictable, so you'll need to be patient.

Finally, start low, go slow, and monitor the show. Be sure your child is started on a low dose. If there is no response after a week or two, increase the dose slowly. Monitor your child's improvement, and when a reasonable response has been achieved, stick with the winning dose. Ask the child's teacher to help assess how well the drug is working.

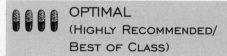

OPTIMAL
(HIGHLY RECOMMENDED/ BEST OF CLASS)

Note: None of these medications are truly optimal, in the sense that their side effects can be serious. But ADHD and ADD are serious conditions that can compromise social and educational development. Therefore the benefits of suboptimal medications may outweigh the risks of no treatment at all.

Ritalin SR (methylphenidate sustained-release)

This long-acting preparation of Ritalin requires only once-daily dosing. Because there may be breakthrough symptoms in the afternoon, some children may find it less effective than regular Ritalin. But it's worth trying, since once-daily dosing is more convenient and may save your child the embarrassment of requiring a second dose to be given in school.

Warning: All stimulants (including Ritalin, Dexedrine, Cylert, Adderall, and Desoxyn) have side effects that include insomnia, weight loss, poor appetite, nausea, rapid heart rate, and hallucinations. Some cause slow growth due to appetite suppression.

Ritalin SR should be used with extreme caution in children with high blood pressure or epilepsy. It should not be used in combination with MAOIs, and it may increase the effects of antidepressants, Coumadin, and Dilantin.

The drug should be introduced at very small doses, and the child should be monitored for at least two weeks before the dose is increased. If acceptable behavioral changes are noted, no increase in dose is necessary. Overdosage of stimulants in children produces signs of social withdrawal, weepiness, and sleepiness. A "zombielike" state usually means too much medication—and implies overdosage.

Dexedrine Spansules (dextroamphetamine sustained-release)
This long-acting stimulant works much like Ritalin. See "Ritalin SR" for warnings, side effects, and approaches to drug therapy.

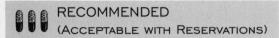 **RECOMMENDED** (ACCEPTABLE WITH RESERVATIONS)

Ritalin (methylphenidate)
This short-acting Ritalin formulation requires twice-daily dosing. See "Ritalin SR" for warnings, side effects, and approaches to drug therapy.

Dexedrine (dextroamphetamine)
This short-acting Dexedrine formulation requires twice-daily dosing. See "Ritalin SR" for warnings, side effects, and approaches to drug therapy.

 DISCOURAGED FOR INITIAL USE (BUT MAY BE REQUIRED IN SELECTED CHILDREN)

Cylert (pemoline)
Serious liver problems have been reported as a side effect in rare cases. See "Ritalin SR" for warnings, side effects, and approaches to drug therapy.

Catapres (clonidine)
This blood pressure medication has been tried in children with ADD or ADHD. It's not a first-line drug for this condition. Side effects include sleepiness, dry mouth, constipation, and fatigue. Do not discontinue this drug suddenly.

Norpramin (desipramine)
This antidepressant has been widely used to treat children with ADHD. Sudden death has been reported in a few children who were taking it. The cause of death is uncertain but is presumed to be toxic effects on the heart. It should be used only if the child does not respond to the stimulants Ritalin or Dexedrine, or if emotional problems or depression are part of the picture.

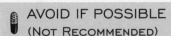 **AVOID IF POSSIBLE** (NOT RECOMMENDED)

Adderall (amphetamine mixture)
No trials that confirm its effectiveness are available.

Desoxyn (methamphetamine mixture)
No large, well-controlled clinical trials are available to confirm its effectiveness.

CHAPTER 5

—

HOME IS WHERE THE HEART IS

Medications for Heart Disease

"Do I really have to take all these pills?" my patients with heart conditions frequently ask. "They make me feel awful. Do you really think they're doing me any good?" When wisely combined and carefully selected, drugs that treat and prevent heart disease can both prolong life and maintain its quality. If you are taking pills for your heart, you'll want them to be nothing less than the best. Few pills have the capacity to be so potent, so problematic—or so life prolonging and protective—as these drugs. Not surprisingly, heart medications are among the most widely prescribed drugs in use today, and a wide range are available. They are frequently combined into multiple-drug regimens or so-called therapeutic "cocktails" to provide many heart-related benefits at once: lowering blood pressure, reducing cholesterol levels, relieving symptoms of chest pain, and improving heart-pumping function.

Life-prolongation benefits have been confirmed for a number of heart pills, including aspirin, the cholesterol-lowering drugs known as the statins, beta-blockers, ACE inhibitors, and estrogen. The most important issue is to determine whether you can benefit from one or more of these medications. If you and your doctor decide that you *are* a candidate for heart medications, the next question is which one or ones are best suited to your specific needs. The MedRANK Checklists in this chapter provide specific recommendations, rankings, and warnings related to prescription drugs used for heart disease.

Although the life-enhancement and -prolongation benefits of heart medications are well established, their potential side effects can range from mild and irritating to serious and life-threatening. A recent British study of almost two thousand hospital patients was conducted to identify the drugs that are most often associated with adverse reactions. It found that pills used to treat heart disease—among them diuretics, blood pressure pills, drugs used to treat abnormal heart rhythms, and the like were more likely to cause quality-of-life impairment and side effects requiring hospitalization than any other group of drugs. Smaller studies conducted in nursing homes and other hospitals across the country have confirmed this finding.

☺ Diuretics ("water pills").

Of the estimated 58 million Americans who have high blood pressure, a significant percentage are treated with thiazide diuretics, or so-called "water pills." The good news is that these diuretics have been shown to reduce the risk of stroke in patients who have high blood pressure. Adding to their attractiveness, they are inexpensive—dirt cheap, to be exact—and have a proven track record in lowering blood pressure in many patient groups, including the elderly. Diuretics are used not only for treating high blood pressure but for improving symptoms associated with congestive heart failure—a condition in which the pumping action of the heart muscle deteriorates to the point of causing fluid to back up in the lung.

As useful and inexpensive as these widely endorsed medications are, you should be aware that they also have the potential for producing undesirable side effects. Especially if they are not monitored carefully or if they are used at high doses, water pills can cause potassium loss, elevate blood cholesterol levels, and make diabetes more difficult to control. If they cause your body to lose enough potassium, you may experience weakness, muscle cramps, nausea, and dizziness. Consequently, if these symptoms appear while you are taking a diuretic, you should consult your physician immediately in order to make dietary modifications that will increase your potassium intake. Alternatively, your physician may prescribe a potassium supplement or a "combination" diuretic that contains an ingredient that protects against potassium loss. All blood pressure–lowering medications, including thiazide diuretics, may cause sexual dysfunction. People may complain of depression and fatigue in an attempt to mask their underlying sexual dysfunction.

The primary advantage of thiazide diuretics is that they are attractively priced and have been shown to be effective in patients with high blood pressure. Some trials, however, suggest that their side effects may be greater than those seen with other blood pressure–lowering medications, such as ACE inhibitors and calcium channel blockers. Finally, although diuretics can lower blood pressure and improve symptoms associated with congestive heart failure (see the MedRANK Checklist "Congestive Heart Failure" on page 95), their life-prolongation benefits have not been convincingly proven.

☺ ACE inhibitors.

ACE inhibitors, which block the manufacture of hormones that constrict blood vessels, are widely used to treat hypertension, either alone or in combination with other blood pressure–lowering medications. Commonly used ACE inhibitors include captopril, enalapril, lisinopril, moexipril, and benazepril. These pills not only lower blood pressure, they treat heart failure and prevent kidney disease in patients with diabetes. As a rule, ACE inhibitors are well tolerated. But you should be aware that up to 25 percent of patients taking such a medication will experience a dry, recurrent cough within six months of starting therapy. This symptom is frequently distressing enough to require discontinuation of the drug. ACE inhibitors are more expensive than diuretics, but they are useful for more conditions, and their side-effect profile is more user-friendly. Compared with water pills, ACE inhibitors tend to preserve sexual function, and they produce no adverse effects on blood cholesterol or sugar levels. They have been shown to *prolong life* in people with congestive heart failure, and they are sometimes used for their prevention benefits in people who have had a heart attack.

☺ *Calcium channel blockers.*

Among the various classes of blood pressure pills, calcium channel blockers probably are the most widely used. Unlike ACE inhibitors and diuretics, which tend to be quite similar from one drug to the next, calcium channel blockers are varied and are therefore more difficult to characterize. These medications block calcium release in the smooth muscle cells that surround the blood vessels, which in turn causes the vessels to relax and lowers blood pressure. But here the similarities stop. Because calcium channel blockers are not created equal, you should be cautioned that they are *not* interchangeable. In fact, each calcium channel blocker is associated with a unique set of advantages and disadvantages.

Over the past few years, considerable controversy has surrounded the safety of calcium channel blockers. But recent recommendations from the FDA and other experts have helped settle the controversy. First of all, be sure that your doctor is using calcium channel blockers only for the *approved* indications. If you find that you are taking a calcium channel blocker for an unlabeled use, you should consult your physician and find out why. In particular, be aware that calcium channel blockers are *not* indicated for the prevention of heart attacks; nor are they desirable in patients who are having or have recently had a heart attack. So-called "short-acting" calcium channel blockers, which are dosed two to three times per day, generally are *not* recommended under any circumstances. If you are taking a short-acting calcium channel blocker —that is, a nifedipine, diltiazem, or verapamil formulation that requires three-times-per-day dosing—you should bring this fact to your physician's attention immediately, so that you can be switched to a long-acting preparation that has to be taken only once daily.

In February 1996, in a position statement published in *The Journal of the American Medical Association*, the FDA endorsed the safety of *long-acting* calcium channel blockers but raised significant concerns about shorter-acting preparations. Consequently, the overall trend in calcium-channel-blocker use should be away from short-acting agents and toward once-daily agents, such as Norvasc (amlodipine), which has a more gradual onset of action and is better tolerated. Abrupt withdrawal of calcium channel blockers should be avoided, and the dosage should not be changed without your physician's approval. The most common side effects include constipation, fluid collection in the legs, insomnia, and diarrhea.

Although most calcium channel blockers

are effective for the treatment of high blood pressure, some of them, such as verapamil and diltiazem, can decrease the force of heart contractions, slow impulses traveling through the heart, or decrease the heart rate. These properties make them useful for the treatment of rapid heart rates, but they are *potentially* harmful in people with congestive heart failure and in the elderly. Compared with the calcium channel blockers Calan and Cardizem, Norvasc (amlodipine) has clear safety advantages, especially in patients who have heart failure, angina, and high blood pressure.

Norvasc, which merits the "Good Heart-keeping" seal of approval, does not decrease the force of heart contractions; nor does it slow heart rate. It has been shown to be safe in patients with bad hearts, bad arteries, bad pumps, and bad prognoses. Procardia XL (nifedipine GITS), another widely used calcium channel blocker, has advantages over Cardizem and Calan, but it does not have the "safe haven" status of Norvasc, which is the cleanest blood pressure medication in terms of risk for drug interactions and drug-disease incompatibilities.

☺ *Beta-blockers.*

Beta-blockers, which slow the heart rate and decrease the amount of oxygen the heart uses, are useful for preventing second heart attacks, relieving chest pain caused by angina, and lowering blood pressure. They have been shown to *prolong life* when given to people who have had a heart attack. Beta-blockers also can vary widely in their benefits and side effects. Among their many advantages, they also are approved for treatment of irregular heart rhythms and prevention of migraine headaches.

As is the case with calcium channel blockers, you should not change from one beta-blocker to another without first consulting your doctor or pharmacist. Although many people experience only minor problems with beta-blockers, a significant percentage report fatigue, depression, sleep disturbances, and light-headedness. Not infrequently, these symptoms disappear with continued use of the medication, but if they don't, you should not hesitate to consult your prescribing practitioner. Finally, some beta-blockers, such as Inderal and Lopressor, penetrate into brain tissues and therefore may be more likely to produce fatigue and sleep problems. In contrast, other beta-blockers, such as Tenormin, do not penetrate into the central nervous system and therefore may be better tolerated.

Other possible side effects of beta-blockers include low blood pressure, slow heart rate, and in a very small percentage of patients, congestive heart failure, especially if the drug is being taken at a high dose. You should not take a beta-blocker if you have bronchial asthma, chronic obstructive pulmonary disease, or other respiratory problems that can be worsened by this medication. Special caution also is required when discontinuing beta-blockers, which should never be stopped suddenly. When these drugs need to be stopped, discontinuation should be gradual, over a period of many days. Sudden cessation can cause worsening of chest pain, irregular heartbeat, heart attack, and (rarely) even death. Other withdrawal symptoms may include sweating, palpitations (pounding in the chest), and headache.

Almost without exception, if you are taking a beta-blocker and feel you are unable to tolerate the side effects, you should consult your physician and initiate a withdrawal period that extends for a minimum of one to two weeks. Other options, either within this class or in another drug class, may work better for you. Finally, a number of potential drug interactions are associated with beta-blockers, so if you are taking one, consult your physician to inquire about possible incompatibilities.

☺ *Cholesterol-lowering medications.*

Without question, pills used to lower blood cholesterol represent one of the most significant advances for the prevention of death from heart disease. The relationship between elevated blood cholesterol and increased risk of heart attack is now irrefutable, which means that if you are a woman over 40 or a man over 35, you should get your cholesterol and lipid levels checked every five years. A lipid profile will show your total cholesterol level, and your HDL (good), LDL (bad), and VLDL cholesterol levels, as well as your serum triglyceride (bad lipid) level. Having a high HDL level and low LDL and total cholesterol levels is associated with a lower risk of dying from heart disease.

According to most studies, lowering your total blood cholesterol level by about 25 percent will cut in *half* your risk of complications or death from heart attack or related problems. Put simply, for every one percent reduc-

tion in your total blood cholesterol level, you can achieve a two percent reduction in your risk of developing problems associated with coronary heart disease. These advantages are especially clear in patients who have diabetes, in people with a known history of heart attacks, and in patients with dramatically elevated cholesterol levels, or so-called "familial hypercholesterolemia."

Elevated blood cholesterol remains one of the leading risk factors for developing heart disease and affects about 20 percent of the U.S. population. Unfortunately, only 40 percent of people with harmfully elevated cholesterol levels are receiving adequate treatment. Effective detection and proven medications—primarily with "statin" drugs, such as atorvastatin, pravastatin, and simvastatin—are available, but there are still many unresolved issues in treatment. For example, Whom should we screen? What do we screen for? Which patients should be treated? and What is the best overall approach to treatment?

Several years ago, in an attempt to answer these questions, the National Institutes of Health established the Expert Panel on the Detection, Evaluation, and Treatment of High Blood Cholesterol in Adults. This consensus panel established the National Cholesterol Education Program (NCEP), which issued a report addressing many basic questions related to the screening and treatment of elevated blood cholesterol levels.

The panel established a screening approach for elevated lipid levels and recommended that total cholesterol and LDL levels be measured in the adult population. It urged people to get an HDL (good) cholesterol level reading at the same time, provided accurate means are available. The addition of the HDL cholesterol level to the lipid screening test was based on the finding that low HDL cholesterol (less than 35 mg/dL) is associated with an increased risk for heart disease, while a high HDL level lowers risk. Whether treatment with lipid-lowering agents is indicated for a patient depends, to a great extent, on the degree of elevated total and LDL cholesterol levels and other underlying risk factors that may predispose the patient to heart disease. People who have high cholesterol levels and who also have a history of heart disease, diabetes, stroke, or peripheral circulatory disorders are considered to be in a high-risk category. They are appropriate candidates for aggressive therapy to lower cholesterol levels, even if their levels are only minimally or moderately elevated.

Just how low should your cholesterol be? Each case is slightly different, but as a rule, if you do not have heart disease but your LDL cholesterol is in the range of 160–225 mg/dL, you should have it lowered by diet and/or drugs to less than 130 mg/dL. If you do have heart disease (the arteries to your heart muscles are clogged) or have had a heart attack, your LDL level should be lowered to less than 100 mg/dL. If you have two or more major risk factors for heart disease—these would include smoking, hypertension, diabetes, family history of premature heart disease, male sex, and low HDL cholesterol—you are considered in the next-highest-risk category. If you fall into this group, the decision to use a cholesterol-lowering medication will depend on how high your cholesterol levels are, your age, and other aspects of your medical history.

Life prolongation and health enhancement are important features of cholesterol-lowering drugs. Recent studies have shown that individuals who have very high LDL cholesterol levels and risk factors for heart disease can actually lower their risk for a first heart attack by using the HMG-CoA reductase inhibitor pravastatin (Pravachol). Pravachol, like all the statins, blocks a critical step in the manufacture of cholesterol and thereby lowers blood levels. Other statins, such as atorvastatin (Lipitor) and simvastatin (Zocor) probably can also prevent first heart attacks, even though they currently do not have official FDA approval for this purpose. Finally, it is important to stress that although HMG-CoA reductase inhibitors (statins) represent a major advance in the pharmacological approach to reducing cholesterol levels, any drug therapy program for cholesterol lowering should be accompanied by dietary changes, exercise, and weight reduction, if required. Please see the MedRANK Checklist "Cholesterol-Lowering Medications" in this chapter for rankings of cholesterol-lowering pills.

Aspirin.

A member of the salicylate class, aspirin is one of the most common and cost-effective medications used to prevent stroke and heart disease. Salicylates can also relieve discomfort by inhibiting pain perception and by blocking the formation of chemicals called prostaglandins. Aspirin prevents blood platelets ("clotting cells") from clumping together and forming clots, which explains its usefulness in preventing heart attacks and strokes. More than two hundred over-the-counter preparations contain aspirin, which means that the risk of drug interactions must always be considered.

Life prolongation has been shown for aspirin, which can reduce the risk of death as well as nonfatal, recurrent heart attack in people who already have had a heart attack or who have a history of severe heart disease. But the benefits of aspirin probably also extend to middle-aged adults who have no history of heart disease whatsoever. Accordingly, many expert panels now recommend that all individuals over the age of 50 be placed on low-dose aspirin therapy—some recommend that men over 40 be started—in order to prevent cardiovascular disease. (Low-dose therapy means 81 mg of aspirin per day.)

Practically speaking, if you have had a heart attack or have heart disease, aspirin should be a part of your medication program, unless there are reasons why the drug may not be safe for you. At low doses, the risk of bleeding complications from aspirin is very low, and therefore you should consider using it to prevent heart attacks even if you have no history of previous heart problems. Because elderly patients are at higher risk of bleeding complications from aspirin therapy, they should be watched very closely. Please see the MedRANK Checklist in this chapter for recommendations on aspirin use.

Other clot-dissolving medications, such as dipyridamole (Persantine), ticlopidine (Ticlid), and pentoxifylline (Trental), are much more controversial. Persantine may be helpful for the small group of patients at risk for stroke who have mechanical heart valves, but in the general population, aspirin is much less expensive and more effective for the prevention of stroke and heart attacks. Persantine is an overused medication, and very few people benefit from taking it. Similarly, the effectiveness of Trental, which is used to treat circulatory conditions that cause leg discomfort, is largely determined by selecting the appropriate patient. In the case of virtually all blood-modifying, clot-dissolving medications, you should watch carefully for symptoms that suggest excessive bleeding. If these occur, notify your physician or pharmacist immediately.

☺ *Nutritional supplements.*

Nutritional supplements such as fish oil capsules have been touted to reduce the risk of heart disease. It should be stressed that although the American Heart Association recommends *eating fish* as part of a low-fat diet, it does not endorse the use of fish oil *supplements* to protect against heart disease. Two servings of fish per week has been shown to reduce death from heart disease.

As far as vitamins are concerned, vitamin E has received the most attention for its possible role in reducing the risk of cardiovascular disease. Whether the chronic intake of vitamin E can prevent heart attacks is still a matter of debate. One large study has shown decreased heart attacks from vitamin E, whereas others have not. We do know that a *diet* rich in vitamin E–containing fruits and vegetables protects against heart disease. Vitamin E does prevent oxidation reactions in the body. Although not approved by the FDA for any of the following conditions, unlabeled uses for this vitamin include: skin disorders, night leg cramps, heart disease, and other conditions associated with aging. If you are going to take vitamin E, it is important to tell your doctor or pharmacist so that medication adjustments can be made if required. Remember, too, that common dietary sources of vitamin E include vegetable oils, leafy vegetables, and nuts.

☺ *Blood thinners.*

Almost without exception, medications that are used to alter clotting or that affect other blood components require close physician supervision and, frequently, home monitoring. Although these medications have many useful purposes, including the prevention of blood clots, heart disease, and stroke, when used inappropriately or in excess, their side effects may have serious bleeding complications. The most important class of medications in this group are the so-called "blood thinners" or anticoagulants. When used in a hospitalized patient, they are available as injectable drugs (Heparin), and in outpatient care, as oral medications. Coumadin is the gold-standard oral blood thinner for the prevention of blod clots in people with heart disease.

Blood-thinning medications have been shown to be useful in treating more than thirty clinical conditions, including stroke, heart disease, and disorders of the circulatory system. They exert their benefits by prolonging the amount of time it takes blood to clot. This reduces the risk that a clot will lodge in a major blood vessel, which is the cause of many serious diseases, including strokes and heart attacks. Those who take an "anticoagulant" medication such as Coumadin (warfarin) should understand that its blood-thinning properties have the potential for causing side effects, especially bleeding from the urinary tract and bruising, as well as other problems.

In order to prevent these complications, strict adherence to the prescribed dosage schedule is absolutely necessary, and regular monitoring with blood tests that measure clotting time is required to ensure that the blood thinner is producing its desired effects. If you are taking Coumadin, you should be aware that a number of medications and food products have the capacity to interact with this class of anticoagulant. Some dietary ingredients and drugs will make Coumadin more potent (increased blood thinning), whereas others will decrease its action (lessened anticlotting effect). Consequently, you should tell your doctor or pharmacist if you plan to change your diet or are taking any over-the-counter or prescription medication along with Coumadin.

CHOLESTEROL-LOWERING MEDICATIONS
The Lipid Limbo, or How Low Can You Go?*

 MedRANK Life Prolongation Checklist

⏳ **Pills of Wisdom:** Elevated cholesterol is the most silent of all killers, but also one of the most treatable. Lowering cholesterol has become a national obsession. And for good reason: The data are unambiguous that if your cholesterol level is too high, you may be a walking time bomb. But you can prolong your life by adopting lifestyle changes and, if necessary, taking pills that lower cholesterol levels. So just do it. Get your cholesterol level checked—and don't delay.

Cholesterol-lowering medications, which have to be taken indefinitely, have been convincingly shown to reduce death and complications associated with coronary heart disease, even in people who have never had heart problems. This means that if your cholesterol level is high enough (an LDL level of greater than 160 mg/dL) and you have no risk factors for heart disease, you will still benefit from bringing your cholesterol level down. These drugs also have been shown to "reverse" blockage in arteries that are already damaged or narrowed by atherosclerosis, an age-related process in which cholesterol deposits are laid down, narrowing the arteries that supply blood to the heart.

When it comes to pills for lowering cholesterol levels, don't settle for anything but the best. In this arena, "the statins are what's happenin'." Statin drugs block an important step in cholesterol production, thereby lowering the amount of cholesterol circulating in the blood. The life-prolonging benefits of the statin drugs (also known as HMG-CoA reductase inhibitors) must be appreciated by every middle-aged and older adult.

Remember, too, that dietary changes should be part of any cholesterol-reducing program you undertake. Effective dietary modifications might even reduce your dependence on medications. Your dietary goals should include reducing your cholesterol and saturated fat intake, increasing soy-based foods, consuming plenty of fresh fruits and vegetables, two or more servings of fish per week, the equivalent of no more than one cocktail every day or two *if* you are so inclined, and reducing caloric intake, if appropriate.

Because these drugs dramatically reduce the risk of fatal heart disease, it is essential that you have your lipid levels measured, to see whether you can benefit from them. A cholesterol blood test screens for total cholesterol, LDL (bad) cholesterol, HDL (good) cholesterol, and triglycerides. Whatever pill you take—and some are much more effective than others—you generally will want to get your LDL down to less than 130 mg/dL (if you don't have heart disease but have risk factors) or to less than 100 mg/dL (if you do have a history of coronary heart disease). Specific cholesterol level targets have been set by the National Cholesterol Education Program. Your doctor ought to be familiar enough with them to guide your lifestyle program and design your drug regimen.

Cholesterol lowering is not just for sick people who have had a heart attack, angioplasty, or open-

---

* Dietary intervention, including the reduction of cholesterol-containing foods and saturated fats, should be part of any cholesterol-lowering program. If dietary intervention is successful, pharmacological therapy may not be required. But as a rule, drug intervention will be part of most programs aimed at reducing blood cholesterol levels especially in those with significant elevations in LDL cholesterol.

heart surgery. It's for basically healthy people too, even those with no history of heart problems. Unfortunately, this fact is not widely appreciated. But healthy people who have no previous symptoms or history of heart disease but who have one or more risk factors for heart disease, and an LDL (bad) cholesterol level in the (moderately elevated) range of 155–230 mg/dL, will benefit from these medications. Studies show that women, in particular, are under-treated when it comes to cholesterol reduction.

Men who have had a heart attack and have a so-called "normal range" LDL level of 125–175 mg/dL will also benefit from having their LDL cholesterol reduced to less than 100 md/dL. In addition, people who have had coronary artery bypass grafts can keep their grafts clot-free for longer periods by using statins to lower their cholesterol. Finally, people who have had a heart attack and have LDL levels higher than the "normal" range will clearly benefit from lipid reduction. (These drugs should not be used during pregnancy.)

How effective are these drugs? As a rule of thumb, you will reduce your risk of a fatal heart attack by one percent for every one percent decrease in your LDL level. The more effectively a pill lowers cholesterol levels, the more prevention it will give you. Although many of the drugs discussed in this MedRANK Checklist can lower cholesterol levels significantly, you usually will get maximal life-prolonging results—as well as more convenience, comfort, and effectiveness—by using the most potent medications available.

Currently, Lipitor is the most potent cholesterol-lowering drug at approved FDA doses. It not only lowers LDL levels more than other drugs, it lowers triglyceride levels as well, which is an added benefit in some people. Zocor is probably the second most potent agent at approved doses, and Pravachol is a very close third. If a *single* cholesterol-lowering drug can meet your needs, so much the better: You can avoid the risks of multiple medication usage and prevent the side effects associated with add-on drugs, or what I call the "add-on blues." You will definitely want to avoid the second-line drugs such as niacin, cholestyramine, bile-acid binding resins, and fibric acids, because their side effects can be very troublesome.

How low can your cholesterol levels go? Generally speaking, the lower the better. But as a rule, if you do not have heart disease, you probably do not have much to gain from getting your LDL below 130 mg/dL, while if you do have heart disease, your target should be 100 mg/dL. Again, I want to stress that you should try to meet your cholesterol target point by using only *one* lipid-lowering drug, because adding a second-line cholesterol-reducer will usually catapult you into the discomfort zone.

In ranking cholesterol-lowering pills, potency, convenience, life prolongation, and effectiveness are the primary considerations.

 OPTIMAL
(HIGHLY RECOMMENDED/
BEST OF CLASS)

HMG-CoA REDUCTASE INHIBITORS ("STATINS")

Lipitor (atorvastatin)

When a medication *is* required to lower blood cholesterol levels, this is my drug of choice. It is the newest of the statin drugs and the most *potent* for reducing LDL and total cholesterol levels. With maximum doses of Lipitor, cholesterol reductions of up to 60 percent have been reported. At the lowest dose (10 mg per day), cholesterol levels can be reduced by up to 39 percent.

Lipitor has other advantages. It can also lower levels of the lipid fraction known as triglycerides. Although the precise role that triglycerides play in causing heart disease is not known, many people have elevations in both cholesterol and triglyceride levels. Lipitor may have a special advantage in these individuals. In short, potency, combined with cholesterol and triglyceride reduction, makes Lipitor the leader of the statin pack. Lipitor also increases HDL (good) cholesterol levels.

Over the long haul, the statins are the best tolerated of the lipid-lowering medications and therefore should be used as the initial drugs of choice in almost all patients. Side effects include mild, temporary gastrointestinal symptoms, muscle aches, rashes, sleep disturbance, and headache. Only 10–15 percent of patients who start these drugs have to discontinue them because of complications.

As a drug class, the statins can also cause inflammation in the muscles. This complication may be more common with statins such as Mevacor (see page 86). Muscle inflammation is more common when statins are used in conjunction with other drugs, including Lopid (gemfibrozil), erythromycin, Sandimmune (cyclosporine), Sporanox, or niacin.

POSTMENOPAUSE ESTROGEN REPLACEMENT

Prempro
Premarin

Hormone replacement therapy with estrogen (or combined estrogen/progestin) is advised in postmenopausal women, because the risk of death from coronary heart disease—including heart attacks—can be reduced by almost 50 percent. (Please see the full discussion of estrogen replacement in the MedRANK Checklist "Estrogen" on page 301.)

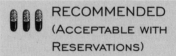

RECOMMENDED
(ACCEPTABLE WITH RESERVATIONS)

HMG-CoA REDUCTASE INHIBITORS

Zocor (simvastatin)

At currently recommended doses, this statin is probably the second most potent cholesterol-lowering drug, after Lipitor. Zocor can lower LDL cholesterol by as much as 37 percent (at maximum doses). It has been shown to prevent heart attacks and death in men and women with total cholesterol levels of 210–310 mg/dL, who also had a history of heart attacks or chest pain (angina) caused by coronary heart disease. This drug may be useful in familial hypercholesterolemia.

Zocor is an excellent drug, but at currently approved doses, it does not appear to be as potent as Lipitor; nor does it have as many FDA-approved indications as Pravachol. Please see "Lipitor" for other features and warnings that apply to all the statins.

Pravachol (pravastatin)

This very-well-studied drug is approved not only for cholesterol reduction but also for the *primary prevention* of heart attacks. This means it will prevent heart attacks in people who have no history of heart disease. At maximal doses, it lowers LDL cholesterol levels by 32 to 34 percent. It may be useful for familial (genetic) hypercholesterolemia. Pravachol has more FDA-approved indications than any of the other statin drugs. (Please see "Lipitor" for other features and warnings related to statins.)

BLOOD PRESSURE–LOWERING PILLS

Cardura (doxazosin)

This blood pressure medication appears to have a slight effect on lowering cholesterol levels in people with high blood pressure. It does not have an FDA indication for cholesterol lowering. If you have high blood pressure and you need, let's say, a 9–11 percent (very minimal) reduction in your LDL level, it may be worth asking your doctor if this drug is right for you, especially if you also have symptoms associated with an enlarged prostate.

DIETARY MEASURES

Soy Protein

A diet in which one-third to one-half of all animal protein intake is replaced with soy protein—in the form of tofu, soy milk, soy burger, or soy flour—can reduce LDL cholesterol by about 13 percent. Vitamin fortification may be necessary.

Fruits and Vegetables

A diet rich in fruits and vegetables (which contain the antioxidants vitamin E plus beta-carotene) is associated with a reduced risk of heart disease.

Fish

One to two servings of fish per week reduces the risk of coronary heart disease by 25 percent. This dietary approach appears to be much more effective than consuming fish oil capsules containing marine n-3 fatty acids.

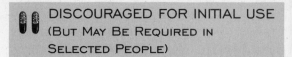

DISCOURAGED FOR INITIAL USE (BUT MAY BE REQUIRED IN SELECTED PEOPLE)

HMG-CoA REDUCTASE INHIBITORS (STATINS)

Mevacor (lovastatin)

By no means should Mevacor be discounted. After all, it was the first HMG-CoA reductase inhibitor to be approved, and its cholesterol-lowering properties are reasonable. But the newer drugs that have more potency (Lipitor) or expanded indications (Pravachol, Zocor) have outflanked Mevacor.

Although muscle-related side effects (myopathy), including muscle weakness and pain, have been seen with all the statins, the incidence may be higher with Mevacor. Finally, Mevacor may be less convenient than other statins because it must be taken with meals.

Lescol (fluvastatin)

This least potent of the statin drugs produces only 20–25 percent reductions in LDL cholesterol, as opposed to 50 percent reductions with some of the other statins (Lipitor). This inferior potency profile makes it less desirable than other drugs.

BILE-ACID BINDING RESINS

Questran (cholestyramine)
Prevalite (cholestyramine)
Colestid (colestipol)

People find these "bile-acid binding" resins ("one scoop, one poop") very difficult to take on a regular basis, with reported discontinuation rates as high as 35 percent. These drugs require multiple daily dosing, which makes them particularly inconvenient, especially compared with the statins. Their gastrointestinal symptoms, including constipation, gas, nausea, belching, and bloating, can be quite disturbing. If you take them just before meals, they may be more tolerable. Metamucil sometimes helps. These resins should not be used as primary agents but as add-on medications for the small group of people whose cholesterol levels do not respond to a statin alone.

Niacin (nicotinic acid)

This is another drug that is not very patient-friendly, with a side-effect profile that most people find intolerable. Niacin can cause gastrointestinal distress, flushing, itching, blurred vision, high blood sugar, and worsening of ulcer disease. Discontinuation rates as high as 40 percent are reported. Liver toxicity has been reported with the sustained-release preparation of niacin. The potential advantage of niacin is that it increases HDL (good) cholesterol more than any other drug.

NUTRITIONAL SUPPLEMENTS

Vitamin E

This vitamin may help protect slightly against the chest pain associated with heart disease and probably prevents heart attacks.

Beta-carotene

No benefit is documented.

Fish oil capsules

No benefit is documented.

 AVOID IF POSSIBLE (NOT RECOMMENDED)

Lopid (gemfibrozil)

This "fibric acid" drug is of limited usefulness, and caution is required. Its main claim to fame is that it can lower LDL, increase HDL, and lower serum triglycerides. But in some cases it produces "paradoxical" increases in LDL, which can be undesirable.

More gastrointestinal problems, including gallbladder surgeries, are seen with Lopid than with other lipid-reducing medications. It should be limited primarily to people who have Type III, IV, or V hyperlipidemia, with very high triglyceride levels. Lipitor may be preferable in these patients.

Use of this drug is not recommended, unless absolutely necessary. First, no consistent, convincing body of medical evidence shows a reduction in fatal heart attacks in those taking gemfibrozil. Second, users of this drug have about twice the risk of developing gallstones and/or requiring surgery for gallstones. Third, a 36 percent increase in deaths unrelated to cardiac causes was reported in one study. Finally, the reduction in cholesterol levels is only modest compared with the statins.

Lorelco (probucol)

The statins are much more effective and raise HDL (good) cholesterol levels better than Lorelco. This drug should not be used with clofibrate since there are no additional advantages from using the combination, which can even lower HDL (good) cholesterol.

Atromid-S (clofibrate)

This drug, which should be avoided, is similar to gemfibrozil (Lopid) and should be used only in people who have elevated triglyceride levels and who have failed to get results with niacin or gemfibrozil. Men with elevated cholesterol levels who took Atromid-S had a higher rate of gallbladder surgery and an increased death rate from cancer. Discontinuation rates are as high as 35 percent.

SHOULD YOU BE ON CHOLESTEROL-LOWERING DRUGS?

  MedRANK Life Prolongation and Enhancement Checklist

Pills of Wisdom: The National Cholesterol Education Program (NCEP)'s guidelines for lipid management suggest that cholesterol lowering be part of a program that addresses multiple risk factors for heart disease. Dietary modifications should be tried first. But you can also prevent death from heart disease by lowering your blood cholesterol levels by using statin drugs. In order of potency, the statins include Lipitor, Zocor, Pravachol, Mevacor, and Lescol. In people whose cholesterol levels do not respond to dietary changes, these are the drugs of choice for cholesterol reduction. Some of these pills may be better than others. (See the MedRANK Checklist "Cholesterol-Lowering Medications" on page 83 for specific recommendations and comparisons.)

If you are a man over the age of 35 or a woman over 40, get your cholesterol levels checked. As part of this blood test, you will get results for your total cholesterol level, an LDL (bad) cholesterol level, an HDL (good) cholesterol level, and a triglyceride (bad) level. These levels and your medical history will determine whether you can reduce your risk of having a fatal or nonfatal heart attack. If you are over 75 and have no history of heart disease, you probably do not need to take medications to lower your cholesterol level.

The target LDL cholesterol levels are as follows: (1) If you have no history of atherosclerosis and no risk factors for heart disease, cholesterol lowering should be implemented if your LDL level is greater than 190 mg/dL, and your level should be lowered to less than 160 mg/dL; (2) if you have no history of atherosclerosis, but you have two or more risk factors for heart disease, cholesterol lowering should be initiated if your LDL is greater than 160 mg/dL, and your LDL level should be lowered to less than 130 mg/dL; (3) if you have a history of atherosclerosis or heart disease, cholesterol lowering should be initated if your LDL is greater than 130 mg/dL, and your level should be lowered to less than 100 mg/dL.

To summarize, if dietary changes fail to bring your cholesterol levels into an acceptable range, *you may benefit from a statin drug if:*

- You are healthy, do not have any history of atherosclerosis or coronary heart disease, do not have any risk factors for heart disease (i.e., smoking, obesity, a sedentary lifestyle, high blood pressure, diabetes), and your LDL cholesterol level is **greater than 190 mg/dL.** Use diet and/or statins to lower your LDL cholesterol level to **less than 160 mg/dL.**
- You are healthy, you have two or more risk factors (smoking, high blood pressure, diabetes, a sedentary lifestyle, obesity) for heart disease,

and your LDL cholesterol level is greater than **160 mg/dL.** You can reduce your risk of a first heart attack by about 30 percent if your LDL cholesterol is lowered to **less than 130 mg/dL.**

- You have definite atherosclerotic heart disease (that is, you have had a heart attack, you have angina, you have had a test showing narrowing of the arteries to your heart, your electrocardiogram or stress test suggests you have heart disease, or something of that sort), *and* your LDL

cholesterol level is **greater than 130 mg/dL.** You can reduce your risk of death from heart disease by about 35 percent by lowering your LDL cholesterol to **less than 100 mg/dL.**

- You have had heart surgery for a coronary artery bypass graft, and your LDL cholesterol level is **greater than 130 mg/dL.** You can reduce the risk of your heart grafts "closing off" or clotting by getting your LDL down to **less than 100 mg/dL.**

ASPIRIN FOR LIFE PROLONGATION*

  MedRANK Life Prolongation and Enhancement Checklist

Pills of Wisdom: It's simple. It's quite safe. It's certain. Aspirin, which has the ability to reduce blood clot formation at very low—and, therefore very safe—doses, is now widely used for preventing complications and death due to heart attacks and strokes. Aspirin can benefit many groups of people, including those who have never had heart disease, as well as those who have.

Unfortunately, despite the well-recognized benefits of aspirin, many individuals fall through the cracks, and their physicians never advise them to take aspirin. As a result, they are denied the health-promoting and life-prolonging benefits of an inexpensive and safe drug. Many studies are still ongoing, but the general consensus is reflected in the following list of eligible candidates.

Finally, remember that aspirin is a medication, and that more than 130 over-the-counter medications contain it as an ingredient. Aspirin can cause drug interactions, so it is important to inform your physician if you plan to take aspirin along with other medications.

You probably should be on aspirin if:

- **You are a man or woman 50 or older and have no history or symptoms of heart disease (primary prevention).** Many experts recommend low-dose (81 mg/day Bayer Aspirin, low-strength) aspirin for all individuals who are 50 or older. Given the low risk of bleeding associated with low-dose aspirin, this is a reasonable strategy for reducing the risk of a first heart attack, especially in men. I recommend starting aspirin in men at the age of forty. The role of aspirin for prevention of first heart attacks in *women* is less clear, especially since women (1) are likely to be on hormone (estrogen) replace-

* Aspirin is a drug. Never start long-term aspirin use without the approval of your physician. The drug should not be taken by people with bleeding problems or known allergies to the medication.

ment therapy, which itself exerts a powerful protective effect against heart disease, and (2) have a higher risk of bleeding strokes.

Clearly, though, if you are over 50 and have one or more of the risk factors for heart disease (smoker, obesity, a sedentary lifestyle, high blood pressure, diabetes, elevated cholesterol), you should ask your physician to consider your suitability for chronic, low-dose aspirin therapy to prevent heart disease.

- **You have had one or more heart attacks.** Aspirin (81–162 mg/day) is recommended to reduce the risk of another heart attack. This recommendation applies to people who have had a heart attack even if they are less than 50 years of age. If you have had a heart attack and currently have not been advised by your physician to be on aspirin, find out why not as soon as possible.

- **You have had chest pain (angina) caused by coronary heart disease.** If you have not had a heart attack but have had angina (symptoms usually caused by insufficient blood or oxygen supply to the heart muscle), you should ask your physician to consider your suitability for chronic aspirin therapy (81–162 mg) to prevent heart disease. Studies suggest you will reduce your risk of death from heart attack and other vascular problems.

- **You have not had a heart attack, but you have been told by your doctor that you have coronary heart disease.** You are a candidate for using 81–162 mg aspirin per day. Coronary heart disease is a condition that applies to people who have had tests (angiograms, scans, EKGs, or treadmills) showing that "deposits" in their heart vessels are probably causing symptoms like chest pain, shortness of breath, and related problems.

- **You have had a coronary angioplasty.** If you have had your heart vessels "opened up" with a coronary angioplasty (also known as a PTCA), long-term aspirin therapy (160–325 mg/day) is recommended, primarily because of its effect on coronary heart disease. It's not clear whether aspirin will prevent recurrent blockage in vessels that have been opened up, but it does have an overall positive effect on coronary heart disease, and therefore is advised. Consult with your doctor if you have had this procedure but have not been advised to take aspirin.

- **You have had a coronary artery bypass graft.** Aspirin (325 mg/day or a higher dose) is advised for people who have had a coronary artery bypass. One study has shown that the addition of dipyridamole (Persantine) may be better than aspirin alone.

- **You have a prosthetic (artificial) heart valve or valvular heart disease.** You are likely to be taking a blood thinner called warfarin (Coumadin). This is appropriate. Some experts recommend adding aspirin to Coumadin, but because aspirin increases risk of bleeding (as does Coumadin), combining the two drugs is potentially dangerous. Therefore aspirin should never be taken along with Coumadin without physician approval. The role of aspirin in patients with diseased or replaced heart valves should be decided on a patient-by-patient basis.

- **You have had a minor stroke or transient ischemic attack.** Aspirin can prevent strokes and the "temporary" strokes called transient ischemic attacks (TIAs). The dose of aspirin that protects people against stroke is not universally agreed upon, but it is in the range of 30–1,300 mg per day. The point is, if you have a blockage of the vessels that lead to the brain (cerebrovascular disease), have had a carotid endarterectomy (a cleaning out of deposits in vessels leading to the brain), or a history of minor strokes or TIAs, you should consult your doctor about the benefits and risks of aspirin in your particular case.

- **You have a strong family history of cancer of the colon or multiple polyps of the colon.**

Studies have shown that aspirin reduces the risk of colon cancer in high-risk populations, although not approved for prevention of colon cancer.

PREVENTING A FIRST HEART ATTACK
"Cocktails" for Cardiac Prevention

 MedRANK Life Prolongation and Enhancement Checklist

 OPTIMAL
(HIGHLY RECOMMENDED/
BEST OF CLASS)

☀ **Pills of Wisdom:** First things first. Get your blood cholesterol levels checked as soon as possible, if you (a) are a woman 35 or older, or a man 40 or older; (b) are a postmenopausal woman; (c) have coronary heart disease risk factors (smoker, obesity, elevated cholesterol, a sedentary lifestyle, high blood pressure, diabetes); (d) have had a hysterectomy (your uterus has been surgically removed); (e) have had someone in your family die at a young age from either a stroke or a heart attack; or (f) have diabetes.

Second, if you have any of the aforementioned heart disease "risk factors," begin a lifestyle-modification program—smoking cessation, weight reduction, and so on (see Chapter 21)—under your doctor's supervision. Lifestyle modifications can reduce the need for certain medications.

At least three medications have the potential for preventing a first heart attack. They include aspirin, estrogen (in women), and cholesterol-lowering drugs. The "cocktail" approach to heart disease prevention follows.

HMG-CoA REDUCTASE INHIBITORS (STATINS)

Lipitor (atorvastatin)
Zocor (simvastatin)
Pravachol (pravastatin)

The *life-prolonging* benefits of cholesterol-lowering medications, especially the statin drugs, must be appreciated by *every* middle-aged and older adult. Cholesterol-lowering medications, which have to be taken indefinitely, have convincingly been shown to reduce coronary heart disease.

Used over the long haul, the statins are the best-tolerated of the lipid-lowering medications and therefore should be the initial drugs of choice in almost all patients. Side effects include mild temporary gastrointestinal symptoms, muscle aches, headache, rashes, sleep disturbance, and headache. Pravachol is the only drug *approved* by the FDA for preventing a first heart attack. Nevertheless, other statins such as Lipitor and Zocor most likely also can reduce the risk of a first heart attack through their effects on cholesterol reduction.

Anti-Platelet ("Blood-Thinning" or "Anti-clotting") Drugs

Aspirin

Many experts recommend low-dose aspirin (81 mg/day of Bayer Aspirin, low-strength, or any other aspirin preparation) for *all* individuals who are 50 or older. Given the low risk of bleeding associated with low-dose aspirin, this is a reasonable strategy for reducing the risk of first heart attacks, especially in men. The role of aspirin for the prevention of first heart attacks in women is less clear, especially since women (a) are likely to be on hormone (estrogen) replacement therapy, which itself exerts a powerful protective effect against heart disease, and (b) have a higher risk of bleeding strokes.

Postmenopause Estrogen Replacement

Premarin (estrogen)
Prempro (estrogen plus progesterone)

Hormone replacement therapy is advised in postmenopausal women, in whom the risk of death from coronary heart disease—including heart attacks—can be reduced by almost 50 percent. (Please see the full discussion in Chapter 19.)

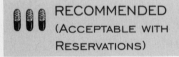 RECOMMENDED (ACCEPTABLE WITH RESERVATIONS)

Dietary Measures

Vitamin E

Full doses (400 to 1000 International units) of vitamin E help protect slightly against the chest pain associated with heart disease, and may reduce the risk of heart attack.

Soy Protein

A diet in which one-third to one-half of all animal protein is replaced with soy protein—in the form of tofu, soy milk, soy burger, or soy flour—can reduce LDL cholesterol by about 13 percent. Vitamin fortification may be necessary.

Fruits and Vegetables

A diet rich in fruits and vegetables (which contain the antioxidants vitamin E plus beta-carotene) are associated with a reduced risk of heart disease.

Fish

One to two servings of fish per week reduces the risk of coronary heart disease by 25 percent. This dietary approach appears to be much more effective than consuming fish oil capsules containing marine n-3 fatty acids.

Multivitamins

The "homocysteine theory" of heart disease suggests a strong link between high homocysteine levels and atherosclerosis. In individuals prone to high blood levels of homocysteine, an optimal intake of 3 to 3.5 mg of B_6, 350 to 400 mg of folic acid, and 5 to 15 mcg of B_{12} is recommended. Many multivitamins contain these amounts, which are sufficient to lower homocysteine levels and, possibly, reduce progression of heart disease.

DRUGS THAT WILL PROLONG YOUR LIFE BY PREVENTING A RECURRENT HEART ATTACK

 MedRANK Life Prolongation and Enhancement Checklist

 Pills of Wisdom: If you have had a heart attack, you can reduce the risk of additional heart attacks by taking the three medications listed in the "Optimal" category. The life-prolonging trio you ought to consider includes: aspirin, a beta-blocker, and a statin (if indicated, and if dietary changes haven't produced the desired cholesterol reduction). ACE inhibitors may also be helpful.

If you have had a heart attack and are not taking these medications, *you should ask your physician why they have not been prescribed on your behalf.* You may be told that you are not a "suitable" or appropriate candidate for therapy with these drugs, or that you have a "contraindication"—that is, there is something about your condition or there is some other medication you are taking that may be harmful in combination with one of these drugs. In any event, these drugs can have a dramatic impact on disease reduction and life prolongation, so you ought to investigate your suitability for their benefits.

OPTIMAL (HIGHLY RECOMMENDED/ BEST OF CLASS)

ANTICLOTTING DRUGS

Aspirin

If you have had a heart attack, aspirin (81–162 mg/day) is recommended to reduce the risk of another heart attack. This recommendation applies even if you are less than 50 years of age. If you have had a heart attack and currently have not been advised by your physician to be on aspirin, find out why not as soon as possible.

HMG-CoA REDUCTASE INHIBITORS (STATINS)

Lipitor (atorvastatin)
Pravachol (pravastatin)
Zocor (simvastatin)

The *life-prolonging* benefits of cholesterol-lowering medications, especially statins, must be appreciated by everyone who has had a heart attack. Specifically, people (most of the studies have been done on men) who have had a heart attack and have an elevated or even "normal range" LDL (bad) cholesterol level, between 125 and 175 mg/dL, will benefit from having their LDL cholesterol reduced to less than 100 mg/dL.

BETA-ADRENERGIC BLOCKING AGENTS (BETA-BLOCKERS)

Tenormin (atenolol)

Beta-blockers can prolong life in people who have had a first heart attack, with studies showing a 25 percent reduction in deaths due to subsequent heart attacks. Unfortunately, less than 40 percent of eligible patients receive these drugs. Be sure you don't fall through the cracks.

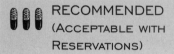

RECOMMENDED
(ACCEPTABLE WITH RESERVATIONS)

ACE INHIBITORS

Accupril (quinapril)
Altace (ramipril)
Capoten (captropril)
Prinivil (lisinopril)
Vasotec (enalapril)
Zestril (lisinopril)

If you have had a heart attack and, as a result, were diagnosed as having congestive heart failure, you can prolong your life and prevent worsening heart failure by taking an ACE inhibitor. Even if you *don't* have heart failure, ACE inhibitors have been shown to prevent recurrent heart attacks by a small degree.

POSTMENOPAUSE ESTROGEN REPLACEMENT

Premarin (estrogen)
Prempro (estrogen plus progesterone)

Hormone replacement therapy is advised in postmenopausal women, in whom the risk of death from coronary heart disease—including heart attacks—can be reduced by almost 50 percent. (Please see the full discussion in Chapter 19.)

BETA-BLOCKERS

Blocadren (timolol)
Lopressor (metoprolol)

See "Beta-Adrenergic Blocking Agents" in the "Optimal" category.

DISCOURAGED FOR INITIAL USE
(BUT MAY BE REQUIRED IN SELECTED PEOPLE)

BETA-BLOCKERS

Inderal (propranolol)

See "Beta-Adrenergic Blocking Agents." Use of Inderal is discouraged because it may have more side effects than other beta-blockers listed in "Optimal" and "Recommended" categories.

AVOID IF POSSIBLE
(NOT RECOMMENDED)

CALCIUM CHANNEL BLOCKERS (SHORT-ACTING)

Calan (verapamil)
Cardizem (diltiazem)
Procardia (nifedipine)

The *short-acting* calcium channel blockers should *not* be used in patients with heart disease and, for that matter, should be avoided in general. You are probably taking a short-acting calcium blocker if you are taking Cardizem, Calan, or Procardia more than once a day.

Note: Procardia XL, Norvasc, Cardizem CD, and Calan SR are *not* short-acting calcium channel blockers—they are long-acting (safer) preparations. Ask your doctor if you require clarification. The long-acting calcium channel blockers—in particular, Norvasc (amlodipine)—although not shown to prevent recurrent heart attacks, can be used safely in people with heart problems.

DRUGS THAT WILL PROLONG LIVES OF PEOPLE WHO HAVE CONGESTIVE HEART FAILURE*
("Water on the Lungs," "Fluid in the Lungs," "Weak Heart," "Bad Heart Pump," "Congestion in the Lungs")

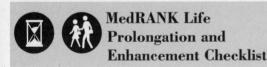 **MedRANK Life Prolongation and Enhancement Checklist**

Pills of Wisdom: Congestive heart failure (CHF) is a condition in which the pumping action of the heart deteriorates to the point where fluid backs up into the lungs. If the heart muscle is sufficently incapacitated—due to poor blood supply or previous heart attacks—the force of the heart's muscular contractions may no longer be able to keep up with the body's demands for oxygen. When this happens, symptoms such as fatigue, shortness of breath, excessive sleepiness, and weakness take over. Eventually, fluid backs up in the lungs, which leads to poor exercise tolerance and severe shortness of breath. Currently, CHF is the most common cause of hospitalization and death for people with chronic heart disease.

For many years, there was very little we could do about congestive heart failure, except reduce the severity of the disabling symptoms with drugs such as digoxin and water pills. Although these medications lessened the symptoms, they did not prolong the lives of people with CHF. Now the prognosis for people with CHF has brightened dramatically as a result of ACE inhibitors—medications that open up the peripheral vessels, reduce the load on the heart, and allow better pumping action. In fact, people with CHF now can have their lives prolonged by years. ACE inhibitors must be used at sufficiently high doses to produce these life-prolonging effects. For the most part, they are quite safe and reasonably priced.

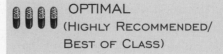 **OPTIMAL**
(HIGHLY RECOMMENDED/ BEST OF CLASS)

ACE INHIBITORS

Accupril (quinapril)
Altace (ramipril)
Capoten (captropril)
Prinivil (lisinopril)
Vasotec (enalapril)
Zestril (lisinopril)

These pills are also used for hypertension. But ACE inhibitors can delay or halt the progressive worsening of the heart muscle's pump function. They prevent unfavorable changes in heart chamber architecture that can lead to poor pumping, inadequate blood output from the heart, and fluid congestion in the lungs. ACE inhibitors must be used at appropriately high doses to achieve improvements in survival. Prolonged survival has been seen in studies using Vasotec, Capoten, and Altace.

---

* Certain medications can counteract the favorable effects of the Optimal and Recommended drugs, or cause worsening of the heart's pumping function. These drugs should be avoided if possible, since they can worsen your heart condition, and increase the risk of sudden death.

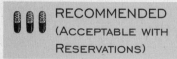

RECOMMENDED
(ACCEPTABLE WITH RESERVATIONS)

VASODILATORS

Hydralazine
Isosorbide Nitrate

These older medications, to a great extent, have been replaced by ACE inhibitors. Nevertheless, there is considerable evidence that the combination of these two drugs can prolong survival of people with CHF. This combination should be considered in patients who, for one reason or another, cannot tolerate the "Optimal" ACE inhibitors.

DIGITALIS DRUGS

Lanoxin (digoxin)

Digoxin has been used for a long time to treat people with CHF. It appears as if it does have a favorable effect on their *symptoms*. But a recent study of 7,500 patients suggests that digoxin does *not* improve survival; nor does it worsen survival. It does, however, appear to reduce the need for hospitalization in people with CHF.

DIURETICS (WATER PILLS)

Thiazide Diuretics
Hydrochlorothiazide
Chlorthalidone
Loop Diuretics
Furosemide
Bumetanide
Ethacrynic acid
Toresemide

Potassium-Sparing Diuretics
Triamterene
Spironolactone
Amiloride

Diuretics do *not* prolong life in patients with CHF. They do, however, improve their *symptoms*. These symptoms include shortness of breath, fatigue, and leg swelling. Diuretics should be added to ACE inhibitors if better symptom relief is required.

DISCOURAGED FOR INITIAL USE
(BUT MAY BE REQUIRED IN SELECTED PEOPLE)

BETA-ADRENERGIC BLOCKING AGENTS (BETA-BLOCKERS)

Carvedilol

Although not approved for the treatment of heart failure, this medication may improve survival in some patients with CHF who are already being treated with an ACE inhibitor, digoxin, and a diuretic. Additional research to determine its effect on CHF is needed.

CALCIUM CHANNEL BLOCKERS
Norvasc (amlodipine)

Although not approved for the treatment of heart failure, one study suggests this medication may improve survival in some patients with CHF (those who do not have blocked arteries) who are already being treated with an ACE inhibitor, digoxin, and a diuretic. Additional research is needed to clarify its possible role in treating certain patients with CHF.

AVOID IF POSSIBLE
(NOT RECOMMENDED)

ANTI-ARRHYTHMIC DRUGS

Tambocor (flecainide)
Rythmol (propafenone)
Ethmozine (moricizine)
Quinaglute (quinidine)

These drugs are used for serious, life-threatening heart rhythm problems. They are potentially dangerous and should be prescribed only by a cardiologist. They can potentially decrease survival in some patients with CHF.

NONSTEROIDAL ANTI-INFLAMMATORY DRUGS (NSAIDs)

Motrin
Ansaid
Voltaren
Anaprox
Naproxen
Others

These drugs can make heart failure worse and and should not be used unless absolutely necessary.

CALCIUM CHANNEL BLOCKERS (SHORT-ACTING)

Verapamil
Diltiazem

These drugs can make heart failure worse and should not be used.

BETA-BLOCKERS (HIGH DOSES)

At *high* doses, these drugs can make heart failure worse and should not be used.

MEDICATIONS FOR CHEST PAIN (ANGINA) CAUSED BY HEART DISEASE

 MedRANK Life Enhancement Checklist

Pills of Wisdom: There are many causes of chest pain, many of them not related to heart disease. But if you have been diagnosed as having *angina*, it means your chest pain is coming from the heart. It is usually caused by the vessels going into spasm or, more commonly, by a narrowing of the arteries that supply the heart muscles due to fat deposits in the walls. Frequently, people need more than one medication to control their angina pain. The three main drug classes used for relief of angina symptoms include nitroglycerin formulations, calcium channel blockers, and beta-blockers. Some are better choices than others.

If your pattern of angina pain changes, you should consult your doctor at once. Increasing severity of pain, more frequent episodes, and pain that is accompanied by nausea, vomiting, or sweating are all cause for concern. Angina pain is a warning sign that not enough oxygen is getting to your heart muscle. You may need additional medications or a procedure to open up your arteries to improve the blood supply to your heart.

OPTIMAL
(Highly Recommended/
Best of Class)

Beta-Adrenergic Blocking Agents (Beta-blockers)

Tenormin (atenolol)
Corgard (nadolol)

Tenormin is highly recommended. The beta-blockers are excellent drugs to treat angina, and they also can prolong life in people who have had a first heart attack. Studies show a 25 percent reduction in deaths due to subsequent heart attacks in people taking beta-blockers. Consequently, if you have had a heart attack and need relief of angina, these drugs are an excellent option (i.e., a "smart drug") that can kill two birds with one stone.

Calcium Channel Blockers (long-acting)

Norvasc (amlodipine)

Norvasc, a long-acting calcium channel blocker, is approved for the treatment of angina caused by spasm of the heart arteries (vasospastic) and for angina caused by narrowing of the arteries due to heart disease (chronic stable angina). It is especially recommended for patients who need treatment for their chest pain and who also have congestive heart failure. Although this medication is not indicated for treatment of heart failure, it is the only calcium channel blocker that is approved by the FDA for *safe* use in such patients. Because Norvasc is also indicated for treating high blood pressure, if you have angina *and* high blood pressure, this may be the "smart drug" for your situation. Consult your physician for more information.

Nitrates (for acute angina treatment)

Nitroglycerin (sublingual)
Nitrostat

This is the classic, proven, and effective way to treat the sudden, acute chest pain associated with an angina attack.

Nitrates (for angina prevention)

IMDUR (isosorbide mononitrate)

With the convenience of once-daily dosing, Imdur is well-suited for the *prevention* of angina.

Nitrates (skin patches or topical creams)

Nitro-Derm
Nitro-Dur
Nitrodisc
Transderm Nitro
Minitran

These patches, which are applied once daily, are approved for the *prevention* of angina chest pain. You may have a preference, depending on the adhesive and patch sizes.

Anticlotting Drugs

Aspirin

If you have angina, you should ask your physician to consider your suitability for chronic aspirin therapy (81–162 mg) to prevent complications of heart disease. Studies suggest if you fall into this category, taking aspirin may reduce your risk of heart attack and other vascular problems.

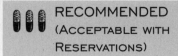

RECOMMENDED
(ACCEPTABLE WITH RESERVATIONS)

NITRATES

ISMO (isosorbide mononitrate)

With twice-daily dosing, this drug is recommended for the prevention of angina chest pain.

Monoket (isosorbide mononitrate)
Isordil (isosorbide dinitrate)
Sorbitrate (isosorbide dinitrate)

These are good drugs for preventing angina. They have to be given every six hours, which is less than optimal as far as convenience goes.

BETA-ADRENERGIC BLOCKING AGENTS (BETA-BLOCKERS)

Inderal (propranolol)
Lopressor (metoprolol)

Beta-blockers are excellent drugs to treat angina. Like Tenormin and Corgard, Lopressor and Inderal are approved for the treatment of angina. But because they are fat soluble and therefore are more likely to distribute into central nervous system tissue, many experts feel they are more likely to cause side effects, such as sleepiness, drowsiness, sleep problems, and fatigue. As a result, they are not as strongly recommended as Tenormin, which may have a more user-friendly side-effect profile. (They also can prolong life in people who have had a first heart attack.)

CALCIUM CHANNEL BLOCKERS (LONG-ACTING)

Cardizem CD (diltiazem)
Dilacor XR (diltiazem)
Tiazac (diltiazem)

These diltiazem-based drugs are excellent drugs for angina. They do, however, have the potential to inhibit the pumping action of the heart and to slow the heart rate. Sometimes this is a benefit, sometimes not. Their safety profile in patients with complicated heart conditions, especially CHF, is not as well established as it is for Norvasc.

Procardia XL (nifedipine SR/GITS)

Procardia XL is an excellent drug for high blood pressure and angina, but its safety profile in patients with complicated heart conditions is not as well established as it is for Norvasc. It also is more likely to cause leg swelling than many other calcium channel blockers.

 ## DISCOURAGED FOR INITIAL USE
(BUT MAY BE REQUIRED IN SELECTED PEOPLE)

CALCIUM CHANNEL BLOCKERS (LONG-ACTING OR EXTENDED-RELEASE)

Calan SR (verapamil)
Isoptin SR (verapamil)
Verelan (verapamil)

Although approved for treatment of angina, these calcium channel blockers can slow heart rates and inhibit heart pumping more than most other calcium channel blockers. This may present problems, especially in older patients who have congestive heart failure, and in people who have complicated heart conditions. The safety profile of long-acting verapamil drugs in patients with complicated heart conditions is not as well established as it is for Norvasc.

Cardizem SR (diltiazem)

Twice-daily dosing makes this drug not as convenient as other formulations of diltiazem (see "Recommended").

NITRATES

Topical Nitroglycerin

This nitroglycerin ointment must be applied every 4–8 hours, which is less than optimal as far as convenience goes. The nitroglycerin skin-patch delivery system is usually better tolerated (see "Optimal").

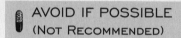

AVOID IF POSSIBLE
(NOT RECOMMENDED)

CALCIUM CHANNEL BLOCKERS (SHORT-ACTING OR GENERIC)

Verapamil (generic)
Calan (verapamil)
Isoptin (verapamil)
Cardizem (diltiazem)
Diltiazem (generic)
Procardia (nifedipine capsules)

Avoid. These short-acting or generic calcium calcium blockers are potentially harmful and have no role in the current treatment of angina chest pain.

CHAPTER 6

THE PRESSURE IS ON

Medications for High Blood Pressure

"I'm not sure what's worse, taking these medications or living with high blood pressure," complains a middle-aged executive. "My doctor has been trying all these different pills. I've been switched from one drug to another, and nothing seems quite right. Some make me sleepy, one made me cough, another made my feet swell, and the last one drove my sex life into hibernation. There's got to be a pill out there that will work."

With more than fifty different medications (including combination pills) available to treat high blood pressure, there will almost always be a pill that is tailor-made for treating your high blood pressure. When you and your doctor find that pill, stick with it. Silent, but potentially very deadly if left untreated, high blood pressure (also called hypertension) is one of the few medical conditions that are very easy to detect and that can be treated effectively before vulnerable organs such as the heart and brain sustain irreparable harm.

Put simply, an ounce of treatment for high blood pressure is worth a ton of cure for heart disease and stroke. High blood pressure ranks as the leading risk factor for heart disease and is arguably the most common reason for American adults to visit their doctor and receive a prescription medication. Cardiovascular disease is the leading cause of death in the United States; of these deaths, about 85 percent are caused by heart attacks and about 15 percent are due to stroke.

There has been a steady decrease in death from cardiovascular disease over the past thirty years, much of it attributable to the improved detection and treatment of high blood pressure. Remember, hypertension is frequently the "entry point" to a continuum of potential problems. In some respects, you can see it as a warning condition. But more important, you can do something about it—and in the process steer your health in the right direction.

Life prolongation in people with hypertension is best accomplished by constructing an individualized program that combines prevention and treatment approaches aimed at improving overall cardiovascular health. The treatment program usually will consist of medications to lower blood pressure along with lifestyle changes to lessen other risk factors for heart disease. These lifestyle changes include—when indicated and necessary—increasing physical exercise, restricting salt, reducing excessive alcohol intake, decreasing intake of fat and cholesterol, ceasing smoking, and losing weight. From a medical perspective, they also may include taking pills for blood cholesterol reduction, improving blood sugar control (if you have diabetes), and undergoing prevention therapy with aspirin and estrogen (if you are a woman).

☺ *Blood Pressure: To Treat or Not to Treat.*

When should high blood pressure be treated with pills? When are lifestyle modifications and nondrug therapy sufficient? What are the target "numbers" for normal blood pressure? The answers to these questions depend, to a great extent, on your needs as an individual, on your age, on the presence of other risk factors, and on whether you have other, associated cardiovascular problems that may benefit from versatile medications used for blood pressure control.

For all practical purposes, normal blood pressure is 120/80 mm Hg (millimeters of mercury). The top number is the systolic blood pressure, and the bottom number is the diastolic blood pressure. Broadly speaking, your blood pressure is considered high if your lower number is greater than 85 or your top number is greater than 160. Some people have what is called isolated systolic hypertension, which means their lower number is normal but their systolic reading is greater than 160. This condition also requires treatment, especially in the elderly. If your diastolic reading is less than 90 mm Hg but greater than 80 mm Hg—and you have no risk factors for heart disease—it is acceptable to try *nondrug* treatment for three to six months. If your blood pressure is still elevated after that point, medications should be started. If you have risk factors for heart disease and your diastolic blood pressure is greater than 90 mm Hg, you probably should start on medications at the outset. In general, if your blood pressure is lower than 120/80, don't worry. Many athletes have low pressures, which can be a sign of cardiovascular fitness. For a logical approach to blood pressure control with medications, review "A Five-Step Program for Optimal Blood Pressure Control," in this chapter.

☺ *Best and Worst Pills for High Blood Pressure.*

Once your physician decides you need pills to control your high blood pressure, which ones are the best and safest? Again, the answer depends on your specific needs. In general, though, if you are started on a medication but your doctor has to keep raising the dose to get adequate control, you probably ought to be switched to another class of medications. The fact is, for reasons we can't always predict, some people respond very nicely to one class of blood pressure pills but not to another. If possible, your doctor should try to find a *single* drug that will control your blood pressure rather than use two or more medications. But there are situations when two or more drugs are necessary or even advantageous. Remember, the success of your blood pressure pills is a matter not only of the "numbers" but of how well you *feel*. You will be able to evaluate these issues simply by completing the Action Plan Side Effect Checklist and the Four-Point Quality of Life Survey on pages 375 and 376. Finally, it should be stressed that you should never discontinue a blood pressure pill without your physician's approval.

What pills are you most likely to get from your doctor? And more important, which pills *should* you be getting? Because treatment for this condition is usually, but not always, a life-long journey, you ought to be started on nothing less than the best. Before starting a drug for a lifetime, you and your doctor should weigh the advantages and disadvantages of all the options. For a drug-by-drug comparison, consult the MedRANK Checklist "The Pressure's Off" on page 105.

☺ *Diuretics, or "water pills," are the most widely used drugs to initiate treatment and maintain adequate blood pressure in people with hypertension.*

Although they have been shown to reduce death from stroke, their routine use has been tarnished by several findings. First, at higher doses, diuretics increase the risk of sudden death from heart disease in people who have abnormal electrocardiograms and, perhaps, in diabetic patients. Also at higher doses, they can increase cholesterol levels and make it more difficult for people with diabetes to control their blood sugar level. Because of these

shortcomings, I *don't* recommend diuretics as first-line treatment for high blood pressure. If you require anything above a low dose (12.5–25 mg) of hydrochlorothiazide, I recommend that you ask your doctor to switch to another class of blood pressure–lowering medications. In addition, if you are taking Lanoxin (digoxin) or if you have an abnormal heart rhythm, diabetes, elevated cholesterol level, or gout, ask your physician whether another class of drugs may serve you better. My opinion is that your doctor will find one that will.

☺ *Beta-blockers have also been shown to reduce the risk of stroke and death from heart disease.*

Because beta-blockers such as Tenormin, Lopressor, and Inderal prevent recurrent heart attacks, they are especially useful ("versatile") if you have high blood pressure and have also had a previous heart attack. Their downside is their side effects, which include fatigue, impotence, decreased sex drive, depression, and nightmares. If you have depression, asthma, heart failure, or sleep problems, you probably are better off on another medication. Among the beta-blockers, Tenormin and similar medications are the best tolerated.

Some blood pressure–lowering drugs are used for off-label indications. For example, the fifteen medications in the beta-blocker class have been approved by the FDA for more than twenty uses or indications, as well as unlabeled uses. Beta-blockers such as Inderal (propranolol) may have a tendency to cause *more* side effects than other drugs in the same class, such as Tenormin (atenolol), but they also have more indications.

☺ The calcium channel blockers are a diverse class of blood pressure–lowering medications.

Among them, I generally do not recommend the long-acting Calan or Cardizem formulations unless you need to have your heart rate slowed down as well. In susceptible individuals, these medications can cause congestive heart failure. Side effects vary considerably from one calcium channel blocker to another. For example, some calcium channel blockers (like Calan) are more likely to cause constipation than others. Others (like Procardia XL and Plendil) are more likely to cause fluid retention and make your legs swell.

Always ask your doctor if switching to another drug is appropriate. For example, if you are taking the calcium channel blocker Cardizem CD and have been experiencing gastrointestinal problems such as gas, constipation, or diarrhea, you may want to ask your doctor if another calcium channel blocker, such as Norvasc, may be less likely to produce these side effects. All in all, Norvasc seems to provide the greatest number of benefits with the least risk. If your doctor feels a calcium channel blocker is right for you, Norvasc may be the logical choice.

☺ ACE Inhibitors are widely used because they are safe and, for the most part, user-friendly.

The most troublesome side effect is cough. Half of those who experience this problem have to be discontinued from the drug. If you have congestive heart failure, diabetes, and high blood pressure, ACE inhibitors are for you. Most of the drugs in this class are quite similar. I recommend any of the once-daily formulations.

☺ Pills and Pitfalls.

It is estimated that 40 million Americans are currently taking drugs to treat high blood pressure. Unfortunately, taking these medications is not always a picnic. Of the 85 percent who should be taking them—as well as the people with high blood pressure we haven't detected yet—many are taking suboptimal medications that are inconvenient, cause troublesome side effects, impair sleep, and wreak havoc on sexual function. In high doses they may be downright bad for the person's health.

Of those who are taking pills for hypertension, as many as 15 percent (or 6 million) may be taking them unnecessarily and are excellent candidates for step-down therapy, a gradual, monitored discontinuation of medications, as recommended by the Joint National Committee V Guidelines for Hypertension. You should always discuss this option with your doctor. The likelihood of your being able to discontinue or reduce the dose of your blood pressure pills is greater if you are taking only a single antihypertensive medication *and* if you implement one or more of the lifesyle modifications discussed above. In other words, if you exercise more, lose weight, and reduce excessive alcohol consumption, you may be able to reduce your need for medications.

THE PRESSURE'S OFF
Medications for High Blood Pressure

  MedRANK Life Prolongation and Enhancement Checklist

Pills of Wisdom: Forty million Americans have high blood pressure, and you or a family member may be one of them. Hypertension, a silent killer, is an important risk factor for heart disease and stroke. Many hypertensive people get inadequate treatment and follow-up, which has enormous public health implications. Appropriate treatment of high blood pressure with medications can prevent heart disease and prolong life.

The initial approach to reducing mild elevations in blood pressure is lifestyle modification, including weight loss, smoking cessation, reduction of alcohol intake, and exercise. If these nonpharmacological approaches are not effective within 3 to 6 months, your physician should prescribe a medication to lower your blood pressure.

There are many classes from which to choose. The good news is that two classes of blood pressure medications—diuretics and beta-blockers—have been shown to reduce death from stroke. The bad news is, these medications can produce troublesome side effects. Many physicians believe that two other classes —although they lack the same body of evidence—the ACE inhibitors and calcium channel blockers, may be more quality-of-life preserving. Decisions regarding choice of blood pressure medication have become quite controversial as a result.

Unfortunately, no blood pressure medication is perfect, and the majority of them have side effects that may have a negative impact on your quality of life. Because high blood pressure is usually treated for many years, the medication your physician selects for you today must stand the test of time. Consequently, subtle but important variations between drugs can make all the difference between a tolerable life and one characterized by insidious, festering side effects.

Naturally, the choice of a blood pressure pill must always be tailored or customized for the individual person. But even within the range of your targeted choices, there will be some pills you'll like and some you won't. Some will make you feel good, and others won't. Some will tend to work over the long haul, and others will require add-on medications to get the job done. Some will preserve your sexual function, and others won't. Some will elevate your blood cholesterol, and others won't. This section will help you make those distinctions.

Even though calcium channel blockers and ACE inhibitors have not yet been shown to prolong life in patients with high blood pressure, they, along with the diuretics and beta-blockers, are nevertheless considered by most physicians as initial drugs of choice for hypertension. This MedRANK Checklist attempts to identify those blood pressure pills within each class that have the lowest incidence of side effects, are safest and easiest to take, have the lowest risk of drug-drug interactions, and have special advantages over similar medications.

If one blood pressure medication is not working for you, try to replace it rather than add on a new medication to your regimen, if possible. Ask your physician to substitute a pill from a different class for the drug you have been taking. So often, physicians simply add pills to existing pills, even though drug replacement would produce equivalent results with fewer pills.

OPTIMAL
(HIGHLY RECOMMENDED/
BEST OF CLASS)

CALCIUM CHANNEL BLOCKERS (LONG-ACTING)

Norvasc (amlodipine)

This drug has a smooth ride. It is a very well tolerated and popular blood pressure pill, with a low discontinuation rate. It is safe, has no clinically significant drug-drug interactions, and can be used safely even if you have other medical conditions, including heart disease or diabetes.

It is highly effective and appears to work reliably in many different groups of people with hypertension, including the elderly and African Americans, as well as middle-aged and younger adults. It is relatively preserving of sexual function, including sex drive in men and women and erectile function in men.

Overall, if your doctor feels you should be on a drug in the calcium channel blocker class, this once-daily pill is the top of the line—a blood pressure pill for a lifetime. Among all the calcium channel blockers, Norvasc has passed the "crash test" for safe use in people with congestive heart failure (poor contracting function in the heart muscle). Studies show it can be used safely in very ill people with heart problems, and for this reason, it carries my "Good Heartkeeping" seal of approval.

ACE INHIBITORS

Vasotec (enalapril)
Zestril (lisinopril)
Prinivil (lisinopril)
Univasc (moexipril)

Monopril (fosinopril)

Many doctors use ACE inhibitors as their first choice for treating blood pressure in younger and middle-aged people. They are preserving of sexual function and are especially useful in people who have diabetes and whose urinalysis shows they are "spilling protein."

As mentioned in Chapter 5, ACE inhibitors *prolong* life in people with congestive heart failure and are prescribed to prevent worsening of heart pumping function in people who have had a heart attack. Used in the right patient, these drugs can be a life-saver, literally.

The downside of the ACEs is that up to 20 percent of people (especially women 60 years or older) develop a persistent dry cough (sometimes worse at night) that is troublesome enough to require discontinuation of the medication. In addition, for controlling blood pressure, ACE inhibitors tend to be less effective in the elderly and in African Americans. Consequently, other blood pressure pills—especially Norvasc—may be more suitable for these groups. How well ACEs work over the long haul without requiring the addition of other blood pressure pills is still not entirely clear. Finally, ACE inhibitors can produce drug interactions, especially with NSAIDs and with diuretics of the potassium-sparing variety.

BETA-ADRENERGIC BLOCKING AGENTS (BETA-BLOCKERS)

Tenormin (atenolol)
Sectral (acebutolol)
Beta-blockers are effective drugs for treating high blood pressure, but their side-effect pro-

file is *not* quite as friendly as the ACEs or the calcium channel blocker Norvasc. In particular, side effects such as fatigue, sleepiness, decreased sex drive (in men and women), sleep disturbances, and depression have been reported with the beta-blocker class.

Tenormin and Sectral are preferred options in this drug class because they may be less likely to cause these symptoms than other beta-blockers. This may be because they don't penetrate into the central nervous system as well as the other medications in this class. Tenormin has FDA approval for high blood pressure, angina, and prevention of recurrent heart attacks. Sectrol has been shown to lower cholesterol levels—although most beta-blockers appear to raise cholesterol levels. Beta-blockers should be avoided—by *some* people with heart failure or diabetes and by people with excessively slow heart rates, lung conditions such as asthma, reactive airway diseases, or chronic obstructive lung conditions. Beta-blockers should never be discontinued suddenly, because they can cause worsening of chest pain in people with angina.

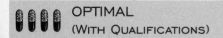

OPTIMAL
(With Qualifications)

DIURETICS ("WATER PILLS")

Lozol (indapamide)
Zaroxolyn (metolazone)
Hydrochlorothiazide (generic)

The use of thiazide diuretics—more commonly referred to as "water pills"—as a first choice for treating high blood pressure is very controversial. I personally recommend *against*

them as a first choice, an opinion shared by many physicians and hypertension experts. On the other hand, many national organizations and high blood pressure experts strongly support diuretics as a first-line blood pressure drug.

They are included in this "Optimal with Qualifications" category only because they have been shown to reduce death rates in people with high blood pressure, are very cheap, and have been shown to be effective for systolic hypertension. In addition, many expert panels (the Joint National Commission on Detection, Evaluation, and Treatment of High Blood Pressure—JNC-V) passionately endorse the diuretics as first-line treatment for high blood pressure.

Diuretics are best used at low doses. It is clear that their safety and benefits are enhanced if used in low doses. When diuretics are prescribed in moderate to high doses, they can potentially increase the risk of death, especially in people who have had a heart attack, who have abnormal EKG patterns suggesting heart disease, and who are at high risk for abnormal heart rhythms. Diuretics also can elevate your blood cholesterol level, especially when used in combination with beta-blockers.

The principal drawbacks of diuretics include a long list of side effects: loss of sex drive, impotence, muscle cramps, potassium loss, fatigue, weakness, elevated cholesterol level, elevated blood sugar, and many others. The diuretics Lozol and Zaroxolyn may be less likely to produce some of these side effects than hydrochlorothiazide and are therefore Optimal in this class.

❚❚❚ RECOMMENDED
(ACCEPTABLE WITH RESERVATIONS)

THIAZIDE DIURETICS

Diuril (hydrochlorothiazide)
Esidrix (hydrochlorothiazide)
HydroDIURIL (hydrochlorothiazide)
Hygroton (chlorthalidone)

See discussion of diuretics in "Optimal with Qualifications" category.

COMBINATION DIURETICS

Aldactazide
Maxzide
Moduretic
Dyazide

These combination pills have the advantage of preventing loss of potassium. They are recommended especially for people who are taking Lanoxin (digoxin) and would like the convenience of avoiding potasssium supplementation, which can be quite unpalatable. These combination pills are also recommended for people who are known to have abnormal heart rhythms that are sensitive to potassium loss. For additional information, see the discussion of diuretics in the "Optimal" category.

ANGIOTENSIN II ANTAGONISTS

Cozaar (losartan potassium)
This is the first "angiotensin II receptor antagonist" to be approved by the FDA for treatment of high blood pressure. It appears to be about as effective as most ACE inhibitors. Like ACE inhibitors, studies suggest it is less effective in African Americans, and accordingly, it may be less effective in the elderly as well.

Cozaar's principal advantage over the ACE inhibitors—at least based on initial short-term studies—is that it does not produce the troublesome cough associated with ACE inhibitors. But it can cause potassium levels to rise. A recent study suggests that Cozaar, like the ACE inhibitors, may *prolong* life in people with CHF. Unfortunately, it does not have the confirmed life-prolongation benefits of ACEs for people who have had a heart attack, and for people with diabetes. I would reserve this pill for people who are unable to tolerate an ACE inhibitor because of the cough.

BETA-BLOCKERS

Cartrol (carteolol)
Zebeta (bisoprolol)
Corgard (nadolol)
See discussion in "Optimal" category for beta-blockers.

CALCIUM CHANNEL BLOCKERS (LONG-ACTING)

Plendil (felodipine)
Plendil is a good but not optimal drug for blood pressure, because it can cause such side effects as leg swelling, dizziness, and headache with greater frequency than the calcium blocker in the "Optimal" category.

Cardizem CD (diltiazem)
Dilacor XR (diltiazem)
Tiazac (diltiazem)
These diltiazem-based, long-acting preparations are approved for high blood pressure.

They do have the potential for inhibiting the pumping action of the heart, and for slowing the heart rate. Sometimes this is a benefit, sometimes not. Their safety profile in patients with complicated heart conditions is not as well established as it is for Norvasc. They should be considered second-line calcium channel blockers.

Procardia XL (nifedipine SR/GITS)

Although it is an excellent drug for high blood pressure, Procardia XL's safety profile in patients with complicated heart conditions is not as well established as it is for Norvasc. It also is more likely to cause leg swelling than many other calcium channel blockers. Procardia XL is very effective and should be considered for people who have very high blood pressure that is resistant to other calcium channel blockers or blood pressure–lowering drugs.

Adalat CC (nifedipine)

This is another long-acting calcium channel blocker with properties similar to those of Procardia XL.

ACE INHIBITORS

Accupril (quinapril)
Altace (ramipril)
Capoten (captropril)
Lotension (benazepril)
Mavik (trandolapril)

Some of these drugs may require twice-daily dosing and therefore are not ranked as highly as those listed as Optimal. Capoten has been shown to be effective in preventing the progression of kidney disease in people who have diabetes and are "spilling protein."

PERIPHERAL ALPHA-BLOCKERS

Cardura (doxazosin)

Approved for high blood pressure and for prostate problems, this pill is recommended especially for people who have high blood pressure as well as an enlarged prostate that is causing urinary symptoms such as decreased flow.

 DISCOURAGED FOR INITIAL USE (BUT MAY BE REQUIRED IN SELECTED PEOPLE)

CALCIUM CHANNEL BLOCKERS (LONG-ACTING OR EXTENDED RELEASE)

Posicor (mibefradil)

This new calcium blocker is used to treat high blood pressure and angina. Although it is an effective drug, it has a higher risk of drug interactions and heart-related side effects than other calcium blockers such as amlodipine. Posicor should not be taken in conjunction with astemizole (Hismanal), cisapride, or any of the statins, including Zocor, Lipitor, Pravachol, Mevacor, Lescol, or Baycol. It should be used cautiously in people who are taking beta-blockers.

DynaCirc (isradipine)

Twice-daily dosing is sometimes required, which can compromise compliance.

Calan SR (verapamil)
Isoptin SR (verapamil)
Verelan (verapamil)

Although approved for the treatment of high blood pressure, these calcium channel blockers can slow the heart rate and inhibit heart pumping more than most any other calcium channel blocker. This may present problems, especially in older patients who have congestive heart failure, and in other people who have complicated heart conditions. The safety profile of long-acting verapamil drugs in patients with complicated heart conditions is not as well established as it is for Norvasc. Constipation is a common, troubling side effect from verapamil-based calcium blockers.

Cardizem SR (diltiazem)

Twice-daily dosing is not as convenient as other formulations of diltiazem.

Cardene SR (nicardipine)

Flushing and headache are common. Twice-daily dosing is inconvenient.

ANGIOTENSIN II RECEPTOR ANTAGONISTS

Hyzaar (losartan potassium and hydrochlorothiazide)

This combination drug provides no particular advantages, except that it is more potent than Cozaar alone. (See the Recommended category for Cozaar).

PERIPHERAL ALPHA-BLOCKERS

Hytrin (terazosin)

This drug sometimes has to be taken on a twice-daily basis, which makes it less convenient than Cardura. It has similar advantages and indications.

BETA-ADRENERGIC BLOCKING AGENTS (BETA-BLOCKERS)

Lopressor (metoprolol)

This drug is indicated for high blood pressure. Unlike Tenormin, Sectral, Corgard, Kerlone, and others, Lopressor is fat soluble and therefore is more likely to penetrate into central nervous system tissue. For this reason, many experts feel it is more likely to cause such side effects as sleepiness, drowsiness, sleep problems, and fatigue. As a result, it is not as strongly recommended as Tenormin (see Optimal), which tends to have a more user-friendly side-effect profile.

Blocadren (timolol)

Twice-daily dosing makes this drug less convenient.

COMBINATION DRUGS

Lotrel (amlodipine/benazepril)
Zestoretic (lisinopril/hydrochlorothiazide)
Vaseretic (enalapril/hydrochlorothiazide)
Lotensin (benazepril/hydrochlorothiazide)
Capozide (captopril/hydrochlorothiazide)
Ziac (bisoprolol/hydrochlorothiazide)

Combination pills are discouraged. They contain two prescription ingredients, thereby potentially increasing the risk of drug interactions and side effects. It is also more difficult to adjust the dose of specific ingredients.

AVOID IF POSSIBLE
(NOT RECOMMENDED)

BETA-BLOCKERS

Inderal (propranolol)
Levatol (penbutolol)
The use of Inderal is discouraged because it may have more side effects than the beta-blockers listed in the Optimal and Recommended categories.

CALCIUM CHANNEL BLOCKERS
(SHORT-ACTING OR GENERIC)

Verapamil (generic)
Calan (verapamil)
Isoptin (verapamil)
Cardizem (diltiazem)
Diltiazem (generic)
Procardia capsules (nifedipine capsules)
Cardene (nicardipine)
Avoid these short-acting or generic calcium blockers. They are potentially harmful and have no role in the current treatment of high blood pressure.

PERIPHERAL ALPHA-BLOCKERS

Minipress (prazosin)

Avoid this drug. Its side effects, such as low blood pressure, are a problem.

CENTRALLY ACTING DRUGS

Aldomet (methyldopa)
Amodopa (methyldopa)
Catapres (clonidine)
Tenex (guanfacine)
Wytensin (guanabenz)
Avoid these drugs. They have too many side effects and no special advantages.

PERIPHERALLY ACTING DRUGS

Reserpine (generic)
Serpalan (reserpine)
Hylorel (guanadrel sulfate)
Avoid these drugs. They have too many side effects and no special advantages.

VASODILATORS

Apresoline (hydralazine)
Hydralazine (generic)
Loniten (minoxidil)
Avoid these drugs. They have too many side effects and no special advantages.

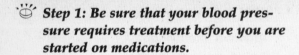

A FIVE-STEP PROGRAM FOR OPTIMAL BLOOD-PRESSURE CONTROL

Step 1: Be sure that your blood pressure requires treatment before you are started on medications.

1. High blood pressure should not be diagnosed on the basis of a single measurement.
2. Blood pressure for most "healthy" people is about 120/80. Blood pressure of 140/90 mm Hg or greater justifies treatment.
3. An initial elevated reading should be confirmed on at least two subsequent doctor visits over a week or several weeks (unless your systolic is greater than 210 mm Hg and/or your diastolic is greater than 120 mm Hg, in which case *immediate* therapy is justified).
4. When a blood pressure reading is obtained, two or more measurements separated by two minutes should be recorded and averaged. If the first two readings differ by more than 5 mm Hg, additional readings should be obtained.
5. Measurements should be taken after five minutes at rest. It is important to ensure that you have not ingested caffeine, a phenylpropanolamine-containing compound, or smoked cigarettes thirty minutes prior to measuring your blood pressure.
6. Blood pressure characterized by systolic readings in the 130–139 mm Hg range and diastolic in the 85–89 mm Hg range should be rechecked in one year. Systolic readings in the 140–159 mm Hg range or diastolic readings in the 90–99 mm Hg range should be confirmed within two months. Systolic readings in the 160–179 mm Hg range or diastolic readings in the 100–109 mm Hg range require evaluation and referral to a definitive source of care within one month.
7. The presence of kidney, heart, or neurological problems is an indication for evaluation, prompt referral, and treatment.

Step 2: Try a three-to-six-month trial of nonpharmacological (that is, no-drug) therapy if you are diagnosed as having mildly to moderately high blood pressure. The following lifestyle modifications are known to reduce blood pressure:

1. Go on a weight-reduction program if you are overweight.
2. Limit your alcohol intake to less than 1 oz. per day of ethanol (24 oz. beer, 8 oz. wine, or 2 oz. 100-proof whiskey).
3. Do regular aerobic exercise.
4. Reduce your sodium intake to less than 2.3 grams of sodium, or approximately 6 grams of sodium chloride.
5. Stop smoking.
6. Reduce your dietary intake of saturated fats and cholesterol.

☺ **Step 3: If the measures listed in Step 2 produce inadequate blood pressure control, then lifestyle modifications should continue but medications should be started.**

1. The initial pill of choice for high blood pressure is controversial, but in general, unless cost is an absolute deterrent, a calcium channel blocker, an ACE inhibitor, or a beta-blocker is recommended. The drugs should be started at the lowest recommended daily dose. See the MedRANK Checklist in this chapter for specific recommendations.
2. When cost is the *sole* barrier, therapy with a thiazide diuretic or beta-blocker is indicated.
3. If an inadequate response is observed, it is preferable to stay on the same agent but increase the dose—if no side effects are observed at that dose.
4. If side effects are observed at any dose, substitute another medication, or reduce the dose of the drug and start an additional agent at a low dose.

☺ **Step 4: Your doctor may want to send you home with an automated blood-pressure-monitoring device. This non-invasive device may be useful in the following situations:**

1. Office or "white-coat" hypertension (that is, your blood pressure is repeatedly elevated in the office or clinic but is repeatedly normal in other environments).
2. Unexplained drug resistance (that is, your pills aren't working).
3. Unexplained blood pressure changes at night (episodic hypertension).

☺ **Step 5: If you have been well controlled on a single medication for more than a year, it is not unreasonable to discontinue the medication gradually under a doctor's supervision. If you have lost weight, stopped smoking, and increased your exercise, elimination of your blood pressure pill—or at least a dose reduction—may be possible.**

1. The step-down approach includes the gradual elimination of a drug, or a dose reduction, if the blood pressure is controlled for more than a year.

CHAPTER 7

—

UP THE DOWN STAIRCASE

Medications for Depression, Insomnia, Anxiety, Schizophrenia, and Other Psychiatric Problems

"Why should I take my Elavil?" a depressed patient protested to me fifteen years ago. "This drug makes me feel worse than my disease. Am I crazy or what?" Not at all. This patient, like so many others, was right on the money. For many years, the drug landscape for psychological disorders was as depressing as the mental illness itself.

For the most part, all we had was a sad list of rather barbaric options—Elavil, Valium, and Thorazine—for the treatment of depression, anxiety, and schizophrenia, respectively. Elavil produced intolerable side effects such as sleepiness and dry mouth, Valium put people to sleep for the week rather than for the night, and Thorazine turned people into walking zombies. Tricyclic antidepressants (TCAs), such as Tofranil, Sinequan, and Pamelor, were anything but user-friendly. Although they worked, users paid a steep price in side effects and risking dangerous drug interactions. In fact, TCAs were so toxic to the heart that emergency departments dur-

ing the 1980s were overrun with suicide victims who had intentionally ingested these dangerous medications.

For many, these drugs were an ordeal worse than the disease itself. People frequently became dependent on them or found them intolerable. Especially at the higher doses, Thorazine, Valium, and Elavil produced side effects that were so disruptive to quality of life that many people let their mood disorders go untreated and sought "refuge" in the symptoms of their disease. Put simply, the potential benefits of these pills didn't justify the known risks and downsides, especially for those with mood disorders of only mild to moderate severity.

In the past twenty years, all of this has changed. It's fair to say that *One Flew Over the Cuckoo's Nest* is behind us—especially when it comes to the treatment of depression. As more targeted and patient-friendly drugs have been developed for psychiatric problems, hundreds of thousands of people have come out of Dr.

Caligari's closet. They now actively seek out pharmacological solutions for mood alterations that, only a decade ago, would have swirled around the trash bin of therapeutic nihilism. The new psychiatric medications have relatively low "noise levels"—that is, they have minimal side effects, are convenient to take, and produce fewer symptoms than the disease itself. The end result: People actually *want* to stay on these medications for long periods.

With respect to patient-friendly medications, the greatest advances have been made in the treatment of depression (Prozac, Zoloft, Paxil), insomnia (Ambien, melatonin), schizophrenia (Risperdal, Zyprexa), and obsessive-compulsive disorder (Paxil, Zoloft). Few will argue that these pills have improved overall quality of life in people suffering from psychiatric disease. Prozac, Zoloft, and Ambien have even become household words among the young, the old, and the restless.

☺ *Antidepressants. The reasons for the evolution of Prozac nation are quite clear. Moodwise, the threshold for using these drugs has been lowered to limbo levels by the new class of antidepressants known as selective serotonin-reuptake inhibitors (SSRIs).*

To explain in broad neurochemical brush strokes: Decreased levels of the neurotransmitter serotonin appear to be linked to symptoms of depression. The SSRIs *increase* the amount of serotonin in brain synapses, elevate mood, improve outlook on life, and energize people, while producing minimal, well-tolerated side effects. They are better targeted at specific brain receptors controlling

mood than were older medications. Other new antidepressants, including Serzone and Effexor, are also effective, but on the whole they do not appear to be as convenient, smooth, or safe as the "big three." Similar advances have been made for drugs used to treat anxiety and insomnia.

Antidepressants are now so user-friendly that for most mood-related conditions, the benefit-to-risk ratio clearly favors drug therapy. The mood-stabilizing and depression-easing effects of the drugs Zoloft, Prozac, and Paxil are really quite remarkable, especially considering their tolerability. These and other SSRIs have now been approved or are widely used off label for: depression associated with seasonal affective disorder (SAD), prevention of panic attacks, depression associated with the premenstrual period (premenstrual dysphoria), postpartum depression, obsessive-compulsive disorders, and many other conditions.

☺ *The signs of depression are unmistakable, and the toll the condition takes on personal and business life is potentially devastating.*

Sadness, crying spells, excessive sleeping or eating, declining libido, and withdrawal—these are the telltale signs and symptoms of depression. If you or a family member has these symptoms, you should act sooner rather than later, because drug therapy can now get you out of the woods. Generally speaking, drug therapy is required for most individuals whose depressive symptoms are severe enough to compromise work, sleep patterns, or social activities.

☺ *One of the most important questions surrounding SSRIs is: Are these drugs overused?*

Maybe, but maybe not. Better living through chemistry does not, and should not, play favorites. Hundreds of thousands of people whose chemical makeup predisposes them to high cholesterol levels take drugs to reduce their risk of heart disease. What is so different about those with a chemical predisposition to depression taking SSRIs to reduce their risk of psyche-scorching melancholy? Probably, there is very little difference.

Still, it is valid to ask whether these pills have become such a permanent part of our personal and collective pharmacology that we've lost sight of which mood swings are serious enough to be treated with drugs, and which ones are a normal part of life and should simply be left alone. Have the SSRIs become quick fixes? Many experts would say, "Yes, these drugs are ubiquitous, and we have lost perspective." They would argue we have taken the path of least resistance by pressing pills into service for every minor psycho-perturbation that ails us.

Yet these market-driven icons of personal pharmacology can lift the veil of moroseness and improve outlook on life. As a result, they have extended their sphere of influence beyond depression per se and into a more nebulous group of individuals who are not clinically depressed but who suffer from the angst-making miseries of modern life. The majority of people currently using SSRIs would never satisfy the strict diagnostic criteria for major clinical depression. But they are benefiting from these drugs nevertheless. For example, SSRIs reduce symptoms of mental and physical distress associated with the premenstrual period, or "premenstrual dysphoric syndrome," which is characterized by severe agitation, depression, and low self-esteem during the five-to-seven-day period preceding menstruation. Although not specifically approved by the FDA for this problem, SSRIs are widely used to alleviate these symptoms.

☺ *There are no easy answers to the question of when to use these medications. After all, depression doesn't begin at one serotonin level and suddenly disappear at another.*

It's all about the gray areas—about whether we perceive life as dark gray or light gray, and whether that perception causes us enough psychological pain to seek help. To a great extent, our suitability for antidepressant therapy depends on whether the friction-causing events in our external world (divorce, disappointment, disability, and death) and the neurotransmitters that make up our internal chemistry combine to produce symptoms that are disabling enough to get in the way of "normal" functions. Most of us exist somewhere on the spectrum between light and dark, between life-blinding joy and joy-blinding sadness, between the suicidal tendencies of Nicolas Cage in *Leaving Las Vegas* and the "What, me worry?" smiling face of *Mad* man Alfred E. Neuman. For us, the need for antidepressant therapy is frequently based on very subjective criteria.

☺ *From a practical perspective, pharmacology must follow our need to function, day in and day out.*

If you are having trouble functioning, the
first step is to find out whether you are depressed. Symptoms of depression include
sadness, low self-esteem, lethargy, feelings of
worthlessness, difficulty sleeping, sudden
weight changes, crying spells, difficulty concentrating, asocial behavior, extreme agitation, and withdrawal. Ask yourself: Are you
sleeping well enough? Are you sad too much
of the time? Do you have recurrent feelings
of worthlessness, guilt, or low self-esteem?
Have your eating patterns changed to the
point of gaining or losing an excessive
amount of weight? Have you stopped having
fun or wanting to have fun? Has your sex
drive changed dramatically or disappeared?

☺ *Although the need for antidepressants
is frequently very clear, in many situations it is not.*

Ultimately, starting an SSRI antidepressant
should be a collaborative decision made by
your physician, with your input. If your depressive symptoms have made day-to-day
functioning a problem, an antidepressant
should be strongly considered. If you do start
one, be sure you are started on the lowest possible dose. Then see how you feel. But be patient—it's not unreasonable to wait four to six
weeks before deciding whether your dose
should be increased. Once you start an antidepressant, you should be willing to make a
nine-to-twelve-month commitment before considering discontinuation. It may take that long

for you to experience the full benefit of an SSRI
at a particular dose. Discontinuation should be
considered if your depression is primarily *situational,* and if you have experienced only *one*
episode of the "blues" in your lifetime.

☺ *If your depression recurs after discontinuation, more likely than not you
need to be on an SSRI permanently.*

As much relief as these pills can offer, SSRIs
are not perfect. They have side effects to be
considered, including anxiety, insomnia, agitation, gastrointestinal problems, sexual dysfunction, and potential drug interactions.
Some side effects, such as diarrhea and gastrointestinal disturbances, may be transient
in nature and go away after a few weeks.
Always consult with your physician to evaluate any side effects you suspect may be serious. Finally, because of the many drug
interactions with this antidepressant class,
you should always consult with your physician if you are taking, or planning to take, an
over-the-counter medication, an antihistamine, or any other drug used to treat psychiatric disorders, especially a monoamine
oxidase inhibitor (MAOI).

☺ *Amphetamines are medications that
stimulate the central nervous system.*

They are used to treat deficit disorders (like
hyperkinetic disorders in children) within the
context of total treatment programs that also
include psychological, educational, and social
guidance. Ideally, these medications should
be employed for the short term only, as part of
an overall treatment program. When used to

treat obesity, these drugs have produced erratic results, and they should always be accompanied by appropriate changes in diet and exercise. The use of amphetamines to improve athletic skills or mental alertness, or to stay awake, is dangerous and illegal.

These drugs should never be shared with other individuals, and their potential for causing drug dependence should be emphasized. Even over-the-counter diet aids, such as phenylpropanolamine (PPA-containing compounds) are not without their risks. When taken in excessive doses, PPA-containing compounds can cause elevated blood pressure, rapid heartbeat, and insomnia. PPA is contained in a number of over-the-counter diet aids and should be taken only as recommended on the package insert. When phenylpropanolamine is consumed with excessive amounts of caffeine—two or more cups of caffeinated coffee—excessive elevations in blood pressure have been reported.

☺ Schizophrenia. Drug therapy for this chronic, disabling condition has made major strides.

The old warhorse drugs such as Haldol, Thorazine, Mellaril, and Navane produced results but were associated with devastating side effects: Movement disorders, drowsiness, and other problems created a troubling undertow. Recently, medications that bind to specific brain receptors thought to be involved in schizophrenia have been developed. Risperdal and Zyprexia are the most promising and should be tried as an initial approach. Although not all people will respond to these medications, those that do will be spared many of the side effects of the older medications. Clozaril, which also shows more targeted activity against brain receptors, is more difficult to use because it can lower the white blood cell count to potentially dangerous levels. Blood counts must be monitored in all people who are prescribed this medication.

☺ Obsessive-Compulsive Disorder is a condition that is being recognized with increasing frequency.

Obsessive-compulsive disorder (OCD) is characterized by inappropriate, excessive ritualization of routine activities, recurrent disturbing thoughts (obsessions), and/or a chronic fixation with meaningless activities (compulsions), such as hand-washing, excessive neatness, or arranging objects in a line, that interfere with normal daily function. Drug therapy can reduce or eliminate such obsessions and compulsions and thereby improve quality of life and productivity in useful, life-enhancing activities.

SSRIs are now considered the safest drugs for long-term maintenance of people with this condition. Anafranil and Luvox also have been used for OCD, but they are less convenient or produce more side effects than Zoloft and Paxil.

☺ Anxiety, Insomnia, and Panic Attacks. Antianxiety medications, such as benzodiazepines, are now available in preparations that have shorter half-lives than they used to.

Benzodiazepines with shorter half-lives are eliminated from the body within a matter of hours and therefore are less likely to produce lingering symptoms such as sedation, confusion, and memory loss, reducing the risk of prolonged drowsiness, falling in the elderly, and hip fractures. But it must be stressed that these drugs are associated with a high risk of side effects, drug interactions, and withdrawal symptoms. Consequently, they must be taken precisely as prescribed.

Widely prescribed for many uses, both indicated and off-label, drugs belonging to the benzodiazepine class are used to treat sleep disorders and panic attacks and to provide short-term relief of symptoms associated with anxiety. The many drugs in this class include alprazolam (Xanax), triazolam (Halcion), chlordiazepoxide (Librium), diazepam (Valium), oxazepam (Serax), and lorazepam (Ativan).

☺ *One of the most widely prescribed benzodiazepines, Xanax, is used to treat panic disorders. Yet it is a double-edged sword: Like other medications in this class, it has the potential for causing drug dependence.*

The combination of euphoria, relaxation, and anxiety reduction it produces has seduced many long-term users, most of whom have found it difficult to discontinue the drug. It should always be used under a doctor's close supervision. If your doctor has prescribed Xanax on your behalf for a period extending beyond one week, find out why.

Although Xanax may be used for short-term relief of anxiety symptoms, safer drugs (SSRIs) with little risk of physical dependence should be used to prevent recurrent panic attacks. Halcion is not recommended because it can cause short-term memory loss and rebound insomnia.

Benzodiazepines such as temazepam (Restoril) and triazolam (Halcion) are used as sedative-hypnotics. They are indicated for treatment of insomnia and, preferably, should be used only for short periods of time—no more than one to two weeks. Ambien, one of the newer medications for insomnia, is preferred over Halcion, Ativan, and Serax because it *may* have a lower risk of physical dependence and appears to preserve normal sleep architecture. Consequently, sleep may be more restorative with this medication. Long-term use of Ambien is generally not recommended and requires regular medical reevaluation. Whenever possible, attempts should be made to find alternative, nondrug therapies for patients who have chronic sleeplessness.

☺ *The so-called "long-acting" benzodiazepines, such as Valium, Librium, and Dalmane, should be avoided in the elderly population—and probably in other people as well.*

The risk associated with using long-acting benzodiazepines in the elderly appears to be substantial. *Long-acting* means that these drugs remain in the system for long periods of time and have the potential to cause prolonged periods of fatigue, mental confusion, and sedation, which can be harmful in this vulnerable population. Most geriatric experts recommend that long-acting benzodiazepines be avoided entirely in the elderly population. Drugs with shorter half-lives, such as Ativan and Restoril, can be used with much lower risk.

Nevertheless, it should be recognized that benzodiazepines, as psychotropic drugs, are widely used in the geriatric population for the treatment of anxiety disorders and insomnia. Although reasonably effective and safe over the short term, you should be aware that these drugs can cause drowsiness, changes in mental function, and impaired coordination because of their depressive effects on the central nervous system.

☺ If you have been on a benzodiazepine for a long period of time, you cannot suddenly discontinue it.

Because benzodiazepines can produce physical dependency, abrupt cessation will produce withdrawal symptoms such as irritability, anxiety, increased heart rate, agitation, and other uncomfortable physical sensations. If you feel the medication is no longer needed, consult with your physician, and initiate a plan of gradual withdrawal that, generally speaking, should occur over a period of several weeks. Gradual tapering increases the likelihood that the drug can be discontinued without experiencing troublesome side effects.

It should be stressed that the decision to discontinue use of a benzodiazepine may be difficult. After all, you may know somebody who has been taking one of these drugs for many years and who seems to depend on it for behavioral or emotional stability. On the other hand, these drugs are sometimes started for management of short-term, situational problems and then become permanent parts of a drug regimen unnecessarily. Not infrequently, you may even be unaware that physical or psychological addiction has occurred. These cases can be difficult because you may believe the drug is still required for symptomatic relief. You should carefully evaluate with your physician or pharmacist the original reasons for prescribing the drug in the first place. If symptoms related to anxiety or abnormal sleep patterns are well controlled, it is certainly appropriate to consider very gradual elimination or dose reduction.

So-called psychoactive medications, which are used to treat neuropsychiatric conditions such as depression, pain, insomnia, anxiety, and other mental disorders, are a vital part of medical therapy for both middle-aged and older Americans. Like cardiovascular medications, these drugs not only have the potential to improve quality of life and stabilize symptoms associated with chronic and episodic illness, they also have the capacity to produce serious and sometimes even life-threatening side effects. Accordingly, the drugs in this chapter should always be taken *exactly* as prescribed and always with physician supervision.

MEDICATIONS FOR DEPRESSION
Things Are Looking Up

MedRANK Life Enhancement Checklist

Pills of Wisdom: Medications are the cornerstone of treatment for major depression. Even when depression is related to a situational or life crisis, antidepressant medications may be required for up to a year, after which gradual discontinuation, in combination with counseling, may be considered. However, if a major depressive episode recurs within two years, long-term therapy may be necessary and appropriate. Depression asssociated with seasonal affective disorder (SAD) may respond to light therapy and to the antidepressant Zoloft.

Antidepressants are now widely used in all ages and demographic groups. Over the past decade, there has been a gradual shift away from drugs in the tricyclic class (like Elavil) and toward selective serotonin reuptake inhibitors (like Prozac, Zoloft, and Paxil). Although not universally approved for the following conditions, SSRIs are also used to treat premenstrual dysphoria (depression associated with premenstrual syndrome), OCD (obsessive-compulsive disorder), seasonal affective disorder (SAD), postpartum depression, and panic disorders.

Whether you really need an antidepressant is ultimately up to your physician, who should always be encouraged to start with the lowest dose possible. Side effects associated with the SSRIs include agitation, tremors, headache, nervousness, insomnia, agitation, increased anxiety, and sexual dysfunction. Some side effects, such as diarrhea and gastrointestinal disturbances, may be transient and will go away after you have been on the medication for a few weeks. Consult your physician if you suspect your side effects may be serious. Finally, there are many drug interactions with this class, and therefore you should always consult with your physician if you are taking or planning to take an over-the-counter medication, an antihistamine, or another drug used to treat psychiatric disorders, especially a monoamine oxidase inhibitor (MAOI).

Among antidepressants, there are better choices and less desirable choices. The SSRIs Zoloft, Prozac, and Paxil are considered by most experts to be the initial drugs of choice for the treatment of mild to moderate depression. Some individuals may respond better to one agent versus another, and this may require some trial and error. Unfortunately, people whose severe depression is not responsive to an optimal or recommended drug may need to shift to a medication in the "Discouraged" or "Avoid" category. In such cases, consultation with a psychiatrist is absolutely necessary, since these drugs tend to be more toxic and are associated with many side effects.

 OPTIMAL
(HIGHLY RECOMMENDED/ BEST OF CLASS)

SELECTIVE SEROTONIN-REUPTAKE INHIBITORS (SSRIs)

Zoloft (sertraline)

Zoloft is recommended as an initial choice, because it appears to have a lower risk of producing drug-drug interactions and tends to be slightly less stimulating than Prozac and slightly less sedating than Paxil. Because drug interactions seem to be less of a problem with Zoloft, it is preferred for people who take multiple medications.

Prozac (fluoxetine)

This effective SSRI may be especially appropriate for people who are overweight, since the drug has mild appetite-suppressant properties. Because it may be a bit more stimulating than Zoloft or Paxil, it may be slightly less advantageous in people who have insomnia as a prominent, disabling symptom of their depression. On the other hand, it may be preferable for people who require stimulation to treat their symptoms. Because drug interactions may be more of a problem with Prozac than with Zoloft, people on multiple medications may be able to reduce the risk of drug interactions by switching to Zoloft. Prozac is more likely to cause side effects such as agitation and muscle tremors.

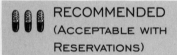

RECOMMENDED
(ACCEPTABLE WITH RESERVATIONS)

SELECTIVE SEROTONIN-REUPTAKE INHIBITOR (SSRI)

Paxil (paroxetene)

As effective as Prozac, and Zoloft, Paxil may be slightly more sedating.

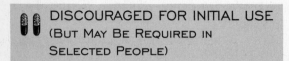

DISCOURAGED FOR INITIAL USE
(BUT MAY BE REQUIRED IN SELECTED PEOPLE)

Remeron (mirtazapine)

Currently, it is difficult to recommend Remeron as a *first-line* antidepressant, although it may eventually be shown to be one. Unfortunately, there are no published studies comparing the effectiveness of this drug with the SSRIs.

This one-daily drug increases the release of serotonin and norepinephrine in brain synapses. It appears to work as well as tricyclic antidepressants such as Elavil. Temporary sleepiness occurs in about half of people who take the drug. Other side effects include increased appetitite, weight gain, constipation, dry mouth, and dizziness. Excessive drowsiness may occur if Remeron is taken with alcohol or benzodiazepines. Drug interactions may occur.

Serzone (nefazodone)

Consider Serzone only as an alternative to the Optimal and Recommended SSRIs. The twice-daily dosing is not optimal, and interactions can occur with Halcion, Xanax, Seldane, and Hismanal. Side effects include headache, drowsiness, dry mouth, nausea, dizziness, sexual dysfunction, and other symptoms. Overall, better-established drugs are preferred as the initial choice.

TRICYCLIC ANTIDEPRESSANTS

Elavil (amitriptyline)
Sinequan (doxepin)
Surmontil (trimipramine)
Pamelor (nortriptyline)
Tofranil (imipramine)
Ventyl (nortriptyline)
Tipramine (imipramine)
Endep (amitriptyline)

These drugs have significant side effects, especially in the elderly. They have what are called *anticholinergic effects,* which means they can cause dry mouth, blurred vision, and trouble with urination, especially in older individuals. Cardiac disturbances can occur, and overdose can be fatal. But if SSRIs are not successful in treating depression, these medications may need to be used.

OTHERS

Desyrel (trazodone)

Desyrel is not recommended as a stand-alone antidepressant. Its use should be reserved for people who require sedation at night because of the stimulatory effects of SSRIs.

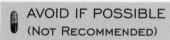

AVOID IF POSSIBLE
(NOT RECOMMENDED)

Effexor (venlafaxine)

Effexor is discouraged as an initial choice for several reasons. The twice-daily dosing is not optimal; persistent increases in blood pressure may be seen with higher dosages; and drug interactions may occur. Its side effects include headache, nausea, insomnia, nervousness, and sexual dysfunction. Use it only if the "better" drugs are unsuccessful.

Wellbutrin (bupropion)

Its three-times-daily dosing is not desirable from a compliance and convenience standpoint. Wellbutrin may cause agitation and has a low risk of sexual dysfunction. Its risk of seizures is greater than with most other antidepressants. It is not the cream of the crop, but may have a role in selected individuals.

INTERMEDIATE-ACTING BENZODIAZEPINES

Xanax (alprazolam)

This drug *is* approved by the FDA for the treatment of *anxiety* associated with depression. Widespread experience with this euphoria-producing benzodiazepine suggests its potential for producing dependency, abuse, and severe withdrawal symptoms. Its use is strongly discouraged.

MAOIs (MONOAMINE OXIDASE INHIBITORS)

Nardil (phenelzine)
Parnate (tranylcypromine)

Warning: These medications can interact with many other drugs, including over-the-counter cold remedies containing the cough suppressant dextromethorphan, SSRIs, tricyclic antidepressants, Demerol, Larodopa, and others. These reactions may be serious and lead to death. Food interactions can also produce severe reactions. People on MAOIs should avoid tyramine-containing products.

OTHERS

Ludiomil (maprotiline)

This drug has an increased risk of seizures.

Vivactil (protriptyline)

Rapid heart rate and low blood pressure may occur more frequently with this antidepressant than with others.

Asendin (amoxapine)

This drug has potentially serious side effects, including movement disorders and a rare but potentially fatal condition called neuroleptic malignant syndrome.

Ritalin (methylphenidate)

Ritalin is not indicated for depression, although sometimes it is used inappropriately for this condition. The abuse potential is high, and many side effects have been reported.

PSYCHOSTIMULANTS

Amphetamines

These are dangerous. Avoid them.

PILLS FOR INSOMNIA
Sleepin' the Night Away*

 MedRANK Life Enhancement Checklist

Pills of Wisdom: Sleep disorders are difficult to diagnose, and their treatment is nothing less than controversial. Yet the importance of pharmacological treatment cannot be overstated, because persistent insomnia is a risk factor for mood disorders such as depression. In fact, successful treatment of chronic insomnia may help prevent major depression. Chronic insomnia has also been associated with an increased risk of automobile accidents, increased alcohol consumption, and daytime sleepiness. In short, this problem is worthy of serious attention.

Whenever possible, nondrug treatment is the preferred *initial* approach for managing insomnia. Lifestyle changes can help, including avoiding coffee, alcohol, and nicotine and eliminating certain prescription medications. The disordered circadian rhythms associated with jet lag are a common cause of sleep irregularities. In addition, insomnia can be a symptom of depression, in which case an entirely different group of medications—an antidepressant such as Desyrel (trazodone), for example—may be required for treatment.

Other behavior-modification techniques have also been shown to work. You should go to bed only when you are sleepy, and you should use your bedroom only for sleep and sex and not for reading, watching television, working, or other activities. You should try to get out of bed at the same time each morning, no matter how much sleep you have had the night before. You can also try to restrict the amount of time you spend in bed to the actual amount of time you spend sleeping, even if you aren't sleeping enough. Over time, in this "sleep-restriction" therapy, you can gradually increase the amount of time allowed in bed, as you spend more time sleeping.

If medications are required, the best options currently available include Ambien, melatonin, Restoril, and certain antidepressants such as Desyrel. But getting to sleep with the help of a sleeping pill does not necessarily mean you are getting a good night's sleep. Drugs used to treat sleep problems, especially the benzodiazepines, can alter sleep architecture in unfavorable ways. In particular, they can reduce the length of time you spend in stage III and stage IV sleep—the "deeper" portions of the sleep cycle—and as a result, they can decrease the restorative value of sleep in those stages.

The sedative effects of other "sleeping" medications—like Valium, Librium, and Dalmane—can last for such a long time that you will still be drowsy the next day. In the elderly, the drowsiness may be serious enough to increase by almost threefold the risk of falling and breaking a hip. On the other hand, ultrashort-acting sleepers such as Halcion are associated with short-term memory loss, daytime anxiety, and rebound insomnia. Unfortunately, many of these medications can produce physical dependence or, when discontinued, withdrawal symptoms.

Many over-the-counter drugs may put you to

* The preferred approach to many sleep problems is nonpharmacological—in other words, methods other than medication use. These include exercising, minimizing daytime naps, regularizing sleep patterns, and avoiding substances that interfere with sleep such as caffeine, alcohol, and other medications. This approach may be more helpful than drugs, which can be associated with dependence and side effects.

sleep but, in the process, also produce such undesirable side effects as prolonged drowsiness, dry mouth, and difficulties with urination. These problems are accentuated in the elderly, and therefore OTC sleep aids are not recommended for this group.

What about melatonin? The news about this relatively safe medication, available without a prescription, appears to be mostly good. But definitive, large-scale studies are still lacking. What we know for now is that the synthesis of melatonin, a hormone produced in the pineal gland in the brain, is stimulated by darkness and inhibited by light. In adults, ingesting 5 mg of melatonin increases the speed of falling asleep, the duration of sleep, and the length of time devoted to rapid-eye-movement (REM) sleep. Studies in elderly people with sleep problems suggest that giving sustained-release tablets (1 or 2 mg per day) can improve the quality and duration of sleep.

Melatonin also appears to have beneficial effects in helping people recover from jet lag, although the exact dose and timing are still to be determined. In the best study evaluating the role of melatonin for jet lag (for individuals traveling eastward across eight time zones), the best results were seen in people who took 5 mg of melatonin at 6:00 P.M. before their departure and at bedtime after their arrival at the final destination. Similar studies, with flight-crew members on round-trip overseas flights, suggest that the best sleep results (fewer symptoms of jet lag and sleep disturbances) are seen when people take 5 mg of melatonin at bedtime upon returning to their point of origin, and then take the same dose at night for the next five days. Interestingly, crew members who started the melatonin three days before returning to their point of origin fared worse in sleeplessness.

Although there are no ideal drugs for sleep disorders, this MedRANK Checklist identifies the safest, most effective pills that will induce sleep, while preserving normal sleep architecture and reducing the risk of drug dependence.

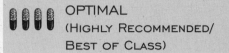

OPTIMAL
(Highly Recommended/ Best of Class)

Nondrug Approaches
See "Pills of Wisdom."

Drug Approaches

Ambien (zolpidem)
This rapidly acting medication is widely prescribed for insomnia. Although claims on its behalf suggest that it has little chance of producing tolerance or physical dependence, the issue is *not* entirely settled. Because it acts on a part of the brain called the GABA-receptor complex, it theoretically carries the same risk as the benzodiazepines. Consequently, use of this drug for longer than four weeks is not advisable.

Ambien appears to preserve normal sleep architecture. Stages III and IV (deep sleep) and REM sleep are maintained, producing more restorative sleep. This medication has been associated with next-day drowsiness, dizziness, and a "drugged" feeling in some people, although mental functions and memory appear to be preserved the day after use.

Melatonin
There is much to say on behalf of this hormone, even though rigorous, scientific studies are not yet available. Its widespread use has produced anectodal reports of its success as a sleeping drug, especially in individuals who need to reset their "biological clock" as a result of time-zone shifting. The possible adverse effects of taking melatonin for long periods simply are not known.

In adults, taking 5 mg appears to increase the speed of falling asleep, the total amount of sleep, and the length of rapid-eye-movement (REM) sleep. Studies in elderly people with sleep problems suggest that sustained-release tablets (1 or 2 mg per day) can improve the quality and duration of sleep.

ANTIDEPRESSANTS

Desyrel (trazodone)

Desyrel, a "sedating" antidepressant, is not approved for sleep disorders, but it is frequently used in patients who have insominia associated with depression, or whose sleep disturbances are caused by the use of an SSRI antidepressant such as Prozac, Paxil, or Zoloft. Some people report a next-day hangover or sedation. The medication can cause priapism (prolonged erection) in men.

This drug is best suited for people with depression and associated sleep problems rather than as a stand-alone sleeping medication. But some sleep experts use Desyrel as their drug of choice for chronic insomnia. Given its low risk of dependence, it should be strongly considered as a drug of choice.

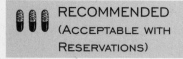

RECOMMENDED
(ACCEPTABLE WITH RESERVATIONS)

BENZODIAZEPINES

Restoril (temazepam)
ProSom (estazolam)
Ativan (lorazepam)

Among the benzodiazepines, these medications have an intermediate duration of action,

which means their "hangover" effects the next day are minimal. Like all benzodiazepines, however, one can develop tolerance and physical dependence on them. They should not be taken with alcohol. Ativan is not FDA approved as a hypnotic (sleeper).

ANTIDEPRESSANTS

Paxil (paroxetine)
Zoloft (sertraline)

The role of SSRIs such as Paxil—as well as Prozac and Zoloft—for sleep disturbances has not been clarified. But when sleep is a prominent symptom of depression, they may play a very useful role.

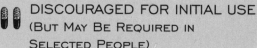

DISCOURAGED FOR INITIAL USE
(BUT MAY BE REQUIRED IN SELECTED PEOPLE)

OTHER HYPNOTICS

Noctec (chloral hydrate)

Chloral hydrate is effective only for short-term use. Physical dependence can occur, and withdrawal of this drug can produce disrupted sleep and nightmares.

NONPRESCRIPTION SLEEP AIDS

Nytol (diphenhydramine)
Unisom (doxylamine)

These nonprescription drugs can cause daytime sleepiness and impairment of the performance skills required to drive and operate machinery. They also have anticholinergic effects, which means they can cause dry mouth, blurred vision, and trouble with urination, especially in older individuals.

Benzodiazepine

Serax (oxazepam)

Better, more quickly acting drugs in this class are available.

 AVOID IF POSSIBLE
(Not Recommended)

Short-Acting Benzodiazepines

Halcion (triazolam)

This drug has received wide attention in the popular press. Its original dosage recommendations were associated with unacceptable side effects. The new lower-dosage recommendations, although improving the safety and adverse side-effect profile of this drug, can still produce memory loss, daytime anxiety, and rebound insomnia.

Long-Acting Benzodiazepines

Valium (diazepam)
Librium (chlordiazepoxide)
Doral (quazepam)
Klonopin (clonazepam)
Dalmane (flurazepam)

These long-acting benzodiazepines should be avoided if possible, especially in the elderly, because they can cause morning-after drowsiness, sedation, and impaired physical performance. Some of these drugs are associated with an increased risk of falling and hip fractures in older individuals. They can produce physical dependence. Better, shorter-acting benzodiazepines are available (see "Recommended" category).

Antidepressants

Elavil (amitriptyline)
Sinequan (doxepin)
Surmontil (trimipramine)

These drugs have significant side effects, especially in the elderly, as well as anticholinergic effects: dry mouth, blurred vision, and trouble with urination.

Others

Barbiturates

These drugs produce tolerance and dependence, and there is a risk of overdosage. Avoid them.

Doriden (glutethimide)
Placidyl (ethchlorvynol)
Xanax (alprazolam)

These drugs produce physical dependence, have abuse potential, and are difficult to discontinue. Better, less toxic drugs are available.

Alcohol

Avoid alcohol as a method to induce sleep. It disrupts the normal sleep architecture.

DRUGS THAT CAN CAUSE INSOMNIA

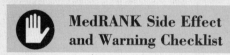 **MedRANK Side Effect and Warning Checklist**

☼ **Pills of Warning:** Some people have insomnia for a very simple reason: They are taking a prescription or over-the-counter medication that is known to cause sleep problems. The following medications have been associated with insomnia.

BLOOD PRESSURE PILLS

Catapres (clonidine)
Inderal (propranolol)
Tenormin (atenolol)
Aldomet (alpha-methyldopa)
Reserpine

ASTHMA MEDICATIONS

Atrovent (ipratropium bromide)
Ventolin (albuterol)
Serevent (salmeterol)
Theo-Dur (theophylline)

DECONGESTANTS

Phenylpropanolamine
Pseudoephedrine

HORMONES

Oral contraceptives
Thyroid preparations
Steroids (prednisone)
Progesterone

CHEMOTHERAPY DRUGS

Medroxyprogesterone
Leuprolide acetate
Goserelin acetate
Pentostatin
Daunorubicin
Inteferon alfa

MISCELLANEOUS

Dilantin (phenytoin)
Nicotine
Sinemet (levodopa)
Quinaglute (quinidine)
Caffeine (OTC products)
    Anacin
    Excedrin
    Empirin
    Cold/cough preparations

CALMING DOWN
Drugs for Anxiety and Panic Attacks*

 MedRANK Life Enhancement Checklist

Pills of Wisdom: The majority of medications used to treat disabling anxiety and/or panic disorders can lead to physical dependence. This is especially true of the benzodiazepine Xanax, which also produces a feeling of euphoria and should be avoided unless absolutely necessary. In some cases, chronic anxiety is a symptom of depression, which is better treated with antidepressants rather than anti-anxiety drugs. Encourage your physician to use the lowest dose of the medication that will work. When you are ready to have the medication discontinued, gradual tapering will produce the best results.

OPTIMAL
(HIGHLY RECOMMENDED/ BEST OF CLASS)

TREAT THE UNDERLYING PSYCHIATRIC DISEASE OR REMOVE THE SITUATIONAL STRESS FACTORS When anxiety is caused or associated with another psychiatric condition, such as depression, panic attacks, or psychosis, it is preferable to treat the underlying condition with the appropriate medication. When anxiety is related to a situational or life crisis, nonpharmacological approaches with counseling may be successful. When anxiety is severe enough to require drug therapy, consider the options listed here. Avoid caffeine, alcohol, and other medications.

SSRI ANTIDEPRESSANTS
(FOR PREVENTION OF PANIC ATTACKS)

Prozac (fluoxetine)
Paxil (paroxetene)
Zoloft (sertraline)

Except for Paxil and Zoloft, these antidepressants are *not* approved by the FDA for prevention of panic attacks. Nonetheless, they are widely and successfully used for this condition. Unlike Xanax, which *is* approved by the FDA for panic attacks, the SSRIs do not produce dependence or have abuse potential. They should be used at the lowest possible dose necessary to relieve anxiety-related symptoms. Although these antidepressants are effective for preventing recurrent panic attacks and episodes of anxiety, they should *not* be used for treatment of anxiety flare-ups or acute panic attacks, which respond best to the benzodiazepines discussed on page 130.

* The preferred approaches in many cases of generalized anxiety is nonpharmacological. Such methods include exercise, counseling, regular sleep patterns, reassurance, and the like. But many people suffer from situational or generalized anxiety that is debilitating enough to require drug therapy. Panic attacks almost always require drug intervention. When medications are indicated, choose the superior, safer choices if at all possible.

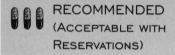

RECOMMENDED
(Acceptable with Reservations)

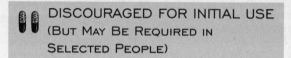

DISCOURAGED FOR INITIAL USE
(But May Be Required in Selected People)

Benzodiazepines (for disabling anxiety disorder and flare-ups of panic disorder)

Serax (oxazepam)
Ativan (lorazepam)

Among the benzodiazepines, these have an intermediate duration of action, which means their "hangover" effects the next day are minimal. Like all benzodiazepines, however, one can develop tolerance and physical dependence on them. They should not be taken with alcohol.

Others

BuSpar (buspirone)

BuSpar, a nonbenzodiazepine antianxiety drug, has two distinct advantages: It does not cause sedation, and it has no known potential for creating dependence or abuse. The downside is that it may take as long as one month to produce its full therapeutic effects. In addition, about 10 percent of patients discontinue BuSpar due to side effects. Some experts question its effectiveness and rapidity of relief, which may not measure up to the benzodiazepines. Finally, its three-times-per-day dosing is less than ideal. Safety is the strong suit of this drug; its convenience and effectiveness remain questionable.

Intermediate-Acting Benzodiazepines

Xanax (alprazolam)

This drug *is* approved by the FDA for the treatment and prevention of panic disorder, as well as anxiety. Despite this official endorsement, widespread experience with this euphoria-producing benzodiazepine suggests that its potential for producing dependence, abuse, and severe withdrawal symptoms may be greater than for other drugs in its class. As a result, *long-term* use of this drug is *not* encouraged, unless necessary. But it can be used effectively—and with less risk of dependence —for a short period of time (3–5 days) in order to get people through the severe symptoms of a panic attack. Once these have passed, the SSRI antidepressants (in Optimal category) are appropriate for long-term prevention.

Long-Acting Benzodiazepines

Valium (diazepam)
Librium (chlordiazepoxide)
Doral (quazepam)
Klonopin (clonazepam)
Tranxene (clorazepate)

These long-acting benzodiazepines should be avoided if possible, especially in the elderly, because they can cause morning-after drowsiness, sedation, and impaired physical performance. Some have been associated with an increased risk of falling and hip fractures in older individuals. They can produce physical dependence. In general, medications with a shorter duration of action (see "Recommended" category) are advised.

OTHERS

Vistaril (hydroxyzine)

This drug is too sedating and is of uncertain value over the long term.

 AVOID IF POSSIBLE
(NOT RECOMMENDED)

SHORT-ACTING BENZODIAZEPINES

Halcion (triazolam)

Its original dosage recommendations were associated with unacceptable side effects. The new lower-dosage recommendations improve the safety and adverse-effect profile of this drug, but they can still produce memory loss, daytime anxiety, and rebound insomnia.

OTHERS

Miltown (meprobamate)
Equanil (meprobamate)

Dependence may be a problem.

ANTIDEPRESSANTS

Elavil (amitriptyline)
Sinequan (doxepin)
Surmontil (trimipramine)

These drugs are associated with significant side effects, especially in the elderly. They also can have anticholinergic effects—dry mouth, blurred vision, and trouble with urination—especially in older individuals.

Alcohol

Avoid alcohol as a method to relieve anxiety.

DRUGS FOR SCHIZOPHRENIA

 MedRANK Life Enhancement Checklist

Pills of Wisdom: Schizophrenia is a serious mental disorder associated with such symptoms as hallucinations, withdrawn behavior, paranoid delusions, and apathy. For many years, the drugs used to treat it were effective but produced undesirable side effects. Newer medications, such as Risperdal and Zyprexa, are effective in a significant percentage of patients and are much more tolerable. They are also quite expensive. To some extent, they have replaced medications such as Haldol and Thorazine as initial drugs to manage symptoms. Haldol can cause movement disorders known as tardive dyskinesia, while Thorazine can cause low blood pressure and sleepiness, among other undesirable side effects. New medications for schizophrenia, such as Clozaril, are less likely to produce movement disorders, but they have a small, but significant, risk of lowering the white blood cell count to dangerously low levels if the medication is not properly monitored.

OPTIMAL
(HIGHLY RECOMMENDED/
BEST OF CLASS)

Risperdal (risperidone)

It's worth trying Risperdal or Zyprexa first. Not all people with schizophrenia respond to this "kinder, gentler" antipsychotic, but those who do tolerate it very well.

Risperdal, along with Zyprexa, appears to be as effective as standard treatments (Thorazine, Haldol) but produces fewer side effects. It seems to improve the so-called "negative" symptoms of schizophrenia, such as withdrawn, uninterested, unresponsive, and apathetic behavior.

Not all patients with schizophrenia will show improvement with Risperdal. But in people who *do* respond, it has the advantage of offering a potentially safer, less sedating profile with fewer long-term side effects than the old warhorses such as Thorazine, Haldol, Mellaril, and Navane.

Sedation, difficulty concentrating, sexual dysfunction, and low blood pressure (especially in the elderly) have been reported. On balance, given the other drug options, Risperdal and Zyprexa seem to offer the best benefit-risk ratio as an initial medication.

Zyprexa (olanzapine)

Like Risperdal, Zyprexa offers substantial promise for schizophrenic patients, especially those with negative symptoms such as apathy and withdrawal. Small studies have shown that Zyprexa was as effective as Risperdal but had a lower incidence of movement-related side effects. As compared with Risperdal,

Zyprexa also has the advantage of once-daily dosing.

This drug is generally well tolerated, but side effects such as weight gain (about 10 to 12 pounds), dizziness, sleepiness, and constipation have been seen.

For now, Zyprexa offers promise. It is a relatively new medication, however, and long-term trials will clarify its role.

RECOMMENDED
(ACCEPTABLE WITH
RESERVATIONS)

Haldol (haloperidol)
Navane (thiothixene)
Trilafon (perphenazine)
Prolixin (fluphenazine)
Stelazine (trifluoperazine)

These medications are the "old standards" for treatment of chronic schizophrenia. But because of their potential for causing disturbing side effects—especially the movement/muscle disorders called "extrapyramidal effects" and tardive dyskinesia—many psychiatrists now prefer an initial trial with Risperdal or Zyprexa, which are largely devoid of these effects. So-called "tardive movement disorders" usually occur after long-term use of these drugs and may persist for long periods, occasionally permanently, even after the drug has been stopped. Sedation is mild to moderate with Haldol; other side effects have also been reported. These medications are recommended with great reservation but also with the understanding that schizophrenia is a serious, debilitating psychiatric condition that requires treatment, even with drugs that have considerable risks and deficiencies.

 ## DISCOURAGED FOR INITIAL USE (BUT MAY BE REQUIRED IN SELECTED PEOPLE)

Clozaril (clozapine)

This drug is frequently effective in people who have failed to respond to Haldol, Thorazine, Mellaril, or related medications. Its effectiveness can be quite dramatic (an important advantage), and its side-effect profile for movement disorders (like tardive dyskinesia) is quite favorable.

Warning: Its principal—and worrisome—downside is the fact that it can cause a sudden drop in the white blood cell count (agranulocytosis) in about 1 to 2 percent of patients, a problem that requires close laboratory monitoring and that can be fatal. As a result of this problem, patients with schizophrenia should first be evaluated on other medications—chosen from among Zyprexa, Risperdal, or Haldol—before starting Clozaril, which some consider a last-resort option. The most suitable patients for this drug are those who have "psychotic" symptoms (delusions, hallucinations, and the like) that have *not* responded to any other medication. If Clozaril is prescribed, regular monitoring of the blood count can reduce the risk of agranulocytosis.

 ## AVOID IF POSSIBLE (NOT RECOMMENDED)

Mellaril (thioridazine)
Thorazine (chlorpromazine)
Serentil (mesoridazine)

Like Haldol, Navane, and Prolixin, these drugs have a long history of successful treatment of patients with schizophrenia. Their principal drawback are their anticholinergic effects, which can be quite disturbing and include dry mouth, memory impairment, confusion, rapid heart rate, sedation, and other symptoms. They can also cause movement/muscular disorders, but not as often as Haldol.

UP, UP, AND AWAY
Drugs for Mania

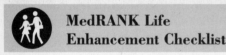 **MedRANK Life Enhancement Checklist**

Pills of Wisdom: Patients diagnosed with depression are generally categorized as having a "unipolar" mood disorder. This is the most common mood disorder. In contrast, people are said to have a bipolar mood disorder if their depressive symptoms have ever been punctuated by one or more *manic* episodes*—excessive agitation, delusions, hyperactivity, and related behavioral symptoms. The drugs listed here are for patients with *bipolar* mood disorder —that is, mania is a prominent feature of their condition.

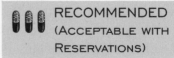 OPTIMAL
(HIGHLY RECOMMENDED/ BEST OF CLASS)

Eskalith (lithium carbonate)

This is the standard treatment for mania and bipolar mood disorder. Lithium can take two to four weeks to work, and as result, a benzodiazepine (Ativan) or an antipsychotic drug (Haldol) may be needed *temporarily* to help control the mania until the lithium kicks in. Lithium has many side effects, among them: hand tremor, thirst, excessive urination, gastrointestinal symptoms, nausea, diarrhea, and sedation. Blood levels must be monitored carefully and regularly, and many drug inter-

actions are known. Interacting drugs include diuretics, NSAIDs, bronchodilators, medications used to treat high blood pressure, and anticonvulsant medications.

RECOMMENDED
(ACCEPTABLE WITH RESERVATIONS)

Benzodiazepines
Restoril (temazepam)
Serax (oxazepam)
Ativan (lorazepam)

These anti-anxiety drugs may have to be combined with lithium to control patients with acute, severe mania—hyperagitation, excessive excitability, and similar behavorial symptoms. Among the benzodiazepines, these medications have an intermediate duration of action, which means their hangover effects are less than with long-acting benzodiazepines. Like all benzodiazepines, however, one can develop tolerance and physical dependence on them.

ANTIPSYCHOTICS

Haldol (haloperidol)

This medication, an old standard treatment for schizophrenia, may be combined with lithium to control patients with acute, severe mania—hyperagitation, excessive excitability,

---

* Please refer to the MedRANK Checklist "Medications for Depression" on page 121 for medications used to treat the *depression* component of manic-depressive mood disorder.

and similar behavorial symptoms. As a rule, this medication should be used *temporarily* (two to four weeks) and only until the lithium kicks in, to prevent further manic episodes.

DISCOURAGED FOR INITIAL USE
(BUT MAY BE REQUIRED IN SELECTED PEOPLE)

Depakene (valproic acid)
Depakote (valproic acid)

These drugs may be used, but generally speaking, *only* in people who cannot tolerate lithium therapy. They are used primarily for people with seizure disorders. These medications can cause nausea, weight gain, abnormal blood counts, and rarely, lethal liver failure.

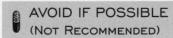

AVOID IF POSSIBLE
(NOT RECOMMENDED)

LONG-ACTING BENZODIAZEPINES

Valium (diazepam)
Librium (chlordiazepoxide)
Doral (quazepam)
Klonopin (clonazepam)
Tranxene (clorazepate)

These long-acting benzodiazepines should be avoided if possible, especially in the elderly, because they can cause prolonged drowsiness, sedation, and impaired physical performance. Some have been associated with an increased risk of falling and hip fractures in older individuals. They can produce physical dependence. In general, benzodiazepines with a shorter duration of action (see Recommended category) are advised as reinforcements for the short-term, temporary treatment of mania.

MENTAL MANGLERS
Drugs That Can Cause Psychiatric Disturbances

 MedRANK Side Effect and Warning Checklist

Pills of Wisdom: Many medications have the potential to produce the symptoms of psychiatric disease, including memory loss, confusion, disorientation, depression, hallucinations, anxiety, nightmares, and many others. This MedRANK Checklist identifies medications that may be causing such symptoms. If you feel a pill you are taking may be responsible for these reactions, notify your doctor at once.

MEDICATIONS AND POSSIBLE REACTIONS

Accutane (isotretinoin)
Depression

Actifed (pseudoephedrine)
Hallucinations, paranoia

Akineton (biperiden)
Confusion, memory loss, disorientation, delirium, auditory and visual hallucinations, fear, paranoia, agitation, bizarre behavior

Aldomet (methyldopa)
Depression, amnesia, nightmares, psychosis

Amipaque (metrizamide)
Confusion, hallucinations, depression, anxiety

Amphetamine-like drugs
Bizarre behavior, hallucinations, paranoia, agitation, anxiety, depression on withdrawal

Anabolic steroids
Aggression, mania, depression, psychosis

Anadrol (oxymetholone)
Aggression, mania, depression, psychosis

Anafranil (clomipramine)
Mania, delirium, hallucinations, paranoia

Anaprox, Naprosyn (naproxen)
Paranoia, depression, anxiety, disorientation, hallucinations

Anavar (oxandrolone)
Aggression, mania, depression, psychosis

Ansaid (flurbiprofen)
Paranoia, depression, anxiety, disorientation, hallucinations

Antabuse (disulfiram)
Catatonia, delirium, depression, psychosis

Anticholinergics and atropine
Confusion, memory loss, disorientation, delirium, auditory and visual hallucinations, fear, paranoia, agitation, bizarre behavior

Anticonvulsants
Agitation, confusion, delirium, depression, psychosis, aggression, mania

Antidepressants, tricyclic
Mania, delirium, hallucinations, paranoia

Antihistamines
Hallucinations

Aralen (chloroquine)
Confusion, delusions, hallucinations, mania

Artane (trihexyphenidyl)
Confusion, memory loss, disorientation, delirium, auditory and visual hallucinations, fear, paranoia, agitation, bizarre behavior

Atabrine (quinacrine)
Mania, paranoia, anxiety, hallucinations, delirium

Ativan (lorazepam)
Rage, hostility, paranoia, hallucinations, depression, nightmares, amnesia, mania

Atropine
Confusion, memory loss, disorientation, delirium, auditory and visual hallucinations, fear, paranoia, agitation, bizarre behavior

Bactrim (trimethoprim-sulfamethoxazole)
Psychosis, depression, disorientation, hallucinations, delusions

Barbiturates
Excitement, hyperactivity, visual hallucinations, depression

Belladonna alkaloids
Confusion, memory loss, disorientation, delirium, auditory and visual hallucinations, fear, paranoia, agitation, bizarre behavior

Benzodiazepines
Rage, hostility, paranoia, hallucinations, depression, nightmares, amnesia, mania

Beta-adrenergic blockers
Depression, confusion, nightmares, hallucinations, paranoia, delusions, mania, hyperactivity

Buprenex (buprenorphine)
Nightmares, anxiety, agitation, euphoria, dysphoria, depression, paranoia, hallucinations

BuSpar (buspirone)
Delirium, mania, panic attack

Caffeine
Anxiety, confusion, psychotic symptoms

Capoten (captopril)
Severe anxiety, hallucinations, insomnia, mania

Cardizem (diltiazem)
Depression, suicidal ideation

Catapres (clonidine)
Delirium, hallucinations, depression

Cephalosporins
Confusion, disorientation, paranoia, hallucinations

Cipro (ciprofloxacin)
Delirium, psychosis

Clinoril (sulindac)
Paranoia, depression, anxiety, disorientation, hallucinations

Clozaril (clozapine)
Delirium

Cocaine
Anxiety, agitation, psychosis

Codeine
Nightmares, anxiety, agitation, euphoria, dysphoria, depression, paranoia, hallucinations

Contraceptives, oral
Depression

Cyclogyl (cyclopentolate)
Confusion, memory loss, disorientation, delirium, auditory and visual hallucinations, fear, paranoia, agitation, bizarre behavior

Dapsone
Insomnia, agitation, hallucinations, mania, depression

Darvon (propoxyphene)
Nightmares, anxiety, agitation, euphoria, dysphoria, depression, paranoia, hallucinations

Demerol (meperidine)
Nightmares, anxiety, agitation, euphoria, dysphoria, depression, paranoia, hallucinations

Depakene (valproic acid)
Agitation, confusion, delirium, depression, psychosis, aggression, mania

Desyrel (trazodone)
Delirium, hallucinations, paranoia, mania

Dexatrim (phenylpropanolamine)
Bizarre behavior, hallucinations, paranoia, agitation, anxiety, depression on withdrawal

Dianabol (methandrostenolone)
Aggression, mania, depression, psychosis

Digitalis glycosides
Nightmares, confusion, paranoia, depression, visual hallucinations

Dilantin (phenytoin)
Agitation, confusion, delirium, depression, psychosis, aggression, mania

Dolophine (methadone)
Nightmares, anxiety, agitation, euphoria, dysphoria, depression, paranoia, hallucinations

Dopar (levodopa)
Delirium, depression, agitation, nightmares, night terrors, hallucinations, paranoia

Elavil (amitriptyline)
Mania, delirium, hallucinations, paranoia

Eldepryl (selegiline)
Hallucinations, mania, nightmares

Ephedrine
Hallucinations, paranoia

Fastin (phentermine)
Bizarre behavior, hallucinations, paranoia, agitation, anxiety, depression on withdrawal

Flagyl (metronidazole)
Depression, agitation, uncontrollable crying, disorientation, hallucinations

Flexeril (cyclobenzaprine)
Mania, hyperactivity, psychosis, delirium

Halcion (triazolam)
Rage, hostility, paranoia, hallucinations, depression, nightmares, amnesia, mania

Histamine H2-receptor antagonists
Hallucinations, paranoia, bizarre behavior, delirium, disorientation, depression, mania

HMG-CoA reductase inhibitors
Depression

Hyoscine (scopolamine)
Confusion, memory loss, disorientation, delirium, auditory and visual hallucinations, fear, paranoia, agitation, bizarre behavior

Inderal (propranolol)
Depression, confusion, nightmares, hallucinations, paranoia, delusions, mania, hyperactivity

Indocin (indomethacin)
Paranoia, depression, anxiety, disorientation, hallucinations

INH (isoniazid)
Depression, agitation, hallucinations, paranoia

Kerlone (betaxolol)
Depression, confusion, nightmares, hallucinations, paranoia, delusions, mania, hyperactivity

Ketalar (ketamine)
Nightmares, hallucinations, crying, delirium

Klonopin (clonazepam)
Rage, hostility, paranoia, hallucinations, depression, nightmares, amnesia, mania

Lariam (mefloquine)
Psychosis, panic attacks, depression

Lioresal (baclofen)
Hallucinations, paranoia, nightmares, mania, depression, anxiety, confusion

Ludiomil (maprotiline)
Hallucinations, agitation, disorientation

Luvox (fluvoxamine)
Mania

Marinol (dronabinol)
Anxiety, disorientation, psychosis

Methyltestosterone
Aggression, mania, depression, psychosis

Mevacor (lovastatin)
Depression

Minipress (prazosin)
Hallucinations, depression, paranoia

Mintezol (thiabendazole)
Psychosis

Morphine
Nightmares, anxiety, agitation, euphoria, dysphoria, depression, paranoia, hallucinations

Motrin (ibuprofen)
Paranoia, depression, anxiety, disorientation, hallucinations

Mysoline (primidone)
Agitation, confusion, delirium, depression, psychosis, aggression, mania

Nalorphine
Nightmares, anxiety, agitation, euphoria, dysphoria, depression, paranoia, hallucinations

Naqua (trichlormethiazide)
Depression, suicidal ideation

Narcotics
Nightmares, anxiety, agitation, euphoria, dysphoria, depression, paranoia, hallucinations

Nardil (phenelzine)
Paranoia, delusions, fear, mania, rage

NeoSynephrine (phenylephrine)
Depression, hallucinations, paranoia, delusions

Nesacaine (chloroprocaine)
Confusion, "doom" anxiety, psychosis, agitation, bizarre behavior, depression, panic

Nonsteroidal anti-inflammatory drugs (NSAIDs)
Paranoia, depression, anxiety, disorientation, hallucinations

Norpace (disopyramide)
Hallucinations, paranoia, panic, depression

Norpramin (desipramine)
Mania, delirium, hallucinations, paranoia

Off (deet)
Mania, hallucinations

Oncovin (vincristine)
Hallucinations

Parlodel (bromocriptine)
Mania, delusions, hallucinations, paranoia, aggressive behavior, schizophrenia, depression

Parnate (tranylcypromine)
Mania or hypomania

Penicillin G procaine
Confusion, "doom" anxiety, psychosis, agitation, bizarre behavior, depression, panic

Pepcid (famotidine)
Hallucinations, paranoia, bizarre behavior, delirium, disorientation, depression, mania

Permax (pergolide)
Hallucinations, paranoia, confusion, anxiety, depression on withdrawal

Placidyl (ethchlorvynol)
Agitation, hallucinations, paranoia

Pondimin (fenfluramine)
Bizarre behavior, hallucinations, paranoia, agitation, anxiety, depression on withdrawal

Pravachol (pravastatin)
Depression

Prednisone, cortisone, ACTH, others (corticosteroids)
Mania, depression, confusion, paranoia, hallucinations

Preludin (phenmetrazine)
Bizarre behavior, hallucinations, paranoia, agitation, anxiety, depression on withdrawal

Procaine derivatives
Confusion, "doom" anxiety, psychosis, agitation, bizarre behavior, depression, panic

Procardia (nifedipine)
Irritability, agitation, panic, belligerence, depression

Pronestyl (procainamide)
Confusion, "doom" anxiety, psychosis, agitation, bizarre behavior, depression, panic

Proventil (albuterol)
Hallucinations, paranoia

Prozac (fluoxetine)
Mania, depersonalization

Quinidine
Confusion, agitation, psychosis

Reglan (metoclopramide)
Mania, severe depression, crying, delirium

Renese (polythiazide)
Depression, suicidal ideation

Ritalin (methylphenidate)
Hallucinations, paranoia

Roferon-A; Intron A (interferon alfa)
Delirium, paranoia, depression, suicidal ideation, anxiety

Rythmol (propafenone)
Agitation, delusions, disorientation, mania, paranoia

Salicylates
Agitation, confusion, hallucinations, paranoia

Sansert (methysergide)
Depersonalization, hallucinations, agitation

Seromycin (cycloserine)
Anxiety, depression, confusion, psychosis

Serpasil (reserpine)
Depression, nightmares

Sulfonamides
Confusion, disorientation, depression, euphoria, hallucinations

Tagamet (cimetidine)
Hallucinations, paranoia, bizarre behavior, delirium, disorientation, depression, mania

Talwin (pentazocine)
Nightmares, anxiety, agitation, euphoria, dysphoria, depression, paranoia, hallucinations

Tegison (etretinate)
Severe depression

Tegretol (carbamazepine)
Agitation, confusion, delirium, depression, psychosis, aggression

Tenormin (atenolol)
Depression, confusion, nightmares, hallucinations, paranoia, delusions, mania, hyperactivity

Tenuate (diethylpropion)
Bizarre behavior, hallucinations, paranoia, agitation, anxiety, depression on withdrawal

Theophylline
Withdrawal, hyperactivity, anxiety, mania

Thiazides
Depression, suicidal ideation

Thyroid hormones
Mania, depression, hallucinations, paranoia

Timoptic (timolol)
Depression, confusion, nightmares, hallucinations, paranoia, delusions, mania

Tofranil (imipramine)
Mania, delirium, hallucinations, paranoia

Tonocard (tocainide)
Confusion, "doom" anxiety, psychosis, agitation, bizarre behavior, depression, panic

Tranxene (clorazepate)
Rage, hostility, paranoia, hallucinations, depression, nightmares, amnesia, mania

Trecator-SC (ethionamide)
Depression, hallucinations

Valium (diazepam)
Rage, hostility, paranoia, hallucinations, depression, nightmares, amnesia, mania

Ventyl (nortriptyline)
Mania, delirium, hallucinations, paranoia

Versed (midazolam)
Rage, hostility, paranoia, hallucinations, depression, nightmares, amnesia, mania

Wellbutrin (bupropion)
Psychosis, hallucinations, agitation, paranoia, catatonia, mania

Xanax (alprazolam)
Rage, hostility, paranoia, hallucinations, depression, nightmares, amnesia, mania

Xylocaine (lidocaine)
Confusion, "doom" anxiety, psychosis, agitation, bizarre behavior, depression, panic

Zantac (ranitidine)
Hallucinations, paranoia, bizarre behavior, delirium, disorientation, depression, mania

Zarontin (ethosuximide)
Agitation, confusion, delirium, depression, psychosis, aggression, mania

Zocor (simvastatin)
Depression

Zovirax (acyclovir)
Hallucinations, fearfulness, confusion, insomnia, paranoia, depression

DRUGS FOR OBSESSIVE-COMPULSIVE DISORDER

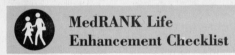

MedRANK Life Enhancement Checklist

☼ **Pills of Wisdom:** Obsessive-compulsive disorder (OCD) is characterized by excessive ritualization of routine activities, recurrent disturbing thoughts (obsessions), and/or chronic fixation on meaningless tasks or activities (compulsions), such as handwashing, excessive neatness, or arranging objects in a line, that interfere with normal daily function. People with this condition are frequently "paralyzed" by these rituals and obsessions and desperately need help.

Medications may normalize their behavior patterns and thereby improve their quality of life and their productivity in useful, life-enhancing activities. When medications are required, the SSRIs Zoloft, Prozac, and Paxil are now considered by most experts to be the initial drugs of choice for the treatment of OCD. All these drugs have the capacity to produce headache, nervousness, insomnia, agitation, increased anxiety, and sexual dysfunction. Many of these symptoms occur during the first few weeks of medication use and then subside. The SSRIs may also be associated with drug-drug interactions.

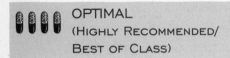

OPTIMAL
(HIGHLY RECOMMENDED/ BEST OF CLASS)

SSRI ANTIDEPRESSANTS

Zoloft (sertraline)

Zoloft is recommended as the initial choice because it appears to have a lower risk of producing drug-drug interactions and tends to be slightly less stimulating than Prozac and slightly less sedating than Paxil. Because drug interactions seem to be less of a problem with Zoloft, it is preferred for people who take multiple medications.

Prozac (fluoxetine)

This very effective SSRI may be a bit more stimulating than Zoloft or Paxil. So it may be slightly less advantageous in people who have insomnia. Because drug interactions may be more of a problem with Prozac, people on multiple medications may be able to reduce the risk of drug interactions by using Zoloft.

Paxil (paroxetene)

As effective as Prozac and Zoloft, Paxil may be slightly more sedating. There is still a potential for drug interactions.

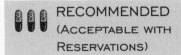

RECOMMENDED
(ACCEPTABLE WITH RESERVATIONS)

SSRIs

Luvox (fluvoxamine)

This drug is *approved* for the treatment of OCD only (not for depression). It may require twice-daily administration for higher doses. It has the same side-effect profile as the Optimal SSRIs. Many drug interactions have been described.

DISCOURAGED FOR INITIAL USE
(BUT MAY BE REQUIRED IN
SELECTED PEOPLE)

TRICYCLIC ANTIDEPRESSANTS

Anafranil (clomipramine)
This drug has significant side effects, especially in the elderly. It also has anticholinergic effects—dry mouth, blurred vision, and trou-

ble with urination, especially in older individuals. Other side effects include sedation and seizures (rare). Multiple daily dosing may be required.

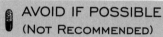 **AVOID IF POSSIBLE**
(NOT RECOMMENDED)

ALL OTHERS

CHAPTER 8

TAKE A DEEP BREATH

Medications for Asthma and Bronchitis

"I'm taking three different inhalers for my asthma, and I'm still wheezing," a patient who had come to the emergency department recently complained. "There has to be a better way." For many people with asthma and lung problems, there is. If you and your doctor emphasize medications that *prevent* recurrent episodes of asthma, you can reduce your dependence on a multiple drug regimen. The key to simplifying your asthma regimen is learning how to use your inhaler(s) appropriately, and complying with your regimen exactly as instructed by your phyisician.

Drugs used to treat common respiratory conditions fall into a number of different categories, including bronchodilators (to open up the airways), antibiotics, inhaled steroids (to reduce inflammation), antihistamines, and decongestants. Although these drugs are generally safe, they do have the capacity to produce both mild and major side effects. The

frequency and severity of those side effects depend on a number of factors, including the dose, the duration of therapy, and the individual's susceptibility. More often than not, many of these drugs are used in combination with other medications to treat asthma, chronic obstructive pulmonary disease, and allergic conditions. Some of them—in particular, the inhaled beta-agonists—have been associated with overuse. Consequently, adhering to your doctor's instructions regarding timing and indications for use is essential for maximizing the drug's benefits and reducing its potential for side effects.

Antibiotics are some of the most important drugs used to treat respiratory problems. Rankings and comparisons of antibiotics used to treat pneumonia, bronchitis, and other respiratory infections can be found in Chapters 13 and 15. Please consult the MedRANK Checklists there for specific recommendations.

☺ *Medications that dilate (open) the respiratory airways and thereby permit air to flow more freely during respiration are called* **sympathomimetic agents.**

These airway-opening drugs can be administered either in tablet form, as is the case with theophylline, or as an aerosolized solution, such as albuterol, salmeterol, and isoetharine. The sympathomimetics dilate (widen) the bronchioles (air sacs) of the lung by relaxing the smooth muscles around the airways and preventing them from having spasms and contractions. This allows better air exchange during breathing. Sympathomimetics thus improve the symptoms of patients whose lung disease is characterized by narrowed airway passages.

The xanthine derivatives, such as theophylline and aminophylline, also make breathing easier by widening certain breathing passages in the lungs. Generally speaking, they can prevent and relieve symptoms of bronchial asthma, but they are not useful for an acute attack. Because of toxicity and side effect problems, the use of theophylline to treat lung conditions, including asthma, has decreased significantly in recent years. Some studies suggest that theophylline may still be overused.

☺ *If you are taking theophylline, it may be worthwhile to consult your physician to see whether you may be better served by an inhaled steroid such as Vanceril or Flovent, or a bronchodilator such as Ventolin (albuterol).*

The trend away from theophylline has been fueled by studies that show that up to 20 percent of people receiving long-term theophylline therapy may have some kind of toxic manifestation. The long-standing controversy over theophylline has centered not only on its problematic side-effect profile but on its effectiveness, especially when compared with other, less toxic medications— inhaled beta-agonists—that are available in aerosolized formulations. At present, it appears clear that theophylline should not be used as a first-line drug for the treatment of mild, intermittent asthma. (Children are an exception and may need theophylline because they may not be very proficient at using inhalers.) Consequently, if you are on theophylline, find out why. In general, an acute worsening of mild asthma symptoms is best managed with a better-tolerated and more rapidly acting beta-2 agonist such as Proventil or Ventolin. If you have mild asthma, you can use these medications on an *as-needed* basis. On the other hand, if your asthma is more severe, you may need to use them on a regular (two to four times per day) schedule.

☺ *If you are taking theophylline for asthma but you have not been given an adequate trial of an inhaled sympathomimetic agent, you should consult with your physician about the possibility of managing your asthma symptoms entirely with an aerosolized preparation.*

Moreover, reliance on sympathomimetics can be reduced significantly by the appropriate use of inhaled corticosteroids. The best *preventive* approach is the use of inhaled steroids.

Although the majority of drugs used to treat respiratory conditions are prescribed by physicians, patients have a great deal of flexibility in terms of how and when these medications are actually used. Many patients use these medications on an as-needed basis—that is, they self-administer these drugs when they feel their symptoms require it. There has been some concern that patient-activated use of bronchodilators can lead to tolerance—that so much of the drug is used that it stops working. The fact is, excessive use of beta-agonist inhalants can produce tolerance. Consequently, these drugs are best reserved for episodic and short-term use, to relieve constriction of the airways. Corticosteroid therapy, preferably through inhalation, is the most effective and appropriate maintenance therapy in patients with asthma.

☺ ***Among the bronchodilators that are currently available, be aware that some inhalers (Ventolin, Proventil, Maxair) can relieve the acute symptoms of an asthma attack, whereas others, such as Serevent (salmeterol) have no role in treating acute symptoms but are used for maintenance therapy only.***

One of the main problems associated with inhaled bronchodilators is suboptimal intake of the inhaled drug and inappropriate use of the inhaler by the patient. A few tips can help. Generally speaking, it is important to shake the aerosol canister before each use. The pressurized inhalation should be administered during the second half of a breath intake,

when the airways are open wider, allowing more extensive aerosol distribution. If you require more than one inhalation dose, you should wait at least one minute between doses. In the case of albuterol, epinephrine, and isoproterenol, the second inhalation should be administered three to five minutes after the first. If these measures fail to provide the usual relief, you should seek medical attention immediately. This could be a sign of worsening asthma, which requires reassessment of therapy. Increasing dose requirements for your bronchodilator also suggests that your condition may be worsening, and that other forms of therapy, including corticosteroids, may be required.

☺ ***Once again, it should be stressed that inhaled corticosteroid preparations, such as Vanceril, Beclovent, Azmacort, and Flovent, represent the primary bulwark of defense against acute asthma attacks.***

These synthetic steroids decrease the number and activity of inflammatory cells, which over the long term may help to relax the smooth muscles in the airways. When inhaled, the effects of corticosteroids are local, and the incidence of side effects is relatively low. It should be emphasized, however, that inhaled corticosteroids are *not* useful for treating *acute* asthma attacks. In other words, they do not provide rapid relief; instead, their primary role is prevention of recurrent asthma attacks and long-term stabilization. Finally, people with severe asthma who are taking corticosteroid inhalants may also be prescribed oral corticosteroids and bronchodilators to provide multiple fronts of attack.

☼ *When asthma symptoms can't be controlled by steroid inhalers and beta-agonists, it may be necessary to use an oral steroid such as prednisone.*

As a rule, you don't need prednisone for more than a week. When using oral steroids to manage acute conditions, such as asthma, allergies, or hives, rapid, short-term tapering courses of steroids are clearly as effective as longer tapering courses. What this means is that if you have been prescribed a course of steroids for a breakthrough asthma attack, you can taper these medications over a three-to-seven-day period. Typically, there is no justification for prolonging tapering over several weeks. Finally, in those patients who have been committed to long-term steroid therapy, every attempt should be made to reduce their dose to less than 10 mg per day, to avoid the bone-wasting complications of long-term therapy.

TAKE A DEEP BREATH
Drugs for Mild or Intermittent Asthma

 MedRANK Life Prolongation and Enhancement Checklist

☼ **Pills of Wisdom:** The most important aspect of drug therapy for mild to moderate asthma is *prevention*. Although some inhalers contain medications (beta-2-selective adrenergic drugs) that can open up the airways when you need quick relief from symptoms, they do very little to *prevent* the long inflammation that produces wheezing, cough, and shortness of breath.

People who have very *mild* disease and require no more than a puff of a bronchodilator every now and then can probably do without inhaled steroids, which are the foundation of asthma prevention. In fact, people with *very mild* cases of asthma do just as well using their airway openers on an *as-needed* basis as they do on a scheduled basis.

On the other hand, if you find yourself requiring more than two puffs a day of a Proventil or Ventolin inhaler, then you should be put on a regular regimen of an inhaled corticosteroid such as Flovent or Vanceril. Judicious use of these steroid inhalers is absolutely essential to prevent recurrent episodes of asthma and will reduce your visits to the emergency department or your physician. Use of an inhaled steroid will also reduce your reliance on oral steroid medications, which can produce undesirable side effects.

Finally, be sure you receive *detailed instructions* for how to use your inhaler. One of the reasons people don't get optimal results from the inhalers is that they don't know how to use them appropriately. This leads to additional—and unnecessary—medication use, as well as added expense.

OPTIMAL
(HIGHLY RECOMMENDED/ BEST OF CLASS)

INHALED BETA-2-SELECTIVE ADRENERGIC AEROSOLS: BRONCHODILATORS ("AIRWAY OPENERS")

Proventil (albuterol)
Ventolin (albuterol)
Maxair Autohaler (pirbuterol)

These inhalers should be used for acute relief of symptoms in people with mild or intermittent asthma. They cannot prevent recurrent attacks but can "rescue" you when wheezing, tightness, shortness of breath, and coughing become intolerable.

Persons who have very mild and intermittent flare-ups of asthma should use these inhalers only when required. In particular, people who have asthma caused by exercise will benefit from these drugs, which can be taken prior to an activity known to trigger an asthma attack.

Don't overuse these airway openers. Equal effectiveness, but less toxicity and fewer side effects, are seen when inhalers are used on an as-needed basis—that is, for relief of acute asthma symptoms. No additional benefits are seen when they are used on a regular basis, especially in people who require less than two puffs of albuterol per day.

If you need more than two puffs per day, regular use may provide some benefit. But if you need more than two puffs per day, your asthma is not being well maintained, and you should be on inhaled *steroids* for preventive maintenance.

Side effects include fast heart rate, palpitations, and shakiness.

LONG-ACTING BRONCHODILATOR

Serevent (salmeterol)

Note: Serevent is a *long-acting* bronchodilator that should *not* be used for the relief of acute (sudden) symptoms of asthma. It does not work immediately and therefore has no role in treating sudden flare-ups. It is especially useful for asthmatics who have symptoms at night, and for maintenance therapy.

ANTI-INFLAMMATORY CORTICOSTEROID AEROSOLS

Flovent (fluticasone propionate)
Beclovent (beclomethasone dipropionate)
Vanceril (beclomethasone dipropionate)

These inhaled steroids, which can eliminate or prevent recurrent attacks of asthma, are essential for people who have mild asthma but require "regular" use of beta-2-selective adrenergic drugs. Experts debate what "regular" use is, but if you use *more than two puffs per day* or one canister per month of a beta-2-selective adrenergic drug, you should probably be on an inhaled steroid aerosol, as well as an inhaled bronchodilator for treatment of flare-ups. Side effects include hoarseness and thrush (*Candida* infection of mouth). It is important to comply with these medications to derive their maximal benefits.

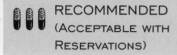 **RECOMMENDED**
(Acceptable with
Reservations)

 DISCOURAGED FOR INITIAL USE
(But May Be Required in
Selected People)

Inhaled Beta-2-Selective Adrenergic Drug

Maxair (pirbuterol)

Same as for inhaled beta-2-selective adrenergic aerosols (in "Optimal" category).

Anti-Inflammatory Corticosteroid Aerosols

Azmacort (triamcinolone acetonide)
Aerobid (flunisolide)

Same as for anti-inflammatory corticosteroid aerosols in "Optimal" category.

Accolate (zafirlukast)

This is the first approved drug in a new class of medications called leukotriene receptor antagonists. It reduces inflammation and constriction of bronchial airways. It is taken twice daily and is used to "maintain" people with mild to moderate asthma. It has the potential for interactions with warfarin, Dilantin, calcium channel blockers, and other medications. Because experience is still somewhat limited with this drug, it should be used only if inhaled corticosteroids prove not to be effective for preventing asthma flare-ups.

Oral Corticosteroids

Prednisone

Oral steroids should be reserved for asthma patients with *moderate* or *severe* disease, rather than for those with mild, intermittent symptoms. On occasion, however, oral steroids will be required for people with milder forms of the disease.

Other Bronchodilators

Atrovent (ipratropium bromide)

Better drugs than this one are available for mild asthmatics. But it may be useful in older patients with chronic lung disease.

Brethaire (terbutaline)

This drug is not as convenient as other inhaled bronchodilators.

Bronchodilator Tablets

Brethine (terbutaline)
Rotacaps (albuterol)
Repetabs (albuterol)
Volmax (albuterol)

These oral bronchodilators do not work as well as inhaled medications.

Others

Intal (cromolyn)
Tilade (nedocromil)

These are not as effective as other asthma drugs. They are used for *preventing* asthma attacks.

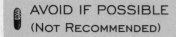

AVOID IF POSSIBLE
(NOT RECOMMENDED)

Theo-Dur (theophylline); many other brand names

This drug is less potent, works more slowly, and has many more side effects than inhaled bronchodilators. It also requires laboratory monitoring. For these reasons, theophylline compounds are not recommended in adults with asthma. They may be necessary in preschoolers and toddlers, who may not take well to inhaled medications.

BREATHE FREE
Drugs for Moderate or Severe Chronic Asthma

  MedRANK Life Prolongation and Enhancement Checklist

Pills of Wisdom: Patients with *moderate to severe asthma* generally require inhaled steroids for preventive maintenance, plus regular use of bronchodilators to help keep airways open. When environmental factors, infections, or other triggers are severe enough to render these two medications less than effective, it may be necessary to take a short (five-to-seven-day) course of oral steroid medications. Oral steroids (prednisone) provide definitive relief for people with severe cases of asthma. Unfortunately, long-term use of these medications can produce many undesirable side effects, including obesity, acne, stomach ulcers, and possibly infection. The use of inhaled steroids, which produce fewer side effects, is the best way to reduce your reliance on oral steroid medications. In *very severe* cases, you may need to be on three or more medications, including oral steroids, inhaled steroids, inhaled bronchodilators, oral bronchodilators, and leukotriene receptor antagonists (Accolate).

 OPTIMAL
(HIGHLY RECOMMENDED/ BEST OF CLASS)

ANTI-INFLAMMATORY CORTICOSTEROID AEROSOLS

Flovent (fluticasone propionate)

These inhaled steroids, which can eliminate or prevent recurrent attacks of asthma, are *essential* for people who have moderate to severe asthma. Not only can they reduce the frequency and severity of attacks, but they can reduce reliance on *other* medications as well. Hence, they are the primary bulwark against recurrent asthma flare-ups.

Virtually everyone who has moderate to severe asthma will need to be on inhaled steroids. If you use more than two puffs per day or one canister per month of a beta-2-selective adrenergic drug, you should probably be on an inhaled steroid aerosol, *along with* an inhaled bronchodilator.

Side effects include hoarseness and thrush (Candida infection of mouth).

Among the inhaled steroids, Flovent is highly recommended for severe cases because it is available in three different dosage strengths and has been shown to reduce reliance on oral prednisone therapy. Flovent has the advantage of providing high inhaled steroid doses, with the convenience of twice-daily dosing.

Beclovent (beclomethasone dipropionate)
Vanceril (beclomethasone dipropionate)
See "Flovent." These inhaled steroid formulations also are excellent, but they do not offer all the options or convenience aspects of Flovent.

INHALED BETA-2-SELECTIVE ADRENERGIC AEROSOLS: BRONCHODILATORS ("AIRWAY OPENERS")

Proventil (albuterol)
Ventolin (albuterol)
Maxair Autohaler (pirbuterol)
These inhalers should be used in combination with inhaled corticosteroids for people with moderate to severe asthma. In patients with moderate to severe symptoms, these inhalers should probably be used on a regular basis. Side effects include heart palpitations and shakiness. People who have asthma caused by exercise will benefit from these drugs.

LONG-ACTING BRONCHODILATOR

Serevent (salmeterol)
Note: Serevent is a *long-acting* bronchodilator. It may be right for you if you experience bad asthma symptoms at night. It is used twice daily on a regular basis, for preventing breakthrough asthma episodes.

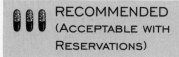

RECOMMENDED
(ACCEPTABLE WITH RESERVATIONS)

ORAL CORTICOSTEROIDS

Prednisone
Oral steroids are appropriate for asthma patients with moderate or severe disease. When inhaled steroids and bronchodilators don't do the job, it's usually time for prednisone.

Although prednisone is the most effective treatment for asthma episodes that don't respond to other medications, it has significantly *more* side effects than other therapies for asthma, including weight gain, elevated blood pressure, bone loss, cataracts, and impaired immune response. If your doctor puts you on steroids, be sure you are rapidly tapered off within seven days, if possible.

INHALED BETA-2-SELECTIVE ADRENERGIC AEROSOLS

Maxair (pirbuterol)
See "Inhaled Beta-2-selective Adrenergic Aerosols" in "Optimal" category.

ANTI-INFLAMMATORY STEROID AEROSOLS

Azmacort (triamcinolone acetonide)
Aerobid (flunisolide)
Same as for "Anti-inflammatory Corticosteroid Aerosols" in "Optimal" category.

DISCOURAGED FOR INITIAL USE (But May Be Required in Selected People)

Accolate (zafirlukast)

This is the first approved drug in a new class of medications called leukotriene receptor antagonists. It reduces inflammation and constriction of bronchial airways. It is taken twice daily and is used to "maintain" people with moderate to severe asthma. It has the potential for causing drug interactions with warfarin, Dilantin, calcium channel blockers, and other medications. Because experience is still somewhat limited with this drug, it should be used only if inhaled corticosteroids are not effective for preventing asthma flare-ups.

Theo-Dur (theophylline); many other brand names

This drug is less potent, works more slowly, and has many more side effects than inhaled bronchodilators. It also requires laboratory monitoring. For these reasons, theophylline compounds are not recommended in adults with asthma, unless they are unresponsive to or fail to comply with other forms of therapy.

OTHER BRONCHODILATORS

Atrovent (ipratropium bromide)

Better drugs than this one are available for patients with severe asthma. But it may be useful in older patients with chronic lung disease.

Brethaire (terbutaline)

This drug is not as convenient as other inhaled bronchodilators.

BRONCHODILATOR TABLETS

Brethine (terbutaline)
Rotacaps (albuterol)
Repetabs (albuterol)
Volmax (albuterol)

These oral bronchodilators do not work as well as inhaled medications.

OTHERS

Intal (cromolyn)
Tilade (nedocromil)

These are not as effective as other asthma drugs. They are used for preventing asthma attacks.

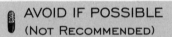

AVOID IF POSSIBLE (Not Recommended)

ALL OTHERS

CHAPTER 9

—

GETTING THE RED OUT

Medications for Allergies and Related Conditions

"How do I stop the itching in my eyes? I can't get a wink of sleep at night," my patients have complained over the years. "And what do I do about my nose? Every spring, it just runs and runs. These allergies are driving me crazy!" Living in Oregon, where seasonal (outdoor) and perennial (indoor) allergies wreak havoc on otherwise healthy people, I am very sympathetic to the misery of allergy sufferers. The bad news is, allergies are an inevitable part of life for about 15 percent of all Americans. The economic costs associated with allergies, including days lost from work, run into the hundreds of millions of dollars. The good news is, effective medications are now available that get the red out, get it out quickly, and keep it out. Not only are the best anti-allergy medications very effective, they are user-friendly and do not produce the drowsiness and dry mouth that plagued the old allergy medications like Benadryl.

Before discussing pills, sprays, and inhalers that work for allergies—and those that don't—I cannot overemphasize the importance of environmental factors in causing allergy symptoms. If you know that you are allergic to pollen, molds, dusts, dogs, cats, or other substances, stay away from these "allergy triggers" (allergens) whenever possible. The causes of year-around indoor allergies can be difficult to identify, so trial and error may be your only recourse. If you notice that your allergies get better on weekends, when you are away from your work environment, something in your workplace may be triggering your symptoms. On the other hand, if your eyes start to itch and your nose begins to run when you are mowing the lawn or playing golf on the weekends, outdoor pollens, ragweeds, and molds may be the culprit.

☺ *The primary bulwark of defense against allergy symptoms includes nasal sprays and oral antihistamines.*

Antihistamines, which block the release of substances that can cause inflammation, are a wide and varied class of medications, with respect to both their indications and their potential for causing side effects. Generally speaking, most antihistamines have proven to be remarkably safe considering their widespread use. The principal concern is the risk of abnormal heart rhythms—which can be life-threatening—associated with the use of the antihistamine Hismanal (astemizole).

In fact, as this book goes to press, the FDA has recommended removing Seldane from the market because of this danger. These heart-related complications are more likely to occur when Seldane or Hismanal is used in combination with other drugs such as erythromycin, ketoconazole, itraconazole, and clarithromycin, all of which can increase blood levels of the aforementioned antihistamines. Although the risk of harm is very small—or nonexistent—when these drugs are used alone, it is difficult to recommend their use, especially since other equally effective antihistamines that do not cause these serious side effects, such as Zyrtec (cetirizine), Claritin (loratidine), and Allegra (fexofenadine), are available.

"Yes, doctor, the medication is helping my allergy symptoms," my patients offered, "but they make me so sleepy." Until a few years ago, this was a very common complaint. The side affects of antihistamines disturbed many of my patients more than the runny nose and itchy eyes had. Some of the most familiar over-the-counter medications, such as Benadryl, Tavist, and Chlor-Trimeton, produce sleepiness and drowsiness in a significant percentage—up to 60 percent—of people who use them. These symptoms can be severe enough to get in the way of normal activities, and therefore I do not recommend these pills for active people who thrive on mental alertness, for people who need to drive cars or operate machinery, or for the elderly.

Fortunately, there are now better, albeit more expensive, alternatives that do not produce these life-compromising side effects. Physicians and manufacturers now frequently divide oral antihistamines into "sedating" and "nonsedating" categories. Among the nonsedating or minimally sedating medications, I recommend Claritin, Zyrtec, and Allegra. Compared to using a placebo pill, Claritin and Allegra—as well as Seldane and Hismanal—can be expected to cause drowsiness in only about 2 people out of 100 who take these medications. Zyrtec can be expected to cause sleepiness in about 8 out of 100 who take it, or a net increase of about 6 percent, compared with such nonsedating drugs as Claritin and Allegra. This is Zyrtec's principal downside, but it is probably not a significant enough blemish to deter your physician from prescribing this antihistamine on your behalf.

🔅 *Although many doctors are concerned about the slight increase in drowsiness seen with Zyrtec, this medication has important cost and clinical advantages over the other antihistamines that, in my view, justify ranking it as Optimal.*

Put simply, Zyrtec provides relief of redness and allergy symptoms very quickly—frequently within an hour. In other words, it gets the red out and gets it out lickety-split. What this means, from a practical, allergy-suffering perspective, is that you may be able to take Zyrtec on an as-needed basis—that is, just on the days when you really need relief.

☼ *If you are tuned in to your body, you can take these pills as soon as you feel your symptoms spinning out of control, and get relief in short order.*

The fact is, in most people, the severity of allergy symptoms varies from day to day, or week to week. Because of this roller-coaster ride, you may not need to take an antihistamine every single day. Unfortunately, most antihistamines, including Claritin, take several hours before their maximal effects have kicked in, which means that the most consistent results are seen with daily administration of the drug. In contrast, because it is so rapidly acting, Zyrtec offers you the flexibility of nipping your allergy symptoms in the bud. Finally, although only 2 percent of people discontinue Zyrtec because of its side effects, if you are one of those individuals who experience drowsiness with it, you can always be switched to Claritin or Allegra. Claritin, Allegra, and Zyrtec also represent safe alternatives with respect to drug interactions and heart problems.

☼ *Regardless of the antihistamine that is selected for you, it is advisable to avoid "shotgun" approaches that use many products simultaneously.*

The risk of side effects and drug interactions is increased dramatically if you are taking antihistamines in combination with antibiotics, decongestants, expectorants, cough suppres-sants, and other over-the-counter medications. The side effects are likely to be even worse in older patients, who are more prone to experiencing fatigue, sedation, mental confusion, and fainting from chronic antihistamine use. Because many different options are available, consult your physician or pharmacist about possible alternatives if your antihistamine fails to relieve symptoms, or if the side effects are more troublesome than you can tolerate.

☼ *If your symptoms are limited to nasal congestion, runny nose, and postnasal drip—so-called rhinitis symptoms—you may first want to try a nasal spray that contains anti-inflammatory medications called corticosteroids, or steroids for short.*

Steroid-containing medications are available not only for oral ingestion or inhalation—an important formulation for asthmatics—but for intranasal administration. Nasal corticosteroids such as beclomethasone, budesonide, and flunisolide shrink swollen nasal tissue caused by allergic rhinitis (like hay fever). Budesonide and beclomethasone sprays are also used to treat nonallergic rhinitis (perennial or continual) in adults. Generally speaking, these medications have minimal side effects and have the advantage of reducing reliance on oral antihistamines, which are also used to treat allergy symptoms involving the nose. Intranasal steroids are most useful for patients whose symptoms are localized to the nasal passages, but unfortunately they have very little effect on patients who have watery, itching eyes as part of their allergic syndrome.

ANTIHISTAMINES FOR ALLERGIES*
Hay Fever, Seasonal Allergic Rhinitis, and Related Symptoms

MedRANK Life Enhancement Checklist

Pills of Wisdom: The symptoms of seasonal (outdoor) and perennial or chronic (indoor) allergies can be debilitating. The aim of therapy is to get the red out and keep it out—to make misery a memory. The primary approach to these problems is *prevention:* avoiding environments, animals, activities, and occupational settings that trigger allergies or make them worse. Unfortunately, this is not always possible. More often than not, when allergy symptoms begin to intefere with our quality of life and daily routine, medications will enter the picture.

Besides avoiding things you are allergic to, the only sure way to relieve your allergy symptoms is to find a drug with which you will comply and that does not create symptoms that are more troubling than those caused by your allergies. When symptoms are limited to the nasal passages (so-called rhinitis), a nasal inhaler containing anti-inflammatory medications (corticosteroids) can be extremely effective. (Please see MedRANK Checklist, "Nasal Sprays for Allergies" on page 159.) When allergy symptoms extend beyond the nose to include runny eyes, itchy skin, and other related symptoms that interfere with sleep, work, or play, an oral antihistamine is often required.

The key to a successful antihistamine is convenience, safety, efficacy, and rapid onset of action. In this regard, not all antihistamines are created equal.

Some (Claritin, Zyrtec, and Allegra) are almost always safe and some (Seldane and Hismanal) have a higher risk for being unsafe. Some antihistamines (Benadryl, Chlor-Trimeton, Tavist-1) have a high likelihood of making you drowsy and sleepy, and others (Claritin, Allegra, Zyrtec) do not. Some antihistamines (Seldane and Hismanal) require caution because of serious drug-drug interactions, and others (Claritin, Allegra, Zyrtec) do not. Some of these pills produce rather rapid relief of symptoms (Zyrtec, Allegra), whereas others do not (Hismanal). These are the kinds of distinctions that will help you and your physician decide which antihistamine will make the misery of allergy a memory for you.

 OPTIMAL
(HIGHLY RECOMMENDED/
BEST OF CLASS)

Zyrtec (cetirizine)

Once-daily dosing improves compliance with this drug. It is the most rapidly acting of all the oral antihistamines—you can expect to see symptom improvement within 60 minutes. Consequently, I recommend it as the initial drug of choice. It has no clinically significant risk of drug-drug interactions, and it is the only antihistamine approved for both outdoor and indoor allergies as well as chronic hives—in this respect, it's a "full service" antihistamine.

----

* Many of the antihistamines in the "Discouraged" category may be familiar to you, because some are available without a prescription. Even though most of these medications are safe under normal circumstances, they can cause drug interactions, and almost without exception, they are less conveniently dosed and are more likely to cause drowsiness, sedation, and dry mouth than the antihistamines listed in the "Optimal" and "Recommended" categories.

There is one special feature with Zyrtec. Because it produces rapid improvement of symptoms, it can be used on an as-needed basis. The only downside is drowsiness and sedation, which is seen slightly more often than with Claritin. On average, about 6 to 7 *more* people out of 100 who take Zyrtec can be expected to have sedation, as opposed to a similar number who take Claritin, which is nonsedating. Zyrtec, nevertheless, has a very low discontinuation rate and can be used safely in people who have asthma.

Claritin
Claritin-D

An excellent antihistamine with the convenience of once-daily dosing and a safety profile equivalent to Zyrtec's, Claritin is a nonsedating antihistamine with no known significant drug-drug interactions. It works less rapidly than Zyrtec and therefore is not particularly suited to being taken on an as-needed basis. Claritin-D contains a decongestant.

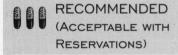

RECOMMENDED
(ACCEPTABLE WITH RESERVATIONS)

Allegra (fexofenadine)

Twice-daily dosing makes this drug less convenient than Claritin and Zyrtec (see "Optimal" category). It has the advantages of an excellent safety profile and no known risk of clinically important drug-drug interactions. The onset of action is fairly rapid—symptoms can start to improve within one to two hours after the pill has been taken. It is a nonsedating antihistamine.

DISCOURAGED FOR INITIAL USE
(BUT MAY BE REQUIRED IN SELECTED PEOPLE)

Hismanal (astemizole)

A once-daily, nonsedating antihistamine, Hismanal is ranked in the Discouraged category because it has been associated with life-threatening cardiac rhythm problems that have led to death. They are more likely to occur when Hismanal is taken along with erythromycin, ketoconazole, or itraconazole. Do *not* take Hismanal with these drugs or with any other medication without first getting the approval of your physician and pharmacist.

Tavist (clemastine)
Tavist-1

Moderately sedating, Tavist requires twice-daily dosing. It has significant anticholinergic side effects that include dry mouth, blurry vision, trouble urinating, and related symptoms. This is only a mild to moderately potent antihistamine.

Optimine (azatadine)

This moderately sedating drug requires twice-daily dosing and has anticholinergic side effects.

Nolahist (phenindamine)

This drug may cause stimulation in children. It requires four or more doses per day—not convenient.

Dimetane (brompheniramine)
Dehist
Bromphen
Veltane

These brompheniramine drugs are slightly

sedating and have mild anticholinergic side effects—dry mouth, blurred vision, drying up of secretions, and difficulty urinating. Dosing is inconvenient, but they are effective antihistamines.

Polaramine (dexchlorpheniramine)
Poladex

These dexchlorpheniramine drugs are similar to the brompheniramine drugs.

Chlor-Trimeton (chlorpheniramine)
Teldrin
Chlor-Trimeton Chlor-Span 12 Hour
Aller-Chlor

These chlorpheniramine drugs are similar to the brompheniramine drugs. Some extended-release formulations can be dosed every 12 hours. Their antihistamine activity is not as potent as the medications listed in the "Optimal" category.

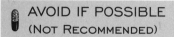 AVOID IF POSSIBLE
(NOT RECOMMENDED)

Benadryl (diphenhydramine); many name brands

The problems with this widely used antihistamine are probably underappreciated by most. Benadryl requires multiple daily dosing, is highly sedating, and produces anticholinergic side effects, which include dry mouth, blurry vision, sleepiness, and difficult urination. It is not recommended for the elderly.

Atarax (hydroxyzine)

Atarax is too sedating and has anticholinergic side effects.

Periactin (cyproheptadine)

Periactin is slightly sedating and requires three doses per day. It produces only moderate antihistamine activity. More effective and potent pills are available.

PBZ (tripelennamine)

This drug is moderately sedating and has moderate potency.

Tacaryl (methdilazine)

This drug requires twice-daily dosing and has anticholinergic side effects.

Temaril (trimeprazine)

This sedating drug requires three-to-four-times-daily dosing—inconvenient. It also produces anticholinergic side effects.

Myidyl (triprolidine)

This mildly sedating drug requires four-times-daily dosing and produces mild anticholinergic side effects.

Phenergan (promethazine)

This highly sedating drug requires three-to-four-times-daily dosing and produces anticholinergic side effects.

NASAL SPRAYS FOR ALLERGIES
Hay Fever, Seasonal Allergic Rhinitis, and Related Symptoms

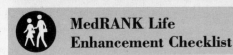 **MedRANK Life Enhancement Checklist**

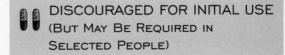 OPTIMAL
(HIGHLY RECOMMENDED/ BEST OF CLASS)

Flonase (fluticasone propionate)
With this drug, once-daily usage is often sufficient. It appears to provide better relief of nasal symptoms than some oral antihistamines. Because of its potency, dosage reduction to one spray per nostril per day may be possible after symptoms stabilize.

RECOMMENDED
(ACCEPTABLE WITH RESERVATIONS)

Note: Most steroid-based nasal sprays are effective. The principal difference among them is dosing frequency, which produces better compliance with some sprays than with others.

Nasacort (triamcinolone acetonide)
Once-daily use.

Beconase AQ (beclomethasone)
Twice-daily use.

Vancenase AQ (beclomethasone)
Twice-daily use.

DISCOURAGED FOR INITIAL USE
(BUT MAY BE REQUIRED IN SELECTED PEOPLE)

Beconase (beclomethasone)
Two to four times daily use.

Nasalcrom (cromolyn sodium)
Three to six times daily use. It may not be as effective as steroid nasal sprays.

CHAPTER 10

<hr>

SKIN DEEP

Pills and Lotions for Skin and Hair Problems

"I've been using this steroid cream for more than six months, and my rash isn't any better" is a common complaint about medications used to treat skin problems. Medicated creams, lotions, and gels represent a wide and important group of drug-based treatment options. They include products for treating inflamed mucous membranes in the mouth and throat, antibiotics to treat acne, drugs for psoriasis, burn preparations, local anesthetics, and a number of miscellaneous agents, including sunscreens and skin cleansers.

Although these medications can be highly effective for eczema, infections, dandruff, and other skin problems, a few warnings and general guidelines will help you get the most out of them. For example, most of the topical preparations discussed in this chapter should be used sparingly, and if results (that is, symptomatic improvements) are not apparent within a few applications, you should consult your physician or pharmacist. In addition, avoid close contact with eyes or mucous membranes unless otherwise indicated.

☺ *Mouth and throat products include mouth-cleansing agents, saliva substitutes, and tannic acids, which are used to provide temporary relief of the pain, burning, and irritation associated with cold sores, canker sores, and fever blisters.*

In general, over-the-counter mouth and throat products, including lozenges, mouthwashes, and sprays, are used to relieve symptoms associated with sore throats and upper respiratory tract infections. These agents, which do *not* cure infections, include Vicks Throat Lozenges, Cepacol, and Scope; they contain a number of active ingredients that provide minimal relief for mild to moderate symptoms. You can read the label and identify ingredients that have specific healing properties suited to your needs. For example, benzocaine is a local anesthetic, whereas cetylpyridinium chloride, eucalyptus oil, benzalkonium chloride, and hexylresorcinol have antiseptic activity. Terpin hydrate is an expectorant that helps promote discharge of mucus from the respiratory tract. Menthol, camphor, cloveoil, and phenol are used for their mild, anti-itch, local anesthetic, and anti-inflammatory properties. Triamcinolone acetonide and hydrocortisone frequently are added for their anti-inflammatory activity. Naturally, if your sore throat is severe or persists for several days, you should consult your physician. Finally, these formulations should not be used for more than two days in children who are three years of age or younger, unless directed by your physician.

☺ *Except for oral antibiotics, most acne medications are intended for external use only.*

They should be kept away from the eyes, eyelids, mouth, mucous membranes, or other areas of highly inflamed or damaged skin. A number of products are available to treat acne, including benzoyl peroxide, benzoic acid, Azelex, Retin-A, topical antibiotics, and other miscellaneous formulations. The best combinations and sequences for using anti-acne medications are listed in the MedRANK Checklist "Acne" on page 164. The most effective acne drugs are available by prescription only, whereas others are available on an over-the-counter basis.

☺ *Some of these products, such as Accutane (isotretinoin), can cause serious side effects—including birth defects—and should be used only under a physician's supervision.*

Most OTC acne products contain some combination of alcohol, resorcinol, antibacterial agents, and other substances used to minimize skin irritation. Severe cases of acne that are resistant to the usual topical preparations may require treatment with oral antibiotics. Severe cases should be monitored by a physician.

☺ *Fingernail and toenail infections caused by fungal organisms are a very common and stubborn problem. As a rule, toenail infections are especially difficult to cure. If not treated aggressively, these cosmetically undesirable infections can smolder for years.*

Currently three antifungal, oral medications are approved for nail infections, which doctors call onychomycosis. Fulvicin (griseofulvin) requires twenty-six weeks of treatment and, therefore, is not recommended. Sporanox (itraconazole) is used for about twelve weeks and can cost up to $950 for a course of therapy. Recently introduced, Lamisil (terbinafine) is used for six weeks ($240) for fingernail infections and twelve weeks for toenail infections ($480). All things considered, it's probably the drug that ought to be used first. But caution and careful consideration are required: All these medications can produce *significant* side effects and potentially serious drug interactions. The decision as to whether the risks and costs justify many weeks of treatment for an infection that is mainly cosmetic and can return must be made by you and your physician.

A number of topical preparations are used to treat psoriasis, including calcipotriene (Dovonex), etretinate, and the psoralens. The psoralens, which act as photosensitizers, reach the skin through the bloodstream and produce a sunburn-like injury. When the skin is exposed to ultraviolet light, the DNA of the skin cells is damaged. If sufficient cell injury occurs, an inflammatory reaction results, which is a prerequisite to healing psoriasis skin lesions. The most obvious symptom is skin redness, which may not begin for several hours and peaks at forty-eight to seventy-two hours. This inflammation is followed over several days to weeks by repair of the skin, which is seen as increased darkening and thickening of the skin layers. These drugs are used to control symptoms of severe and resistant disabling psoriasis that is not responsive to treatment with steroid creams. These medications should always be used under a physician's supervision and exactly as instructed. Methotrexate can produce a number of serious side effects but may be necessary in serious cases of psoriasis.

☞ *A number of antidandruff formulations are available, including Selsun Blue, Polytar, Head and Shoulders, and Ionil. These shampoos are used for the treatment not only of dandruff but of seborrheic dermatitis of the scalp and other skin conditions.*

Their ingredients include tar derivatives, benzocaine, resorcinol, and benzoic acid. Until re-cently, the most effective products included zinc pyrithione or selenium sulfide. We now suspect that dandruff is caused by overgrowth with a yeast (fungal) organism, called *Pityrosporum ovale*. As a result, Nizoral (2 percent ketoconazole) is probably the best medicated shampoo (available by prescription only) for this condition. You can consult the MedRANK Checklist "Dandruff" for comparisons and rankings of shampoos used to treat dandruff.

Although a number of preparations are available, most shampoos are used in a similar manner. You should massage the shampoo into a wet scalp and let it remain there for two or three minutes, followed by a thorough rinsing. You should repeat the application and then rinse thoroughly once again. As a rule, two applications per week for about two weeks will control most mild to moderate cases of seborrheic dermatitis or dandruff. Following these initial applications, you may use these antidandruff agents less frequently —weekly, every two weeks, or even every three to four weeks. Because minor irritation may occur, you should not apply them more frequently than is needed to maintain control. You should be aware that tar derivatives may stain the hair, skin, or fabrics. Finally, avoid contact with eyes and other sensitive areas.

☞ *Steroid creams are highly effective for a number of common skin disorders, including contact dermatitis, eczema, allergic rashes, and seborrheic dermatitis.*

Don't overuse these drugs, because they can cause drying of the skin and acnelike eruptions. For recommendations regarding use of topical steroid preparations, you will want to consult the MedRANK Checklist "More Than One Way to Skin the Fat" on page 164.

A number of topical anesthetics are available for minor skin disorders. Most of these ointments, creams, and gels contain some combination of Xylocaine, benzocaine, lidocaine, and other ingredients. It should be stressed that these drugs are for external use only and should not be used in or around the eyes. Moreover, they can impair your ability to swallow and increase the risk of choking, especially when eating or drinking. Always use the lowest dose possible that provides adequate pain relief. Stop therapy if irritation, rash, or other signs of inflammation develop. If your condition persists and/or fever develops, you should consult your physician.

☼ *Most burn preparations include substances that have anti-inflammatory and antibacterial properties. Among the most popular are mafenide (Sulfamylon) and silver sulfadiazine.*

These medications are usually applied once or twice daily to burned areas. If you are allergic to other sulfa drugs, you may react to silver sulfadiazine. Sunscreens with an SPF of 15 or greater are essential to protect against sun-induced skin cancers.

☼ *The emollients are a diverse group of chemicals. Most are available over the counter and are used to relieve itching and aid the healing of mild eczema, minor wounds, insect bites, and other skin irritations.*

Some are used for diaper rash and chafing. A number of diaper rash products are available, most of which contain some combination of an antimicrobial agent, an astringent, camphor, calcium carbonate, and kaolin. The topical analgesic cream capsaicin is used for temporary relief of pain from rheumatoid arthritis, osteoarthritis, and painful diabetic neuropathy or following shingles. The drug is recommended for external use only, and the onset of relief may take several weeks. Capsaicin is a natural chemical derived from plants; it is believed that it causes the skin to become insensitive to pain by removing pain-transmitting compounds from the nerve endings. The active ingredient is also found in red chili peppers.

☼ *Minoxidil (Rogaine) is a topical solution used to promote hair growth in individuals with male pattern baldness and thinning of the hair. This medication is approved for similar use in women.*

Not all patients respond to this product, although those who do report satisfactory results in a significant percentage of cases. It is important to emphasize that at least four months of continuous use are usually required before you will see evidence of hair growth. Further growth can continue throughout the first year of treatment, even though this new hair growth is not permanent. If you stop treatment with minoxidil, you can expect hair loss to occur within a few months. Be aware that accidental oral ingestion of this medication can produce significant side effects.

A wide number of anorectal and perianal hygiene products are available, most of which are used to treat symptoms associated with hemorrhoids and other inflammatory conditions. No single product appears to be significantly better than any other. Many components are contained in these products, including hydrocortisone, local anesthetics, astringents, antiseptics, and other protectants. You should always follow the manufacturer's instructions to achieve the best results.

Finally, many topical and oral medications can produce skin reactions, including rashes and pigmentation changes. Please consult the MedRANK Checklist "Medications That Can Cause Photosensitivity Reactions" on page 170 for a comprehensive list of such drugs.

MORE THAN ONE WAY TO SKIN THE FAT
Creams and Medications for Acne

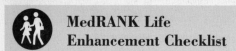

MedRANK Life Enhancement Checklist

Pills and Lotions of Wisdom: Acne is a common disease that affects between 50 and 90 percent of adolescents in the United States. It is caused by a rather complex interaction between chemical factors that affect skin structures and sebaceous follicles and the bacterium *Propionibacterium acnes*, which has been implicated as the causative organism in most cases. The initial approach is to eliminate medications known to cause acne. These include steroids, androgens, and certain birth control pills containing androgenic progestins such as norethindrone and norgestrel. No foods have convincingly been shown to produce acne, and therefore dietary changes are *not* required.

From a practical and treatment perspective, acne is sometimes divided into two categories, obstructive and inflammatory. Obstructive acne is characterized by comedones, which are more commonly referred to as whiteheads (closed comedones) or blackheads (open comedones). Whiteheads and blackheads contain fatty substances and enzymes. When comedones leak their contents into the surrounding skin, they produce an inflammatory reaction, which produces the red, raised pus-filled lesions characteristic of acne. These pustules can produce enough inflammation to cause permanent scarring.

The best approach to acne will depend on whether comedones are present, the severity of the inflammation, and the type of skin lesions. Except for antibiotics, which are taken by mouth in cases of severe, disfiguring acne, most acne treatment plans include medications such as Retin-A or Azelex to eradicate comedones, in combination with other medications that kill the bacteria responsible for inflammatory skin lesions.

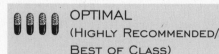

OPTIMAL
(HIGHLY RECOMMENDED/ BEST OF CLASS)

Retin-A (tretinoin, 0.25% gel)

Retin-A is the optimal agent for people with acne that is characterized primarily by whiteheads and blackheads. It helps remove existing comedones and prevents development of future ones. The 0.25 percent gel is well tolerated by most people, but this skin medication *can* produce a *temporary flare-up* of inflammation shortly after it is started. It also increases the risk for sunburn. Retin-A is generally used once daily for several weeks.

Azelex (azelaic acid, 20% cream)

This drug is as effective as benzoyl peroxide or tretinoin, but appears to be *less* irritating to the skin. In fact, the burning, stinging, and redness seen with other acne creams and gels occurs in only a small percentage of people who use Azelex. Like benzoyl peroxide and topical antibiotics, Azelex stops the growth of *Propionibacterium acnes.*

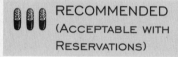

RECOMMENDED
(ACCEPTABLE WITH RESERVATIONS)

Benzoyl Peroxide (generic, 2.5% gel)

Because Azelex (see "Optimal") may have fewer side effects, it is preferred over benzoyl peroxide.

Emgel (2% erythromycin gel)
Erycette (2% erythromycin solution)
T-Stat (2% erythromycin solution)

These antibiotic solutions are used for mild inflammatory acne. They prevent development of new acne pustules but do nothing for current lesions. Consequently, it may take weeks to see results with these antibiotics, which should be *combined* with Retin-A, Azelex, and other forms of therapy.

Doxycycline

With its twice-daily dosing schedule, this may be the most convenient oral antibiotic for acne.

DISCOURAGED FOR INITIAL USE
(BUT MAY BE REQUIRED IN SELECTED PEOPLE)

Erythromycin

This oral antibiotic may be required for severe cases of acne. It can cause gastrointestinal side effects—like nausea and cramping—and its four-times-per-day dosing schedule is not convenient. Oral antibiotics prevent the development of new acne lesions, and therefore it may take six to eight weeks before you know whether you are responding to this form of therapy.

Tetracycline

With four-times-per-day dosing, tetracycline is inconvenient for adolescent lifestyles.

Metronidazole gel

This drug appears to work, but other medications are more established. This drug kills the bacteria responsible for acne. Common side effects include skin irritation, which can be accompanied by redness, stinging, dryness, burning, and allergic reactions.

Spironolactone

This drug is an anti-androgen, and is sometimes used in women with severe acne that has *not* responded to other treatments.

Meclan (meclocycline)

This topical cream gives off a foul sulfurous odor when first applied to the skin.

AVOID IF POSSIBLE
(NOT RECOMMENDED)

Accutane (isotretinoin)

This powerful drug is used for people with very severe cases of acne. One or two fifteen-to-twenty-week courses can bring very bad cases under complete control. But you should be aware that the Academy of Dermatology states that Accutane should never be the initial treatment of acne. Use this drug *only* if your acne has not responded to more standard therapies.

Accutane is a potent teratogen and has caused a number of devastating birth defects. There are very strict guidelines for using it, including a detailed patient consent form, proof of a negative pregnancy test, constant monitoring for pregnancy, and contraceptive use.

Many other side effects are associated with Accutane, most of which are reversible after the medication is stopped.

APPROACHES TO BALDNESS

MedRANK Life Enhancement Checklist

Pills and Lotions of Wisdom: Male pattern baldness is a common condition that can compromise the self-confidence and self-image of young men. The therapeutic arsenal for this condition is limited to Rogaine 2 percent topical solution (minoxidil), which can work in a significant percentage of patients. Men who are most likely to benefit from Rogaine include those under 40 who have been bald for less than ten years and have a balding area that is no larger than 4 inches in diameter. If you are patient and do not expect dramatic results, this topical medication may produce satisfactory results. But you will not see immediate results. Six months of treatment may be required before hair growth is apparent. In addition, new hair growth will continue only if you continue the twice-daily applications.

OPTIMAL
(HIGHLY RECOMMENDED/ BEST OF CLASS)

Propecia (finasteride)

This drug, also used to treat symptoms caused by an enlarged prostate gland, is currently the most effective medication available for male pattern baldness. It is a safe drug, but it should be noted that a small but notable percentage of men taking Propecia will experience decreased libido, impotence, or decreased volume of ejaculate.

RECOMMENDED
(ACCEPTABLE WITH RESERVATIONS)

Rogaine (minoxidil)

Rogaine will work for some people and not for others. The hair growth it produces tends to peak after one year of treatment. After five years, hair growth is still maintained above the original levels. Some users feel that Rogaine prevents the progression of their baldness, but this is difficult to confirm. The only side effect is scalp irritation.

Retin-A (tretinoin)
There is anectodal evidence to suggest that the application of Retin-A to the scalp several minutes before Rogaine is applied may enhance its effectiveness for male baldness.

SOLUTIONS FOR DANDRUFF

 MedRANK Life Enhancement Checklist

 Pills of Wisdom: Our understanding of what causes dandruff has changed over the past few years. It is now thought that dandruff represents an inflammatory reaction in reponse to the yeast (fungal) organism Pityrosporum ovale. Medications that inhibit its growth have been shown to reduce the redness, scaling, and flaking associated with dandruff. Issues of treatment boil down to cost and convenience. Although many shampoos work, Nizoral (2% ketoconazole) produces excellent results and has the advantage of only once-weekly use for dandruff prevention. This antifungal shampoo is as effective as any other approach and is very well tolerated.

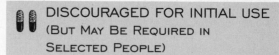 OPTIMAL
(HIGHLY RECOMMENDED/ BEST OF CLASS)

Nizoral (2% ketoconazole)
This antidandruff shampoo produces excellent results and has the advantage of once-weekly use. But it's the most expensive approach to dandruff. Initially, it should be used twice weekly for a few weeks, and intermittently thereafter.

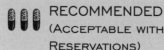 RECOMMENDED
(ACCEPTABLE WITH RESERVATIONS)

Head and Shoulders (1% zinc pyrithione)
Zincon (zinc pyrithione)
Head and Shoulders Intensive Treatment
The active ingredient is effective and well tolerated, and the products are reasonably priced.

Selsun Blue (1% selenium sulfide)
Selsun (2.5% selenium sulfide)
Selenium sulfide 2.5% (generic)
Selenium sulfide can irritate the scalp and discolor the hair.

DISCOURAGED FOR INITIAL USE
(BUT MAY BE REQUIRED IN SELECTED PEOPLE)

Tegrin (1.5% crude coal tar)
This product can irritate the scalp and may cause an unpleasant odor.

STEROID CREAMS AND OINTMENTS FOR ITCHING, DERMATITIS, MILD PSORIASIS, AND ECZEMA

 MedRANK Life Enhancement Checklist

Pills and Lotions of Wisdom: Many skin conditions respond to steroid creams. As a result, steroid creams are probably the most useful topical preparation you can have in your home medicine cabinet. Low-strength creams, such as 1% hydrocortisone, are now available without prescription and can be used for a wide range of conditions, including itching, redness, and scaling caused by eczema, dermatitis, seborrheic dermatitis, and psoriasis.

As a rule, these skin conditions produce red scaly patches on the skin and may be accompanied by itching and thickening of the skin. Topical steroids will reduce the itching, redness, and scaling. The key to steroid creams is to use the least potent preparation that will get the job done. They vary widely in potency; the strongest steroid is five hundred times stronger than the weakest. Generally speaking, you will want to start with a topical steroid that is powerful enough to control the skin condition, then switch to a less potent one (such as 1% hydrocortisone) for maintenance purposes. The sooner you switch to a less potent preparation, the better.

These products are available as solutions, ointments, and creams. As a rule, ointment formulations are more potent than creams and will work best for thick, scaling skin problems. Cream formulations are less greasy and, from a cosmetic point of view, will produce the best results for skin problems on the face. Gels and lotions are more drying than creams. Steroid creams are sometimes prescribed for application two to four times per day, but more often than not, one or two applications will be enough.

The long-term side effects of the more potent steroid creams include drying and atrophy of the skin, acnelike eruptions, and skin discoloration. Using lower-potency steroid creams reduces the risk of cosmetically undesirable side effects. Contact with eyes and the eyelids should be avoided, and superpotent creams should not be used on the face. You should avoid contact with fabrics, chemicals, or other substances known to cause your skin eruptions.

If itching is a prominent part of your problem, you may benefit from an oral antihistamine, such as Zyrtec. Finally, if your skin eruption is severe and extensive, as might be the case with poison ivy, you will achieve rapid, definitive relief by taking oral steroid medications (prednisone) for a period of ten to fourteen days.

STRENGTH OF STEROID CREAMS AND OINTMENTS

WEAKEST

Hytone cream 1.0%
Hytone cream 2.5%
Hytone lotion 1.0%
Hytone lotion 2.5%
Hytone ointment 1.0%
Hytone ointment 2.5%
Hydrocortisone

Pramosone cream 1.0%
Pramosone cream 2.5%
Pramosone lotion 1.0%
Pramosone lotion 2.5%
Pramosone ointment 1.0%
Pramosone ointment 2.5%
Hydrocortisone acetate and
pramoxine HCl 1%

WEAK

Aclovate cream 0.05%
Aclovate ointment 0.05%
Alclometasone dipropionate

Aristocort cream 0.1%
Triamcinolone acetonide

Kenalog cream 0.025%
Kenalog lotion 0.025%
Triamcinolone acetonide

Locoid solution 0.1%
Hydrocortisone butyrate

Locorten cream 0.03%
Flumethasone pivalate

Synalar cream 0.01%
Synalar solution 0.01%
Fluocinolone acetonide

Tridesilon cream 0.05%
Desonide

MODERATELY STRONG

Cordran cream 0.05%
Kenalog lotion 0.1%
Kenalog ointment 0.025%
Flurandrenolide
Triamcinolone acetonide

Locoid cream 0.1%
Locoid ointment 0.1%
Hydrocortisone butyrate

Synalar cream 0.025%
Fluocinolone acetonide

Tridesilon ointment 0.05%
Desonide

Valisone cream 0.1%
Valisone lotion 0.1%
Betamethasone valerate

Westcort cream 0.2%
Westcort ointment 0.2%
Hydrocortisone valerate

STRONG

Aristocort ointment 0.1%
Triamcinolone acetonide

Cordran ointment 0.05%
Flurandrenolide

Elocon cream 0.1%
Elocon lotion 0.1%
Mometasone furoate

Kenalog cream 0.1%
Kenalog ointment 0.1%
Triamcinolone acetonide

Synalar ointment 0.025%
Fluocinolone acetonide

Topicort LP cream 0.05%
Desoximetasone

STRONGER

Aristocort A ointment 0.1%
Triamcinolone acetonide

Cyclocort cream 0.1%
Cyclocort lotion 0.1%
Amcinonide

Diprosone cream 0.05%
Betamethasone dipropionate

Florone cream 0.05%
Diflorasone diacetate

Lidex E cream 0.05%
Fluocinonide

Maxiflor cream 0.05%
Diflorasone diacetate

Maxivate lotion 0.05%
Betamethasone dipropionate

Valisone ointment 0.1%
Betamethasone valerate

VERY STRONG

Cyclocort ointment 0.1%
Amcinonide

Diprosone ointment 0.05%
Betamethasone dipropionate

Elocon ointment 0.1%
Mometasone furoate

Florone ointment 0.05%
Diflorasone diacetate

Halog cream 0.1%
Halog ointment 0.1%
Halog solution 0.1%
Halcinonide

Lidex cream 0.05%
Lidex gel 0.05%
Lidex ointment 0.05%
Lidex solution 0.05%
Fluocinonide

Maxiflor ointment 0.05%
Diflorasone diacetate

Maxivate cream 0.05%
Maxivate ointment 0.05%
Betamethasone dipropionate

Topicort cream 0.25%
Topicort gel 0.05%
Topicort ointment 0.25%
Desoximetasone

STRONGEST

Temovate cream 0.05%
Temovate ointment 0.05%
Clobetasol propionate

Diprolene ointment 0.05%
Diprolene AF cream 0.05%
Betamethasone dipropionate

Psorcon ointment 0.05%
Diflorasone diacetate

Ultravate cream 0.05%
Ultravate cream 0.05%
Halobetasol propionate

MEDICATIONS THAT CAN CAUSE PHOTOSENSITIVITY REACTIONS

MedRANK Side Effect and Warning Checklist

Pills of Wisdom: As the weather becomes warmer and people spend more time outside in the sun, the risk of skin reactions associated with medication use increases. Drug-related skin rashes, which are called photosensitivity reactions, can be due to a number of topical preparations, oral medications, cosmetics, perfumes, and sunscreens. Some of these reactions can persist for weeks, even after the medication is discontinued.

This MedRANK Checklist contains the drugs most commonly implicated in photosensitivity reactions. If you are taking one of them and develop a skin rash, you should notify your physician.

ANTIBIOTICS

Achromycin (tetracycline)
Ancobon (flucytosine)
Cipro (ciprofloxacin)
Dapsone
Declomycin (demeclocycline)
Floxin (ofloxacin)
Fulvicin-U/F (griseofulvin)
Lamprene (clofazimine)
Maxaquin (lomefloxacin)
Minocin (minocycline)
NegGram (nalidixic acid)
Noroxin (norfloxacin)
Penetrex (enoxacin)
Proloprim (trimethoprim)

Pyrazinamide
Sulfonamides
Terramycin (oxytetracycline)
Vibramycin (doxycycline)

ANTIDEPRESSANTS

Adapin (doxepin)
Anafranil (clomipramine)
Asendin (amoxapine)
Aventyl (nortriptyline)
Desyrel (trazodone)
Elavil (amitriptyline)
Ludiomil (maprotiline)
Nardil (phenelzine)
Norpramin (desipramine)
Surmontil (trimipramine)
Tofranil (imipramine)
Vivactil (protriptyline)

ANTIHISTAMINES

Benadryl (diphenhydramine)
Periactin (cyproheptadine)

ANTIHYPERTENSIVE DRUGS

Aldomet (methyldopa)
Capoten (captopril)
Cardizem (diltiazem)
Loniten (minoxidil)
Procardia (nifedipine)

ANTIPARASITIC DRUGS

Aralen (chloroquine)
Mintezol (thiabendazole)
Quinine

ANTIPSYCHOTIC DRUGS

Compazine (prochlorperazine)
Haldol (haloperidol)
Mellaril (thioridazine)
Navane (thiothixene)
Permitil (fluphenazine)
Stelazine (trifluoperazine)
Thorazine (chlorpromazine)
Trilafon (perphenazine)
Vesprin (triflupromazine)

CANCER DRUGS

DTIC-Dome (dacarbazine)
Eulexin (flutamide)
Fluoroplex (fluorouracil)
Folex (methotrexate)
Velban (vinblastine)

DIABETES MEDICATIONS

DiaBeta (glyburide)
Diabinese (chlorpropamide)
Dymelor (acetohexamide)
Glucotrol (glipizide)
Orinase (tolbutamide)
Tolinase (tolazamide)

DIURETICS ("WATER PILLS")

Aquatensen (methyclothiazide)
Diamox (acetazolamide)
Diucardin, Saluron (hydroflumethiazide)
Diuril (chlorothiazide)
Dyrenium (triamterene)
Exna (benzthiazide)
HydroDIURIL (hydrochlorothiazide)
Lasix (furosemide)

Metahydrin (trichlormethiazide)
Midamor (amiloride)
Mykrox, Zaroxolyn (metolazone)
Naturetin (bendroflumethiazide)
Renese (polythiazide)

NONSTEROIDAL ANTI-INFLAMMATORY DRUGS (NSAIDS)

Butazolidin (phenylbutazone)
Clinoril (sulindac)
Dolobid (diflunisal)
Feldene (piroxicam)
Indocin (indomethacin)
Motrin (ibuprofen)
Naprosyn (naproxen)
Orudis (ketoprofen)
Relafen (nabumetone)

SUNSCREENS

Bain du Soleil; Solbar (benzophenones)
Bull Frog; Coppertone (cinnamates)
Coppertone, Tropical Blend (homosalate)
Hawaiian Tropic; Neutrogena (menthyl anthranilate)
PABA-405 Solar Cream (aminobenzoic acid)
Photoplex; Shade UVAGuard (avobenzone)
Tropical Blend; Presun (PABA enters)

OTHERS

Accutane (isotretinoin)
Atromid-S (clofibrate)
Benzocaine
Citrus rind oils
Cordarone (amiodarone)
Fluorescite (fluorescein)
Librium (chlordiazepoxide)
Myochrysine (gold salts)
Norpace (disopyramide)
Oral contraceptives
Oxy 10 (benzoyl peroxide)
Perfumes, shaving lotions, cosmetics, and Sunscreens (6-methylcoumarin)
Perfumes (musk ambrette)
Phenergan (promethazine)
PhisoHex (hexachlorophene)
Quinidine sulfate and gluconate
Retin-A (tretinoin)
Symmetrel (amantadine)
Tegison (etretinate)
Tegretol (carbamazepine)
Temaril (trimeprazine)
Topicort (desoximetasone)
Xanax (alprazolam)

CHAPTER 11

IT'S IN YOUR HEAD

Medications for Stroke, Alzheimer's Disease, Parkinson's Disease, Epilepsy, MS, and Migraine Headaches

"I have a history of stroke in my family," a worried, elderly woman offers during a routine office visit. "Are there any new medications that will prevent me from having one?" Neurological problems such as Alzheimer's disease, Parkinson's disease, stroke, and multiple sclerosis can be devastating for both patients and their families. It is no wonder that so many people have called me, over the years, whenever they read about a new treatment for one of these disabling diseases. They were desperate for something that would treat the disabling pain of recurrent migraine headaches, that would slow the deteriorating visual function caused by multiple sclerosis, or that would improve the memory and cognitive function of a parent with Alzheimer's disease.

For so long, pharmacological therapy for most neurological problems was woefully inadequate. In many cases, all a doctor could do was diagnose the condition and then watch the patient's status decline over time. All of this is changing now. Drug therapy for neuro-logical problems is advancing at a rapid pace, and significant new developments have been made for multiple sclerosis, Parkinson's, Alzheimer's, and migraine headaches.

☺ *Stroke is the third-leading cause of death in the United States and is a major cause of disability in the older population. Although drug therapy and surgical treatments are improving, prevention is still the most effective approach.*

The cornerstone of prevention is to identify risk factors known to cause stroke and to treat them aggressively. These risk factors include high blood pressure, heart disease (including heart attacks), smoking, diabetes, and, possibly, elevated cholesterol levels. All of these conditions depend heavily on medications for both prevention and treatment.

Where should you start? You and your doctor should pay meticulous attention to controlling your blood pressure (see Chapter

6) and identifying medications known to reduce your risk for heart disease (see Chapter 5). Among others, the best pills include aspirin, estrogen, beta-blockers (Tenormin), and cholesterol-lowering medications (Lipitor, Pravachol, and Zocor). Your chances of quitting smoking are improved with nicotine patches (see Chapter 21).

☺ *To maximize the benefits of treating stroke risk factors, you should consult the MedRANK Checklists in Chapters 5, 6, and 21, which rate the best pills for heart disease, cholesterol, high blood pressure, and smoking cessation.*

One major risk factor for stroke is an irregular heart rhythm called atrial fibrillation. It is seen in a small but significant percentage of older people with heart disease after the age of 65. In this rhythm disturbance, the small chambers (atria) of the heart start to beat very fast and irregularly (fibrillation), which can cause blood clots to develop in the wall of the heart. Suddenly, and in an unpredictable fashion, these clots can be dislodged from the heart chamber and travel through the bloodstream to the brain, where they can get "stuck" in a major blood vessel. This cuts off the supply of oxygen to brain tissues and causes a devastating stroke. Unfortunately, in most people, atrial fibrillation is a permanent condition. The good news is, blood-thinning medications are available that will reduce the risk of blood clots from developing in the heart and therefore lower the likelihood of having a stroke.

☺ *The most effective medication for preventing stroke and prolonging life in people with atrial fibrillation is Coumadin (warfarin). If you have been diagnosed with this heart rhythm problem and are not on Coumadin, you should call your doctor and inquire whether you might be a suitable candidate for this medication.*

It can reduce your risk of having a stroke by as much as 45 percent. The main side effect of Coumadin is excessive bleeding, a problem that, to a great extent, can be prevented by carefully monitoring your clotting time with blood tests. If your doctor determines that Coumadin is too risky for you, the next best approach is aspirin therapy, which should be used at a dose of at least 325 mg/day (one full-strength adult tablet), or Ticlid, a drug that prevents clotting. Other medications, such as Persantine, have not been shown to be effective for this problem.

What if you already have had a major or minor stroke and want to protect yourself from additional problems down the road? Frankly, the best approach for preventing subsequent strokes is not entirely clear. To a great extent, prevention depends on whether your stroke symptoms have been caused by significant buildup of plaque in your carotid arteries, which are the main blood vessels supplying the brain. If previous or recurrent strokes are your problem and you are relatively young (less than 70 years of age) and a good candidate for surgery, and your hospital has an excellent team of vascular surgeons, you could probably benefit from an operation called carotid endarterectomy. In this procedure, a neurosurgeon or vascular specialist "cleans up" deposits in your carotid arteries and widens the passages so that blood may flow more freely. This lowers the risk of little clots and deposits dislodging and flowing upstream and cutting off the blood supply to vital brain structures.

☺ *Some people are not good surgical candidates, which usually means they have other conditions that place them at high risk for surgical complications. If you are elderly, or have had only one remote episode of a minor stroke, or your carotid arteries are not sufficiently narrowed or damaged to warrant surgery, your best option for stroke prevention is either aspirin or Ticlid (ticlopidine).*

If your symptoms were mild and disappeared rapidly—this is called a transient ischemic attack, or TIA—aspirin, which prevents clots from developing, is inexpensive and relatively safe. The exact dose is controversial, but between 30 and 325 milligrams per day is the dosage that most physicians recommend. You may use ticlopidine if you are intolerant or allergic to aspirin for one reason or another, are a woman who has had a TIA, or have had a stroke in the past. But ticlopidine has worrisome side effects. It can increase your blood cholesterol, and rarely—sometime between three weeks and three months after starting the medication—it can lower your white blood cell count to dangerously low levels. Consequently, if your doctor puts you on this medication, you should have your blood counts checked every two weeks for the first three months of treatment.

☺ *Alzheimer's Disease. "My mother was just diagnosed with Alzheimer's, and she's starting to lose her memory," explains a concerned daughter. "Are there any medications that will keep her from going downhill?"*

Alzheimer's disease, the most common cause of what is called dementia, affects almost 2.5 million people over the age of 65 in the United States and Canada. Although there are no *cures* on the near horizon, help is on the way. Currently, two medications (Aricept and Cognex) have been approved by the FDA for the treatment of mild to moderate symptoms associated with Alzheimer's disease. From a medication standpoint, the key to prolonging cognitive function—memory, thinking, and orientation—in people with Alzheimer's is to diagnose the condition as early as possible and to begin the patient on drug therapy promptly.

☺ *Of the two drugs available, Aricept is clearly the pill of choice. It is given only once a day, is relatively safe, and produces cognitive improvement or delays deterioration in mental function in up to 68 percent of people with mild to moderate symptoms of Alzheimer's.*

Unfortunately, it is impossible to predict which patients will respond to this drug, so some trial and error is involved. The other approved drug, Cognex, is *not* recommended as initial treatment inasmuch as high doses of it are required, the patient has to take three pills per day, and long-term monitoring of liver function is required. To maximize the benefits you can get from Aricept and understand how the drug works, you will want to refer to the MedRANK Checklist "Pills for Improving Cognitive Function in Early Alzheimer's Disease" on page 178. If a family member has more advanced Alzheimer's, Aricept may produce little if any improvement. At this later stage of the game, many patients develop behavioral problems—including agitation and aggressive behavior—and require treatment with a number of drugs, including antipsychotic medications and, possibly, tranquilizers. See the MedRANK Checklist "Drugs for Managing Behavioral Problems in Alzheimer's Disease" on page 180.

☺ *Headaches are a common problem. The majority are related to chronic, recurrent conditions for which excellent medications are available.*

Tension-type headaches respond to Tylenol or nonsteroidal anti-inflammatory drugs (NSAIDs) such as Aleve, Motrin, or Advil. A small percentage of headaches are caused by serious, life-threatening problems such as brain tumors, bleeding strokes, and infection. Migraine headaches are especially painful and are frequently accompanied by nausea, vomiting, and pain. They frequently begin with an "aura," or "prodrome," consisting of blind spots, flashing lights, and other sensations, although many people with migraine headaches do not have these "classical" warning signs. They are followed by a full-blown headache within 20 to 30 minutes. The headache can last from minutes to hours, and sometimes waxes and wanes over a pe-

riod of days. The exact cause of migraine headaches is still unclear, but sudden relaxation of brain vessels is likely.

☺ *When it comes to treating migraine, it is important to distinguish between pills that work only during the warning phase and are able to nip the headache in the bud, and those that can relieve symptoms even* after *the headache has started.*

Ergotamine tartrate–containing compounds such as Cafergot have been used to *prevent* migraine headaches; generally speaking, they are most successful if taken at the first sign of a migraine attack. If you wait too long, they won't help. Depending upon the nature of your migraine syndrome, this usually means taking Cafergot as soon as you notice flashing lights, blind spots, or flickering objects. These drugs work by reducing the pulsation and relaxation of blood vessels in the brain.

Unfortunately, abuse and dependence may result from long-term use, and these drugs can have unpleasant side effects. In contrast, the drug Imitrex (sumatriptan) is intended for the *treatment* of migraine headaches. It is very effective even during the headache phase. If you are having recurrent migraines that interefere with your daily activities, you will need to be on a medication that offers long-term prevention. The best choices are Inderal, Blocadren, and Calan SR. See the MedRANK Checklists "Migraine Headaches" and "Migraine Headache Prevention" on pages 189 and 191 for comparisons and recommendations.

☺ *Multiple Sclerosis. The source of considerable disability, multiple sclerosis (MS) is a common condition affecting about one in every thousand adults.*

Its symptoms are caused by the progressive destruction of the coverings—called myelin—of nerve fibers in the brain. The gradual erosion of these myelin sheaths is thought to be caused by a number of factors, including genetic predisposition, environmental exposure, and problems with the immune system. Current thinking is that in people with MS the body's immune system inappropriately attacks its own nerve sheaths, in what is called an autoimmune reaction. Much as the fraying of an electrical cord can create short-circuits, nerve impulses to and from the brain are compromised as the myelin deteriorates. This leads to a variety of symptoms, from visual disturbances and tremor to movement problems and urinary complaints. Patients with MS usually have waxing and waning symptoms, but the disease usually progresses over time. When the symptoms peak in severity, this is called an "acute attack" of MS.

☺ *A number of medications are used to treat MS. The best for acute attacks are intravenous steroids, at high doses for three days. This approach is preferred over oral steroids alone.*

Treating MS patients whose symptoms are rapidly progressive can be a problem. The use of cyclophosphamide and ACTH can produce short-term improvement of symptoms.

Clearly, the most important advances are in the area of injectable drugs, which are valuable for patients who have multiple relapses and progressive symptoms. Avonex is considered to be the medication of choice. The most recent medication approved for MS is Copaxone. Although the precise action of the drug is not known, it is thought to work by causing the body's immune system to attack the drug itself rather than the myelin on the nerve cells. MS medications should be prescribed by neurologists who have experience treating people with this condition.

☺ *Nausea, Dizziness, and Motion Sickness. A wide range of medications are available to treat nausea, dizziness, and motion sickness, including Dramamine, Antivert, scopolamine, and Tigan.*

Generally speaking, these drugs act on the central nervous system and are called anticholinergics. Although they are very effective for controlling symptoms associated with nausea and vomiting, it is important that your physician determine the underlying cause of your symptoms before prescribing a medication from this class. Although these drugs are fairly well tolerated, you can expect side effects associated with their anticholinergic properties. These include drowsiness, excitation (especially in children), difficult urination, and dry mouth. Accordingly, these drugs should be used cautiously if you plan to drive a car or perform other tasks requiring mental alertness.

PILLS FOR IMPROVING COGNITIVE FUNCTION IN EARLY ALZHEIMER'S DISEASE

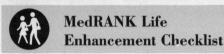

MedRANK Life Enhancement Checklist

Pills of Wisdom: There currently is no known cure for Alzheimer's disease. However, current theories about this condition attribute many of the thought and memory disorders seen in Alzheimer patients to a deficiency in transmission of acetylcholine, a neurotransmitter. Medications that can increase the amount of acetylcholine in brain synapses have been shown to improve cognitive function and memory, as well as behavioral activities related to daily living, in patients with Alzheimer's dementia.

The first drug approved for this purpose, Cognex (tacrine), showed a modest but statistically significant reduction in the mental deterioration of patients with mild to moderate Alzheimer's. Unfortunately, the drug required multiple daily administrations and monitoring of liver function, and it produced a number of side effects. As a result, it was *not* widely accepted as an important advance in treatment.

Aricept (donepezil hydrochloride) is a new medication that appears to offer significant promise for patients who are in the *early* stages of their disease. (It must be emphasized that this drug is not very effective in patients with advanced AD.) It increases the amount of acetylcholine available for nerve transmission by inhibiting the enzyme (acetylcholinesterase) that would normally break down acetylcholine in the brain synapses. In essence, it permits more acetylcholine to "hang around" in the brain synapses for longer periods and thereby compensate for the depletion of acetylcholine-producing enzymes that accompanies Alzheimer's disease. It is a safe medication with convenient once-daily dosing.

Loosely speaking, you can see Aricept as sort of an "STP" for the brain. It doesn't change the underlying loss of neurons, but it does enhance and augment the neurotransmitters that are still available. It is designed to improve memory and thinking during the early and middle phases of AD. It has a much different purpose from medications used to manage the behavioral problems—agitation, disorientation, shouting, and confusion—seen in patients with the advanced disease, which are discussed in the MedRANK Checklist "Drugs for Managing Behavioral Problems in Alzheimer's Disease" on page 180.

The most important issue regarding the use of Aricept is timing. This medication is very time-sensitive, which means its benefits are maximized if the medication is given *as soon as possible* after the diagnosis of AD is made. It is designed to keep people functioning at quality levels and to slow deterioration during the early phases of the illness. This means that if you know an adult with complaints of memory loss, confusion, disorientation, unexplained depression, or loss of spatial orientation in public places, you should seek a medical evaluation for them promptly. Your suspicion of AD should be increased if there is a family history of this disease, which is known to have a genetic basis.

Although Aricept doesn't produce dramatic improvements in *all* people who take the drug, the improvements are *impressive enough* in a significant percentage of people to make this drug a centerpiece of the initial treatment program. Consequently, if the diagnosis is strongly suspected, then Aricept should be started *without delay*. Even if the beneficial effects last only a year or two, the ability to function productively in a family setting for this length of time is more than worth the price. Such psychosocial intervention also has been shown to delay institutionalization.

Remember, the reponse people with Alzheimer's

disease will have to medications can be unpredictable. It's almost always best to begin with low doses and, if one drug is not successful, to discontinue it and try another. If these medications produce side effects of excessive drowsiness, withdrawal, or mental confusion, notify the patient's physician and request an adjustment in dose or, perhaps, a less potent medication.

 OPTIMAL
(HIGHLY RECOMMENDED/
BEST OF CLASS)

Aricept (donepezil hydrochloride)

This time-sensitive medication is best started as soon as the diagnosis of Alzheimer's is made. Best results are seen in people who have mild to moderate dementia of the AD type.

The principal side effects are nausea, diarrhea, and vomiting, but they occur in less than 10 percent of patients. Not all people respond to this drug. Overall, however, about 60 percent of users show some improvement. Those who do respond think better, remember better, and function better than they would have without this medication. There are two doses of the drug, a 5 mg and a 10 mg tablet. The improvement people experience is similar at both dosage strengths, although a few more people respond to the 10 mg tablet than to the lower dose.

In the best-case scenario, with Aricept you can expect a slight to moderate improvement in thinking and memory capacity and a marked slowing in cognitive deterioration for, perhaps, six months to two years. There is not enough experience to know what effects, if any, the drug has beyond that window, but

some people may continue to respond, especially if their disease is not progressing too rapidly. Most people started on Aricept show deterioration if the drug is *discontinued.*

The drug is well tolerated, and few people have to stop therapy. Diarrhea, nausea, and vomiting are the main side effects, but these are usually not severe enough to cause discontinuation.

 RECOMMENDED
(ACCEPTABLE WITH
RESERVATIONS)

Prempro (estrogen and progesterone)
Premarin (estrogen)

There is mounting evidence that women who begin estrogen replacement therapy with menopause may delay the onset of symptoms of Alzheimer's disease. The mechanism for this is unknown, and further studies are required to substantiate this suggestion. But women with a family history of AD should be encouraged to begin hormone replacement, if qualified, in order to take advantage of these possible benefits.

 DISCOURAGED FOR INITIAL USE
(BUT MAY BE REQUIRED IN
SELECTED PEOPLE)

NSAIDs (nonsteroidal anti-inflammatory drugs)

This is a very interesting and *controversial* approach. Considerable evidence suggests that inflammation in the brain plays a prominent role in the nerve degeneration seen in Alzheimer's. The theory that NSAIDs may confer some protection against AD is borne out by the finding of unexpectedly low rates of this disease in people with rheumatoid arthritis, a condition in which NSAIDs are used as a first-line therapy. The use of NSAIDs, or steroids such as prednisone, in patients with AD is *speculative* at this point. Moreover, it should be stressed that NSAIDs can produce many side effects, including life-threatening ulcers and bleeding, in the elderly. Consequently, its benefits may not outweigh the risks. *More information is needed.*

Deprenyl (selegiline)

This antioxidant drug, which has been shown to be effective in preventing deterioration in patients with Parkinson's disease, is currently being evaluated by the National Insititue on Aging and Alzheimer's Disease, to see whether it can retard mental decline in patients with AD.

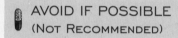

AVOID IF POSSIBLE (NOT RECOMMENDED)

Cognex (tacrine)

Prior to the availability of Aricept, Cognex was the only acetylcholinesterase inhibitor approved for people with AD. There are few, if any, good reasons for using this drug now that Aricept is available. Cognex requires monitoring of liver function tests, it has to be given three times daily, and it produces side effects in a significant percentage of patients. It is unlikely that people who fail to respond to Aricept will respond to Cognex.

Hydergine

This drug has no known benefit in AD.

Persantine

This antiplatelet medication has no known benefit in AD.

Vitamins and Nutritional Supplements

These products have no known benefit in AD.

DRUGS FOR MANAGING BEHAVIORAL PROBLEMS IN ALZHEIMER'S DISEASE*

MedRANK Life Enhancement Checklist

Pills of Wisdom: During later stages of Alzheimer's disease, many people—who by this time may be cared for in an institutional or foster home set-

ting—develop agitation, confusion, disorientation, and related behavioral disturbances. Behavioral disturbances occur in over 90 percent of people with AD, which is the most common cause of psychiatric disease associated with a specific neurological problem. The behavioral problems range from shouting and anger to agitation and sexual assault and can cause tremendous

---

* Behavioral control in patients with Alzheimer's is a tricky and controversial area. In general, medications should be used only if the patient is a potential harm to other individuals or to themselves. Before medications are started, it is important that your physician exclude other causes for the confusion and agitation, which, among other things, can be caused by other medications—or withdrawal from drugs.

distress for patients and their families. If their behaviorial problems are potentially harmful to themselves or others, they usually will need to be treated with medications. Unfortunately, there are no Optimal drugs for managing these problems, and experts disagree on the advantages of one class of drugs over another.

Before using medications, the first step is to evaluate possible environmental factors that may trigger agitation and psychotic episodes. Does the patient have a combative roommate, or is the room too hot or noisy? Treatment should optimize physical activity and social stimulation and use such techniques as validation, encouragement, support, reminiscence, and maintenance of religious identity. Caregiving strategies that optimize communication—"It's not what you say, but how you say it"—are of paramount importance.

Agitation occurs in about 45 percent of people with AD. The manifestations vary widely and include hitting, kicking, pushing, scratching, tearing things, biting, and spitting. Verbal aggression, including threats, accusations, and name-calling, also occur in about 25 percent of patients with advanced AD. Treatment with antipsychotic drugs such as Haldol and Mellaril produces modest but consistent results. Small doses should be tried first, since they can be very effective. Depression is a common problem in AD, and it should be treated if present. The role of benzodiazepines is still not clear. Ativan and Serax can be tried when the primary problems include insomnia, anxiety problems, and tension. Benzodiazepines can cause sedation, paradoxical increases in agitation, confusion, memory loss, and withdrawal symptoms, if stopped suddenly.

Many drugs are currently being evaluated in large, well-designed trials. These include Buspar, Desyrel, Zoloft, Tegretol, Citalopram, Risperdal, and Deprenyl. Early studies suggest these medications may offer excellent, and safer, alternatives to the traditional antipsychotic medications such as Haldol. As results appear, their role will be clarified.

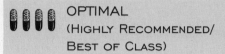

OPTIMAL
(HIGHLY RECOMMENDED/ BEST OF CLASS)

None Available

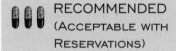

RECOMMENDED
(ACCEPTABLE WITH RESERVATIONS)

ANTIPSYCHOTICS

Haldol (haloperidol)
Trilafon (perphenazine)
Stelazine (trifluoperazine)
Prolixin (fluphenazine)
Navane (thiothixene)

These medications, the "old standards" for treatment of schizophrenia, are also used in low doses to treat behavioral problems in patients with Alzheimer's disease. They can cause disturbing side effects—especially the movement/muscle disorders called "extrapyramidal effects" and tardive dyskinesia. These so-called "tardive movement disorders" usually occur after long-term use, and may persist for long periods—occasionally permanently, even after the drug has been stopped.

Sedation is mild to moderate with Haldol; other side effects have also been reported. These medications are recommended with great reservation, but also with the understanding that severe agitation and disorientation require treatment, even with drugs that have considerable risks and deficiencies. These drugs should be used at the lowest possible dose to achieve results.

BENZODIAZEPINES

Restoril (temazepam)
Serax (oxazepam)
Ativan (lorazepam)

Among the benzodiazepines, these medications have an intermediate duration of action, which means their "hangover" effects are less than with long-acting benzodiazepines. (See "Avoid" category.) Like all benzodiazepines, however, one can develop tolerance to and physical dependence on them. These drugs may need to be combined with one of the medications listed under "Antipsychotics" in the "Recommended" category.

ANTIDEPRESSANTS

Desyrel (trazodone)

Studies with the antidepressant trazodone are encouraging. When compared with Haldol in a small group of patients, trazodone was more effective for repetitive behaviors and verbal aggression and was associated with fewer side effects. More clinical trials are currently in progress and will shed more light on the usefulness of this drug.

Zoloft (sertraline)

Small studies have shown this drug is effective for treating depressive symptoms in patients with AD.

ANTI-ANXIETY MEDICATIONS

BuSpar (buspirone)

Experience with this anti-anxiety drug is limited, but small initial studies suggest it can improve behavioral disturbances in people with AD. It has two distinct advantages: It does not cause sedation, and it has no known potential for creating dependence or abuse. The downside is that this medication may take as long as one month to see its full therapeutic effects. In addition, about 10 percent of patients discontinue the drug due to its side effects, which include headache, nervousness, and dizziness. Finally, its three-times-per-day dosing is less than ideal. Safety is the strong suit of this drug; convenience and effectiveness will be clarified in a study to be reported in 1997.

 DISCOURAGED FOR INITIAL USE (BUT MAY BE REQUIRED IN SELECTED PEOPLE)

Mellaril (thioridazine)
Thorazine (chlorpromazine)
Serentil (mesoridazine)

Like Haldol, Navane, and Prolixin, these drugs have a long history of successful treatment for schizophrenia. However, they are also used in low doses to combat, manage, and minimize the agitation, confusion, and disorientation seen in people with Alzheimer's disease and other so-called organic dementias.

The principal drawback of these medications is their anticholinergic side effects, which can be quite disturbing and include dry mouth, memory impairment, confusion, rapid heart rate, and sedation, among others. These medications are more sedating than those in the "Recommended" category, a feature some experts consider an advantage, but which family members of patients with dementia may find undesirable. Also on the downside, however, they may make confusion worse in a significant percentage of patients. These drugs can also cause movement/muscular disorders, but not as often as Haldol.

Risperdal (risperidone)
This fairly new drug has been approved for the treatment of schizophrenia, but no controlled trials are yet available that evaluate its effectiveness with AD. In small trials, however, patients who responded poorly to more conventional drugs such as Haldol did show improvement on Risperdal. More clinical studies are needed to define its role in these patients.

Deprenyl (selegiline)
This drug is primarily used to treat Parkinson's disease, in which it has been shown to delay deterioration of muscle rigidity and other symptoms. Smaller studies in people with AD have found that Deprenyl produced improvements in paranoid delusions, agitation, activity disturbances, anxiety, and phobias. A larger trial completed by the Alz-

heimer's Disease Cooperative Study is due out in late 1997.

 AVOID IF POSSIBLE
(NOT RECOMMENDED)

LONG-ACTING BENZODIAZEPINES
Valium (diazepam)
Librium (chlordiazepoxide)
Doral (quazepam)
Klonopin (clonazepam)
Tranxene (clorazepate)

These long-acting benzodiazepines should be avoided if possible, especially by the elderly, because they can cause "morning after" drowsiness, sedation, and impaired physical performance. Some of these drugs have been associated with an increased risk of falling and hip fractures in older individuals. They can produce physical dependence. In general, medications with a shorter duration of action (see "Recommended" category) are advised.

DRUGS FOR PARKINSON'S DISEASE
Pills for Loosening Up and Getting Rid of the Shakes

  MedRANK Life Prolongation and Enhancement Checklist

Pills of Wisdom: There is no cure for this progressive, debilitating disease, but advances in drug treatment have improved the outlook for most patients. Parkinson's disease is caused by a loss of dopamine-containing cells in a part of the brain called the substantia nigra. This part of the brain is involved

in maintaining posture, facial movements, and other important muscular activities. As dopamine (a neurotransmitter) is depleted, symptoms such as muscle rigidity, tremor, and movement problems appear. During the later stages of the disease, many people develop sudden fluctuations between being very mobile and being immobile, a phenomenon that has been called the "on-off" effect.

Because drugs used to treat Parkinson's must be introduced into the regimen in the proper sequence, and because they have many side effects, consultation with a neurologist is advised. These drugs must be dosed very carefully and combined carefully to produce optimal results. Because neurologists have the greatest experience using these medications, they should be considered optimal prescribers for this condition. The goal of medications is to relieve symptoms, preserve function, and prevent deterioration.

OPTIMAL
(HIGHLY RECOMMENDED/ BEST OF CLASS)

Deprenyl (selegiline hydrochloride)

Although vitamin E, a popular and safe antioxidant, is of no value in Parkinson's, the monoamine oxidase B inhibitor Deprenyl *has* produced excellent results.

At least three well-designed studies now confirm that early use of Deprenyl—as soon as the diagnosis of Parkinson's is made—will delay disability and the need for immediate therapy with levodopa. (See Sinemet CR 50/200, below.) As a result, this drug should be prescribed when Parkinson's disease is first diagnosed. It can cause tremor and impaired muscle movements, especially when used with levodopa, but these side effects will usually respond to lowering the levodopa dose.

Sinemet CR 50/200 (carbidopa/levodopa)

Drugs containing levodopa are the cornerstone of treatment for Parkinson's disease. Sinemet CR is probably the best medication in this class.

A sustained-release preparation, it represents a major treatment advance for people who experience fluctuations in their symptoms when taking the shorter-acting preparation (Sinemet). The more constant blood levels with Sinemet CR 5/200 provide more consistent control of symptoms.

The most important and debated issue concerns the optimal "timing" of levodopa therapy. Some doctors prefer not to use Sinemet CR during the early stages of Parkinson's because the effectiveness of the drug declines dramatically in a large percentage of people after two years of use. On the other hand, some studies show *life prolongation* if levodopa is started early, within one to three years after the onset of symptoms. Deciding when to start this drug is a judgment call that will have to be made by your physician.

Starting this drug *earlier rather than later* is probably advantageous, because as the disease progresses, the benefit from each dose becomes shorter, producing a "wearing off" effect. To some degree, Sinemet CR has helped reduce "on-off" fluctuations, and as a result, it may be preferable to standard Sinemet, which requires three daily doses.

Sudden discontinuation of levodopa drugs is not advisable, since it can cause a worsening of Parkinson's symptoms, fever, rigid muscles, and confusion. As a result, most experts recommend gradually tapering the medication over three to five days if it has to be discontinued.

Side effects associated with levodopa include nausea, vomiting, high blood pressure, movement problems, and hallucinations. Vivid dreams, delusion, and confusion can also occur in the elderly.

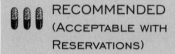

RECOMMENDED
(ACCEPTABLE WITH RESERVATIONS)

Sinemet (carbodopa/levodopa)

To a great extent, Sinemet has been replaced by Sinemet CR. It is not a controlled-release preparation, so the ride is not as smooth in most people. In addition to side effects associated with Sinemet CR, the fluctuations in symptoms are more pronounced with Sinemet than with the controlled-release formulation. See "Sinemet SR" under "Optimal" for additional information about levodopa medications.

Desyrel (trazodone)

Depression frequently accompanies Parkinson's disease and should be treated. Many antidepressants have been evaluated in these patients, and Desyrel appears to be an excellent choice. Experience with SSRI antidepressants such as Prozac and Zoloft is more limited in people with Parkinson's, but one study reports a worsening of symptoms in some who took Prozac.

DISCOURAGED FOR INITIAL USE
(BUT MAY BE REQUIRED IN SELECTED PEOPLE)

Parlodel (bromocriptine)

This drug stimulates the dopamine receptors. It may be particularly helpful in the late stages of the disease, when levodopa treatment becomes less effective.

When used alone, Parlodel is less effective at eliminating the symptoms of Parkinson's than the levodopa drugs (Sinemet SR, Sinemet), but it is less likely to cause move-ment problems and lasts longer. Parlodel can cause excessive lowering of blood pressure, and it can worsen the side effects of levodopa when used in combination.

Permax (pergolide)

Same as above.

Tocopherol (vitamin E analogue)

Antioxidants related to vitamin E have not been shown to reduce progression of symptoms in Parkinson's disease.

AVOID IF POSSIBLE
(NOT RECOMMENDED)

Artane (trihexyphenidyl)

This drug was the mainstay of treatment for many years, but it has been eclipsed by more effective drugs with fewer side effects.

When it is useful, Artane is more likely to control the tremors and drooling associated with Parkinson's disease than the rigid muscles or slow movements. It is not as effective as Sinemet CR, but it may have an added beneficial effect when used in combination with other medications.

Because this drug has anticholinergic properties, it can cause a number of undesirable effects, including memory impairment, hallucinations, dry mouth, constipation, difficulty urinating, and visual problems.

Cogentin (bentropine)

Like Artane, this anticholinergic helps restore balance between dopamine and other neurotransmitters. It may be beneficial when tremor is the primary problem. It has the same troubling side affects as Artane.

Symmetrel (amantadine)

This drug promotes the release of dopamine from degenerated nerve cells. (It is also used to treat influenza.) It may improve muscle rigidity and slow body movements, especially when used with Sinemet. Unfortunately, the benefits of Symmetrel are short-lived, and most people show little reponse after a few months of treatment. Its side effects are similar to those of Cogentin and Artane, but it can also produce ankle swelling and insomnia.

DRUGS FOR EPILEPSY

  MedRANK Life Prolongation and Enhancement Checklist

Pills of Wisdom: Selecting the safest and most appropriate drug to treat a person with epilepsy requires precise characterization of the epileptic disorder. There are many different types of seizures— the International Classification lists more than thirty-six varieties. Some respond very favorably to some medications but not to others. Because an accurate classification of the seizure problem is absolutely necessary, the initial evaluation and drug selection should probably be made by a neurologist or epilepsy specialist.

As a rule of thumb, it is best to treat epilepsy with a *single* medication if possible. Before you are committed to long-term treatment with more than one drug, all reasonable attempts should be made to find a single medication that will control your seizures. If one drug is not effective, an alternative medication should be introduced very gradually. If the alternative drug is working, the original drug should be gradually withdrawn. Only if the attempt to withdraw the first drug is not successful should treatment with both drugs be continued. There are no rigorous studies that convincingly prove the supremacy of one drug combination over another, and therefore trial and error is part of the process.

People with more complicated problems, and especially those who find themselves unresponsive to one medication after another, or who require more than one drug to manage their convulsions, should be seen by a seizure expert called an epileptologist.

Frequently, it is impossible to completely eliminate all seizure activity, in which case you and your doctor will have to accept the persistence of some seizures or their manifestations.

Adding more medications in an attempt to suppress the seizures entirely is frequently counterproductive, because the likelihood of side effects (see the MedRANK Checklist "Side Effects of Drugs for Epilepsy" on page 188) increases dramatically as more medications are prescribed.

Monitoring levels of antiepileptic drugs is part of the treatment program for nearly *all* epileptic patients, but you should be aware that drug levels do not always correlate with clinical results. Regardless of your drug regimen, it is important to balance the adequacy of seizure control with quality of life. Not infrequently, little is to be lost by simplifying the drug regimen and seeing whether the number of seizures is reduced as a result.

Finally, seizure medications do *not* necessarily need to be continued indefinitely. In fact, in more than

60 percent of people who remain free of seizures, the medication can eventually be withdrawn successfully. Some doctors will wait for a two-year seizure-free interval before withdrawing the medication, whereas others will wait for a five-year period. The most cautious approach is to have your medications lowered gradually over a two-to-six-month period. One study, however, showed that discontinuation was just as successful if performed over a six-week period as when tapered over a nine-month period.

Medication withdrawal will be most successful in children who have "benign epilepsy" and in people who have epilepsy of unknown cause (idiopathic). Your odds of remaining seizure-free off medications is greatest if it's been several years since you've had a seizure, if you had very few seizures before control was achieved with medications, and if you have a normal neurological examination.

 OPTIMAL MEDICATIONS

GRAND MAL SEIZURES
Primary Generalized Tonic Clonic

Best Pills:
Dilantin
OR
Depakote
OR
Tegretol

Second-Best Pills:
Mysoline
OR
Lamictal
OR
Phenobarbital

PARTIAL SEIZURE
Including Secondarily Generalized Seizures

Best Pills:
Dilantin
OR
Tegretol
OR
Depakote

Second-Best Pills:
Mysoline
OR
Phenobarbital

Add-on Alternatives:
Neurontin
OR
Lamictal

PETIT MAL

Best Pills:
Zarontin
OR
Depakote

Second-Best Pills:
Klonopin
OR
Lamictal

ATYPICAL ABSENCE, MYOCLONIC, OR ATONIC SEIZURES

Best Pills:
Depakote

Second-Best Pills:
Klonopin

SIDE EFFECTS OF DRUGS FOR EPILEPSY

MedRANK Side Effect Checklist

Pills of Wisdom: Epilepsy is a common disease, and with an estimated 50 million people worldwide suffering from it, the benefits and risks of drug therapy have come under close scrutiny. The objective of drug therapy is to choose a single drug at a dose range that produces no side effects and that can restore normal quality of life through complete seizure control.

This goal is easier to articulate than to accomplish. By their very nature, drugs for epilepsy are designed to act on the central nervous system, and therefore, they have the capacity to produce a wide range of disturbing side effects. It is important that you know what side effects are associated with specific pills so that you can alert your doctor to possible problems and so that, if the side effects are severe enough, you can be considered for an alternative antiepileptic medication.

This Checklist identifies all drugs currently approved for epilepsy and their most important—and serious—side effects.

Dilantin (phenytoin)

Nausea, vomiting, swelling of the gums, depression, drowsiness, acne, coarse facial hair, anemia, blood changes, rash, allergic reactions, liver problems, birth defects, rapid eye muscle movements, dizziness, loss of balance while walking, impaired movement of arms and legs, and paradoxical increase in seizures. Many drug interactions are possible.

Tegretol (carbamazepine)

Double vision, nausea, headache, drowsiness, dizziness, rash, birth defects, severe anemia, serious lowering of white blood cell count, liver problems, and low blood sodium levels. Many drug interactions.

Depakote (valproic acid)

Liver failure, inflamed pancreas, low platelet counts, tremor, weight gain, heartburn, nausea, vomiting, hair loss, leg swelling, birth defects, and brain dysfunction.

Phenobarbitol

Depression, fatigue, decreased pep, insomnia (in children), irritability (in children), hyperexcitability (in children), rash, arthritis, birth defects, liver problems, and tendon contractions.

Mysoline (primidone)

Fatigue, decreased pep, depression, hallucinations, psychosis, decreased sex drive, impotence, rash, low white blood cell counts, low platelet counts, and birth defects.

Zarontin (ethosuximide)

Nausea, decreased appetite, vomiting, agitation, drowsiness, headache, lethargy, skin rash, allergic reactions, severe anemia, and low white blood cell count.

Klonopin (clonazepam)

Drowsiness, drooling, dizziness, sedation, fatigue, aggression (in children), hyperactvity (in children), rash, and low platelet counts.

Neurontin (gabapentin)

Sleepiness, fatigue, rapid eye muscle movements, dizziness, impaired coordination, and gastrointestinal upset.

Lamictal (lamotrigine)

Rash, sleepiness, blurred vision, dizziness, headache, double vision, poor coordination, nausea, and vomiting.

Felbatol (felbamate)

A growing number of cases of severe anemia (aplastic anemia) and life-threatening liver failure have substantially curtailed use of this drug. It should be used only as a last resort— that is, only when all other medications have proved unsuccessful in controlling seizures.

MIGRAINE HEADACHES

 MedRANK Life Enhancement Checklist

Pills of Wisdom: For many years, migraine sufferers had few options. They could take Cafergot-like drugs during the aura, in the hope of aborting the attack, or they could rely on potent narcotic analgesics that placed them at risk for physical dependence. None of these alternatives was really satisfactory. Cafergot produced such side effects as nausea and vomiting, and "narcotic" pain pills put people out of commission for many hours at a time.

Fortunately, important advances have been made in the treatment of migraine headache, the most important of which is Imitrex. This medication, which can be taken as a pill or injected, can provide dramatic relief of pain, even after the headache has started and reached full-blown proportions. Imitrex is safe, does not produce physical dependence, and is recommended as the initial pill of choice in people with moderate to severe migraine attacks.

This MedRANK Checklist includes medications that are useful for treating migraine headaches. If the headaches are severe and recurrent, it will probably be appropriate to use medications to *prevent* further episodes. Pills for migraine prevention are described in the next MedRANK Checklist.

 OPTIMAL
(HIGHLY RECOMMENDED/ BEST OF CLASS)

Imitrex (sumatriptan)

Imitrex has made most previous therapies for migraine obsolete—and for good reason. Imitrex, which can be taken by mouth or injected by the patient, is the best choice for migraine attacks of moderate severity, but it may also be effective against severe attacks. It is more expensive than other therapies but is not associated with physical dependence and produces few of the troubling side effects—nausea, vomiting, drowsiness—seen with Cafergot and similar drugs. For maximal effectiveness, Imitrex should be taken as soon as migraine symptoms are noted. Flushing, a sensation of warm skin, and chest heaviness are the main side effects.

Tylenol (acetaminophen)

Not a big gun, but a safe and effective pain reliever, Tylenol is useful for lessening symptoms in headaches of *mild* and, perhaps, moderate severity. If Tylenol does not provide adequate relief, Imitrex is indicated.

Anaprox (naproxen) and other NSAIDs

The NSAIDs are for mild migraine headaches only. More intense headaches will require treatment with Imitrex. Gastrointestinal side effects include heartburn and indigestion.

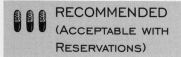

RECOMMENDED
(ACCEPTABLE WITH RESERVATIONS)

Cafergot (ergotamine)

This drug is effective only if you take it as soon as you notice any of the *preliminary signs* that suggest a migraine headache is on the way: flashing lights, "blind spots," and other sensations. Once the headache itself has actually started, Cafergot is of little value. Its side effects limit its usefulness. They are common and include nausea and vomiting. Drug dependence can be a problem with continued use.

D.H.E. 45 (dihydroergotamine)

This drug has to be given by *injection*. It has many of the same side effects as Cafergot, including nausea. Drug dependence may occur.

DISCOURAGED FOR INITIAL USE
(BUT MAY BE REQUIRED IN SELECTED PEOPLE)

Midrin (acetaminophen/isometheptine/dichloralphenazone)

This medication is possibly effective for treating migraine headaches.

Fiorinal (aspirin/caffeine/butalbital)

Although widely used for migraine, this medication is discouraged because it contains barbiturates, which can cause physical dependence, especially with continued use.

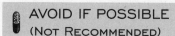

AVOID IF POSSIBLE
(NOT RECOMMENDED)

OPIOID PAIN RELIEVERS

Darvon (propoxyphene)
Tylenol #3 (acetaminophen/codeine)
Vicodin (hydrocodone)

Use of opioid pain relievers is *discouraged* because physical dependence can develop with repeated use. Occasionally, in severe cases, strong pain relievers will be required. But when their repeated use becomes part of the treatment plan, this is a problem. You will either need to develop a pain-relief program using Imitrex and a nonnarcotic pain reliever, or long-term prevention therapy is indicated.

Stadol (butorphanol)

With this nasal spray, drowsiness and confusion may be a problem. *Not recommended.*

MIGRAINE HEADACHE PREVENTION

 **MedRANK Life
Enhancement Checklist**

 Pills of Wisdom: Most people who suffer from migraine headaches will be able to use pain-relieving pills such as Imitrex. (See "Migraine Headaches" on page 189.) But a small percentage of people have *recurrent* headaches that interrupt normal activities. These individuals are candidates for a prevention program. This MedRANK Checklist gives you the best options currently available.

 OPTIMAL
(HIGHLY RECOMMENDED/
BEST OF CLASS)

Inderal (propranolol)
Blocadren (timolol)
Corgard (nadolol)
Lopressor (metoprolol)

These four beta-blockers are no picnic, but they may be required in people with recurrent migraine attacks. Depression and other side effects, including fatigue, nausea, and sexual dysfunction, may be troublesome. Despite their side effects, these drugs appear to provide the best results for migraine *prevention*. Propranolol and timolol have FDA indications for migraine prevention.

 RECOMMENDED
(ACCEPTABLE WITH
RESERVATIONS)

Calan, Isoptin (verapamil)

These medications may be effective and are widely used. They do not, however, have FDA approval for this indication. Side effects include headache, constipation, and weight gain.

 DISCOURAGED FOR INITIAL USE
(BUT MAY BE REQUIRED IN
SELECTED PEOPLE)

Sansert (methysergide)

Sansert is not an ideal drug for migraine prevention. Side effects include weight gain, swelling of extremities, and tissue fibrosis, which may be seen with prolonged (less than 6 months) use.

Elavil (amitriptyline)

This antidepressant is successful in some migraine sufferers. Drowsiness, dry mouth, blurred vision, and other side effects limit its user-friendliness.

AVOID IF POSSIBLE
(NOT RECOMMENDED)

Depakene (valproic acid)

This drug is only moderately effective. Its side effects include hair loss, weight gain, and liver problems. It is not FDA approved for preventing migraine.

CHAPTER 12

GUT WRENCHERS

Medications for
Gastrointestinal Problems

"I've tried everything and nothing makes my heartburn better" is the usual complaint I hear from patients who suffer from chronic indigestion. "But I've heard about these new, powerful drugs," they sometimes go on, "that completely block acid production in the stomach. Are they as good as people say?" The answer is, dramatic improvements have been made in the treatment of stomach ulcers, severe heartburn, abdominal discomfort, and diarrhea. In fact, many of the better drugs available for treating gastrointestinal problems are now available on an *over-the-counter* basis. They include, among others, antacids and antiulcer medications such as Tagamet (cimetidine), Zantac (ranitidine), and Pepcid (famotidine).

☼ *Perhaps the most important point that should be made about OTC drugs used to treat heartburn and similar condi-*
tions is: Don't use them for prolonged periods without a physician's consultation or approval.

For example, you may feel a burning sensation in the pit of your stomach. Maybe you experience it once or twice a week and, along with it, a sour, acid taste in your mouth. Perhaps you are having trouble sleeping, and the pain makes you feel miserable. Although sometimes these complaints are nothing more than simple heartburn, occasionally they indicate the presence of a more severe condition, such as a full-blown stomach ulcer or gastroesophageal reflux disease (GERD). Treating these conditions with frequent doses of OTC medications will not get the job done. The important point is that if nonprescription medications do not relieve your symptoms within a one-to-two-week period, you need a more thorough evaluation by a physician.

☼ *Over the past ten years, we have witnessed dramatic advances in the quality and convenience of drugs used to treat acid-related conditions.*

Antacids have given way to histamine-2 antagonists or H2-blockers. They in turn have been eclipsed by *proton pump blockers*, which are currently the gold standard for suppressing acid production. Before the introduction of H2-blockers such as Tagamet, Zantac, Pepcid, and Axid, which block acid production in the stomach, antacids were the primary defense against ulcer disease. Available in liquid suspension or tablet form, antacids neutralize or reduce stomach acids and inhibit the activity of other digestive enzymes that can be irritating to the stomach.

Antacids still have a role for minor conditions. You can use preparations such as Mylanta-II to relieve the symptoms of an upset stomach, especially if the problem is caused by too much acid secretion. Heartburn, acid indigestion, and sour stomach will respond to these OTC preparations. If you take antacids exactly as directed, they appear to be as effective as Tagamet or Pepcid for the treatment of heartburn. It is important to stress, however, that antacids are not approved for the treatment of stomach *ulcers.*

☼ *Antacids are much less expensive than H2-blockers, but they are much less convenient to take. Clinical experience suggests that most people simply cannot comply with a strict antacid regimen as directed, and consequently the once-daily H2-blockers tend to be associated with better results.*

One of the most important issues surrounding H2-blockers is whether they have lost their edge and whether it might be better just to use "industrial strength" proton pump blockers, such as Prilosec and Prevacid, for most acid-related problems. Actually, it's not time yet to throw H2-blockers out the therapeutic window. They still play a role, especially for long-term preventive treatment in people whose ulcer has already healed and for minor symptoms caused by GERD. Although H2-blockers may not block acid production as completely as proton pump blockers—and will not relieve symptoms as quickly in people with stomach ulcers or reflux problems—they are effective, very safe over the long term, and much less expensive. Proton pump blockers also appear to be safe over the long haul, but this is not as well established as it is for the H2-blockers. A very effective strategy is to use the more powerful and costly proton pump blockers during the most severe stage of your illness—let's say, when your ulcer is active and your symptoms are at their peak—and then "downgrade" to H2-blockers for long-term maintenance.

☼ *Interestingly, antibiotics now are playing an increasingly important—in fact, essential—role in treating stomach ulcers that have not been caused by irritating drugs such as aspirin, Motrin, Naprosyn, Relefan, Daypro, Voltaren, corticosteroids, and other nonsteroidal anti-inflammatory drugs (NSAIDs).*

A significant percentage of people who have stomach ulcers need not only medications to block acid production but antibiotics to kill *Heliobacter pylori,* a species of bacteria identified about ten years ago that has been shown to be responsible for more than 80 percent of ulcers in patients whose ulcer disease is not caused by NSAIDs. The diagnosis of *H. pylori* infection can now be made with a blood test and a simple breathing test. This means that you can probably be spared invasive tests such as an endoscopy before starting drug therapy.

 When ulcers are caused by H. pylori, the goal of treatment is eradication of the organism, which requires a combination of one or more antibiotics plus an H2-blocker or a proton pump blocker such as Prilosec or Prevacid.

There are "more is less" and "less is more" approaches to curing stomach ulcers. Some drug regimens that are used to treat ulcers are inexpensive, but they require up to six weeks of treatment with a combination of more than 250 pills! Good luck. Other, equally effective approaches require you take about 60 pills over a two-week period. The simpler regimens tend to be anchored by the proton pump blockers, and the more complicated regimens are linked to H2-blockers. Needless to say, you will be much more likely to take your pills—and therefore, cure your ulcer—with the leaner, more streamlined regimen. For specific recommendations regarding the best medications for curing stomach ulcers caused by *H. pylori,* see the MedRANK Checklist "Putting Out the Fire: Pills for Stomach Ulcers Caused by *H. pylori* Infection" on page 200.

 The proton pump blockers are not only the most powerful drug class used to treat ulcer disease, they are also the drugs of choice for gastroesophageal reflux disease (GERD), a condition in which stomach acid splashes up into the esophagus.

These medications are generally used in people who have not responded to traditional high-dose therapy with H2-blockers. Other physicians prefer to use proton pump blockers right out of the gate, which is also what I recommend. But Prilosec and Prevacid are much more expensive than H2-blockers; therefore, indications for their use need to be clarified. In general, you are a candidate for Prilosec and Prevacid therapy if you have severe daytime symptoms or a history of erosive ulcerations in your esophagus, or if you have failed full-dose H2-blocker therapy. As you might expect, the proton pump blockers produce excellent results. After four weeks of treatment, about 80 percent of people with severe disease will heal, and more than 90 percent of patients are free from disease after two to three months of treatment.

 One of the most important questions surrounding H2-blockers is how long therapy should be continued. Once the severe phase of your ulcer or GERD is over, how long should you stay on these drugs?

The goal is to relieve symptoms, heal the ulcer, and reduce the rate of ulcer recurrence and complications. If you are young and healthy and have experienced no complications, your treatment period for *H. pylori* ulcers can be as short as two to six weeks. (If your ulcer is not related to *H. pylori*, you will usually be given a prescription for three to six months of medication.) If your symptoms are not relieved promptly after two to three weeks, or you experience the onset of alarming symptoms such as intense pain, vomiting, or dark tarry bowel movements, you should be reevaluated by your physician. As a good rule of thumb, if your symptoms fail to improve within a two-to-three-week period, you need to be reevaluated by your physician. If your ulcer has been complicated by bleeding or other problems, you may need to be on long-term-maintenance treatment with H2-blockers.

PILLS FOR MILD ACID INDIGESTION AND HEARTBURN*

 MedRANK Life Enhancement Checklist

Pills of Wisdom: Virtually everyone has symptoms of "acid indigestion" or heartburn at one time or another. As a rule, these symptoms may indicate minimal reflux (regurgitation) of irritating gastric acid into the esophagus. On occasion, heartburn may indicate more serious disease. The typical symptoms include a burning sensation under your chest bone, which can radiate into your neck and which is relieved promptly by a couple of tablespoons of antacids. Variations of these symptoms can occur.

Some people treat heartburn with nonprescription medications for *long* periods before consulting a doctor. This is unwise, inasmuch as nonprescription drugs are not potent enough to prevent the progression of acid conditions that can lead to ulcers of the stomach and duodenum (peptic ulcers) or of the esophagus (esophagitis). A more severe, and sometimes chronic, form of acid reflux disease, called gastroesophageal reflux disease (GERD), is discussed in the MedRANK Checklist "Pills for Severe Acid Indigestion and Heartburn" in this chapter.

If your symptoms are the result of stomach acids working their way back up and splashing against the lining of your esophagus—a common cause of heartburn—there are a number of things, besides taking medications, that you can do to reduce the severity of your symptoms. First, try the following lifestyle modifications: Elevate the head of your bed at night before going to sleep. Avoid bedtime snacks. Eat foods that have a lower fat content; high-fat foods stimulate acid production by the stomach. If you are a smoker, stop, and if you drink alcohol even occasionally, reduce your intake substantially. Smoking is associated with ulcer disease, and alcohol irritates the lining of your stomach. And if you are taking such stomach-eroding drugs as aspirin or an NSAID, you

* This MedRANK Checklist discusses treatment options for mild symptoms associated with heartburn and sour stomach. More severe acid-related symptoms are discussed in the MedRANK Checklist "Pills for Severe Acid Indigestion and Heartburn" on page 197.

should stop taking them at once, unless you are on very low doses of aspirin to prevent heart disease or some other serious disease—in which case you should report heartburn and similar symptoms to your physician.

Along with making these lifestyle changes, you can use the best drugs discussed in this MedRANK Checklist. These nonprescription products should be used only if you have mild or intermittent symptoms. If your discomfort is not relieved with these pills, or if it persists to any degree whatsoever for more than two weeks, you should be evaluated by your doctor.

OPTIMAL
(HIGHLY RECOMMENDED/ BEST OF CLASS)

Pepcid (Famotidine, 20 mg capsules, available OTC)

An H2-blocker, Pepcid blocks acid production by stomach cells and can provide relief for people with mild heartburn. The OTC dose of this medication, which is one-half the strength of the prescription formulation, is not potent enough to treat ulcers. But it does relieve symptoms of heartburn and "acid stomach" and is preferred over Tagamet, because it is much less likely to cause drug interactions.

Because H2-blockers do not produce immediate relief, you will probably want to use an antacid (see "Recommended" category) for a few days, until the effects of the H2-blocker kick in.

Zantac (Ranitidine)

This drug is also effective and has only a small chance of causing drug interactions.

Axid AC (Nizatidine)

Same as above.

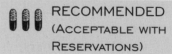

RECOMMENDED
(ACCEPTABLE WITH RESERVATIONS)

Tagamet (Cimetidine, 100 mg OTC capsules)

This is the first H2-blocker that was approved for over-the-counter sale. It blocks acid production by the stomach cells and can provide relief for people with occasional heartburn. But the OTC dose of 100 mg is simply not potent enough to heal ulcers. Consequently, if your symptoms persist despite Tagamet use, you may have a more serious condition than heartburn, one requiring higher doses or more potent medications.

The downside of Tagamet is that compared with the other H2-blockers available for OTC use, Tagamet is much more likely to cause interactions with other drugs. Consequently, Pepcid and Zantac are preferred, especially if you are taking other medications.

ANTACIDS

Extra-Strength Maalox Plus
Mylanta Double Strength

These antacids contain magnesium hydroxide, aluminum hydroxide, and/or simethicone. Generally speaking, two tablets are taken four times daily. Liquid formulations also are available. If an antacid provides rapid relief, the chances are good that your problem is acid-related. However, a good response is not helpful in locating the specific site where excessive acid is causing damage to your gastrointestinal tract, since acid-related discomfort can come from the stomach, duodenum, or esophagus.

Antacids are generally safe, but because of their effects on drug absorption, they can either decrease or increase the potency of many other medications, including blood thinners (Coumadin), seizure medications, and H2-blockers used for ulcer disease. Consult with your pharmacist if you are taking prescription medications and plan to take antacids.

DISCOURAGED FOR INITIAL USE
(BUT MAY BE REQUIRED IN SELECTED PEOPLE)

Alka-Seltzer
Read the label carefully. Many Alka-Seltzer compounds contain aspirin. They should *not* be taken to relieve heartburn symptoms.

AVOID IF POSSIBLE
(NOT RECOMMENDED)

Pepto-Bismol
Aspirin absorption may occur. This medication is intended for diarrhea and is not indicated for treatment of heartburn.

NSAIDs (Motrin, Advil, Aleve, many other OTC and prescription drugs)
Nonsteroidal anti-inflammatory drugs (NSAIDs) can cause erosion and irritation of the stomach lining that is sometimes even severe enough to produce ulcers. These drugs should *not* be used to relieve sour stomach, heartburn, or similar symptoms.

Aspirin
Like the NSAIDs, aspirin can irritate the stomach lining and should *not* be used for treating symptoms associated with heartburn.

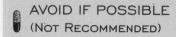
PILLS FOR SEVERE ACID INDIGESTION AND HEARTBURN
(Gastroesophageal Reflux Disease, Acid Reflux Disease, Symptoms of Hiatal Hernia, Intense Heartburn)

MedRANK Life Enhancement Checklist

Pills of Wisdom: Gastroesophageal reflux disease (GERD) is a very common disease whose treatment requires intensive lifestyle changes and drug therapy. Although some degree of acid regurgitates from the stomach to the lower portion of the esophagus in all people, the symptoms of tissue damage (heartburn, sour stomach, stomach pain, and bloating) caused by the irritative effects of stomach acid are what define true GERD. This condition is oftentimes associated with a hiatal hernia, a small pouch that can serve as a storehouse for gastric contents (including acid) and that can come in contact with the lower esophagus.

If your symptoms are mild and infrequent, you may be able to manage with the medications discussed in the MedRANK Checklist "Pills for Mild Acid Indigestion and Heartburn." But when the burning becomes more persistent and severe and fails to respond to OTC H2-blockers and antacids, there is a good chance that the lower end of the esophagus has been severely irritated by the constant regurgitation of stomach acid against the lining of the esophagus. This condition is referred to as esophagitis, or GERD. Sometimes this acid-related damage can erode the lining of the esophagus to the point of producing ulcers, sores that, when extensive, can lead to bleeding and other serious problems.

In addition to drug therapy, people with GERD should implement the following lifestyle modifications: Elevate the head of your bed at night before going to sleep. Avoid bedtime snacks. Eat foods that have a lower fat content—high-fat foods stimulate acid production by the stomach. If you are a smoker, stop, and if you drink alcohol even occasionally, reduce your intake substantially, and if possible, eliminate alcohol consumption completely.

Drug therapy for severe heartburn associated with GERD offers two main options: (1) the H2-blockers, Tagamet, Pepcid, Zantac, and Axid; and (2) the proton pump blockers Prilosec and Prevacid. The proton pump blockers shut down acid production almost *completely* and produce relief much *faster* than the H2-blockers. Stated simply, they are the *gold standard* of treatment. They are also significantly more expensive than H2-blockers, and for this reason, many doctors first try patients on an H2-blocker and reserve drugs like Prilosec and Prevacid for severe cases that have widespread damage in the esophagus. Although this is a reasonable approach, I believe it is preferable to get the job done quickly and definitively, even in milder cases, with one of the proton pump blockers, because they have the most rapid healing rates. The safety of proton pump blockers over the long haul still requires confirmation, although people have used them for years without serious complications.

Once you start a proton pump blocker for this condition, you may be on it forever. Most people have a relapse of symptoms after these drugs are discontinued, so expect to be on a lower "maintenance" dose of a proton pump or H2-blocker indefinitely. There was significant concern, initially, that the long-term side effects and potential toxicity of these drugs were not really known, and, therefore, their long-term use was considered questionable. When these drugs are given to rats in high doses for two years, there is an increased incidence of tumors of the stomach. Fortunately, this toxicity has *not* yet been reported in humans. In fact, more and more studies are showing that proton pump blockers are safe for long-term treatment. Careful evaluation is continuing.

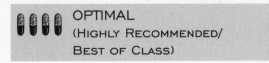

OPTIMAL
(HIGHLY RECOMMENDED/ BEST OF CLASS)

PROTON PUMP BLOCKERS

Prilosec (omeprazole)

This is the first proton pump blocker that was marketed in the United States. Up to 90 percent of people with severe GERD get relief with this drug. Like Prevacid, Prilosec shuts down acid production almost completely, which explains its unparalleled effectiveness for treating acid-related disorders. It can produce healing of severely damaged areas in the esophagus, even when H2-blockers have failed. Prilosec is also approved for the *short-term* treatment of peptic ulcers, producing more rapid healing rates and relief of symptoms than the H2-blockers. This drug also is used in combination with one or more antibiotics to cure stomach ulcers that are caused by infection with the bacterium *Heliobacter pylori*. Occasionally, abdominal pain and nausea are side effects.

Prevacid (lansoprazole)

Prevacid appears to be as effective as Prilosec for the treatment of GERD and peptic ulcer disease. It is also an "Optimal" drug.

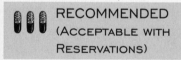

RECOMMENDED
(ACCEPTABLE WITH RESERVATIONS)

H2-BLOCKERS

Pepcid (famotidine)
Zantac (ranitidine)
Axid (nizatidine)
Tagamet (cimetidine)

These H2-blockers are approved for treatment of GERD that is of *mild* to *moderate* severity. Many physicians try one of these medications before using a proton pump blocker. H2-blockers provide symptomatic relief in 50 to 75 percent of people.

There is nothing wrong with trying H2-blockers first, although I recommend starting with the proton pump blockers simply because they produce more rapid relief and more predictable results in a larger percentage of patients. Why save the best for last?

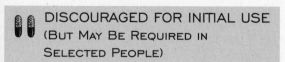

DISCOURAGED FOR INITIAL USE
(BUT MAY BE REQUIRED IN SELECTED PEOPLE)

Propulsid (cisapride)

This medication causes the lower part of the esophagus (the sphincter) to contract, thereby reducing the amount of acid that can enter the esophagus from the stomach. It is used to relieve heartburn symptoms experienced at night and in combination with other medications. It is not particularly effective for daytime symptoms.

Caution is required: Aside from its less-than-ideal effectiveness, Propulsid has other drawbacks as well. It has been associated with rare cases of abnormal heart rhythms that have the potential to be fatal. It should not be taken with drugs known to prevent the breakdown of Propulsid and that thereby increase its toxic effects. Drugs that should not be taken with Propulsid include itraconazole, ketoconazole, erythromycin, clarithromycin, Posicar, and troleandomycin, among others.

Sucralfate

This drug may be useful in some cases but is not the standard treatment for GERD.

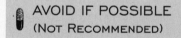

AVOID IF POSSIBLE
(NOT RECOMMENDED)

Urecholine (bethanechol)

This drug has to be given four times daily.

Reglan (metoclopramide)

This drug accelerates emptying of the stomach and stimulates stomach contractions. It is not particularly effective for GERD and is used as an *add-on* for people who have GERD but have failed to respond to conventional treatment. The primary side effects are depression and a movement disorder that can mimic symptoms of Parkinson's disease.

PUTTING OUT THE FIRE
Pills for Ulcers Caused by *H. Pylori* Infection

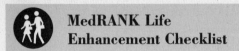 **MedRANK Life Enhancement Checklist**

Pills of Wisdom: The most important recent development in peptic ulcer disease is the discovery that most stomach ulcers that are *not* caused by drugs that irritate the gastrointestinal tract—NSAIDs, aspirin, and others—are actually caused by an *infection* of the stomach lining with bacteria called *Heliobacter pylori*. This hardy organism is unique in that it can survive in the human stomach or duodenum by invading the lining and neutralizing stomach acids with a powerful enzyme it produces.

H. pylori appears to be transmitted by human-to-human contact, and the ulcer it causes is healed by an antibacterial regimen that kills the bacteria. Not surprisingly, the finding that most ulcers are infectious in nature has revolutionized treatment, which now requires antibiotics *as well as* medications that block acid production. The majority of ulcers caused by NSAIDs involve the stomach, whereas *H. pylori* infections can cause ulcers both in the stomach and in the duodenum.

From a practical perspective, the important thing for your doctor to determine is whether your ulcer is caused by *H. pylori* or by an NSAID, excessive alcohol ingestion, steroids, or some other stomach irritant. Blood tests can help confirm the diagnosis of *H. pylori*, but are not helpful in determining whether the organism has been eradicated. Recently, the FDA has approved a noninvasive breath test, the Meretek UBT, that can determine whether *H. pylori* has been eradicated, but it costs about $300. To use this test, all you have to do is drink a liquid and then breathe into a container, which is sent to a laboratory for analysis.

If you have *not* been taking NSAIDs, aspirin, or steroids or drinking alcohol in excessive quantities, and you have symptoms of a stomach ulcer, the chances are greater than 85 percent that your ulcer is caused by *H. pylori* infection. In most cases, if your symptoms are strongly suggestive of an ulcer, it is appropriate for your physician to treat you on an "empirical" basis with an antibiotic and a drug that blocks acid production.

Some regimens for treating *H. pylori*, however, are very complicated and inconvenient and, therefore, compromise patient compliance. The most cumbersome regimens require treatment with four different medications and more than 240 pills for a two-week period. Newer but more costly regimens require only 70 pills to be ingested over a four-week period, which is much more patient-friendly.

Although both approaches work very well, one is clearly more convenient and practical than the other. Health plans that are watching every penny may try to treat you with the cheaper, more cumbersome regimen. If this is the case, you may want to request therapy with the following Optimal regimens.

PILLS FOR ULCERS CAUSED BY *H. PYLORI* INFECTION

 OPTIMAL
(HIGHLY RECOMMENDED/
BEST OF CLASS)

Biaxin (clarithromycin) *plus*
Prilosec (omeprazole) *plus*
Flagyl (metronidazole)

This short-course, low-pill regimen is highly effective. You will need to take only two Biaxin tablets, one Prilosec tablet (20 mg), and two Flagyl (500 mg) tablets per day, for ten days. With a total of 50 pills over ten days, this is probably as simple and effective as it gets for curing *H. pylori* ulcers. The total cost of treatment is about $140.

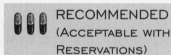 RECOMMENDED
(ACCEPTABLE WITH
RESERVATIONS)

Biaxin (clarithromycin) *plus*
Prilosec (omeprazole) *or*
Prevacid (lansoprazole)

This two-drug treatment is one of the leanest, meanest, and most convenient approaches for curing this disease. Cure rates run 65 to 80 percent, and some physicians add the antibiotic amoxicillin, which raises the cure rates to the 90 percent level.

You will have to take about 70 pills over a four-week period. Each day you take three pills of the antibiotic Biaxin and one Prilosec (40 mg) for two weeks; then one Prilosec (20 mg) per day for an additional two weeks. The cost of a total course of therapy is $280 to $300. This regimen is no more effective than the four-drug cocktail—in fact, it may be slightly less effective—but compliance and convenience are enhanced considerably. The proton pump blocker Prevacid, although not yet FDA approved for *H. pylori* eradication, is as effective as Prilosec.

 DISCOURAGED FOR INITIAL USE
(BUT MAY BE REQUIRED IN
SELECTED PEOPLE)

Flagyl (metronidazole) *plus*
Tetracycline (generic) *plus*
Pepto-Bismol (bismuth subsalicylate)
plus
Zantac (ranitidine)

This regimen is effective and less expensive than the Optimal regimen but is lacking in user-friendliness. Requiring that patients consume 240 pills over a six-week period, this four-drug cocktail is *discouraged* as the initial regimen, despite its $140 price tag.

It doesn't go down easy. Each day of the regimen requires consumption of three tablets of Flagyl, four tablets of tetracycline, eight tablets of Pepto-Bismol, and one tablet of Zantac. Some physicians may substitute amoxicillin for tetracycline. Cure rates run 85 to 95 percent with the four drugs. If you're up to this incredible pill marathon, good luck. If you're not, push your physician to use the Optimal regimen. You'll be happy you did.

PILLS FOR ULCERS NOT CAUSED BY *H. PYLORI* INFECTION

MedRANK Life Enhancement Checklist

Pills of Wisdom: Peptic (acid) ulcers of the stomach or duodenum are generally caused either by infection with *H. pylori* or by the use of drugs that irritate the stomach lining. These drugs include nonsteroidal anti-inflammatory medications (NSAIDs), aspirin, and steroids. Excessive alcohol ingestion can also cause stomach ulcers.

Treatment will depend on exactly what kind of ulcer you have. If *H. pylori* infection is the cause, eradication of the organism with antibiotics and proton pump blockers is the treatment of choice. (See the MedRANK Checklist "Pills for Stomach Ulcers Caused by *H. pylori* Infection" in this chapter.) If your ulcer is not related to *H. pylori* infection, you will need treatment with drugs that block acid production in the stomach.

Among drugs that block acid production, your physician will have the choice of proton pump blockers, such as Prevacid and Prilosec, and H2-blockers, such as Tagamet, Zantac, Pepcid, and Axid. Many physicians and health plans prefer the H2-blockers because they are *less* expensive and get the job done. But the H2-blockers are being replaced by the more expensive proton pump blockers, which provide faster pain relief and healing. In my view, these real-world benefits are significant and therefore justify the additional expense.

Many studies show that people are kept on anti-ulcer medications much longer than needed. As a rule, if your ulcer condition is mild; if it is your *first* episode of ulcer disease; if there are no bleeding complications; and if you have eliminated the cause (NSAIDs, excessive alcohol, or other precipitating factor), you do not have to take maintenance drugs over the long term.

Generally speaking, a six-to-eight-week course of the medications discussed here will be sufficient to heal your ulcer, and additional treatment is not necessary or desirable. On the other hand, if your ulcer has been complicated by bleeding problems; if you continue to pursue drug treatment or a lifestyle that predisposes you to ulcers; or you have recurrent ulcers, you will be better off taking an anti-ulcer drug over the long term, albeit at a *reduced* dose.

This MedRANK Checklist ranks medications that are used to block acid production to treat ulcers not caused by *H. pylori* infection. Several "classes" of drugs are available, but some work more quickly than others and, as a result, are preferred.

OPTIMAL (HIGHLY RECOMMENDED/ BEST OF CLASS)

Prilosec (omeprazole)

This is the top-of-the-line treatment. Prilosec shuts down acid production almost completely and with unparalleled effectiveness. Prilosec is indicated for the short-term treatment of ulcers, in which it produces rapid relief and cures. Overall, about 85 percent of ulcers are healed after two weeks of treatment, and about 95 percent heal within four weeks.

Prevacid (lansoprazole)

Prevacid carries an Optimal ranking for all the same reasons cited for Prilosec.

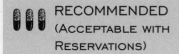

RECOMMENDED
(Acceptable with Reservations)

H2-Blockers

Pepcid (famotidine)

H2-blockers used to be the gold standard for treatment of ulcer disease not associated with *H. pylori* infection, but they are quickly being moved to the back burner. Although H2-blockers produce excellent cure rates, they don't produce healing rates as *rapid* as those seen with proton pump blockers.

But if you are going to be treated with an H2-blocker, I prefer Pepcid. Like the other drugs in its class—Tagamet, Zantac, and Axid—Pepcid blocks acid production and promotes ulcer healing, but with a lower risk for causing drug interactions.

Zantac (ranitidine)
Axid (nizatidine)

These H2-blockers are as effective as Pepcid but may have a slightly increased risk for causing drug interactions. If you are not taking any other drugs with which interactions may occur, they are recommended as highly as Pepcid.

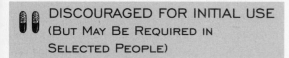

DISCOURAGED FOR INITIAL USE
(But May Be Required in Selected People)

Tagamet (cimetidine)

There is no disputing that this drug works. In fact, Tagamet achieves healing rates comparable to those for Pepcid and Zantac. But it may interact with Valium, Coumadin, and Dilantin.

Tagamet rarely causes reversible impotence and breast enlargement in men. For these reasons, it is the least preferred of the H2-blockers.

Cytotec (misoprostol)

This drug is less effective than both H2-blockers and proton pump blockers. With its four-times-per-day dosing schedule, it is much less convenient than other therapies. It also produces diarrhea in a significant percentage of people.

The main indication for Cytotec is to *prevent* gastric ulcers in people who are on long-term treatment with NSAIDs. It is recommended especially for people at high risk, including the elderly and people with a previous history of ulcer disease, who absolutely require NSAIDs as part of their treatment plan for a pain-related condition.

Antacids

Extra-Strength Maalox Plus
Mylanta Double Strength

Antacids contain magnesium hydroxide, aluminum hydroxide, and/or simethicone. Generally speaking, two tablets are taken four times daily. Liquid formulations also are available.

These drugs are no longer the preferred approach for treating ulcer disease. Antacids are generally safe, but because of their effects on drug absorption, they can either decrease or increase the potency of many other medications, including blood thinners (Coumadin), seizure medications, and H2-blockers used for ulcer disease. Consult with your pharmacist if you are taking prescription medications and plan to take an antacid.

AVOID IF POSSIBLE
(NOT RECOMMENDED)

Alka-Seltzer

Read the label carefully. Many Alka-Seltzer compounds have aspirin. These should *not* be taken to relieve heartburn symptoms.

Pepto-Bismol

Aspirin absorption may occur. This medication is intended for diarrhea and is not indicated for the treatment of heartburn.

NSAIDs (Motrin, Advil, Aleve, many other prescription and OTC drugs)

Nonsteroidal anti-inflammatory drugs (NSAIDs) can cause erosion and irritation of the stomach lining that sometimes is even severe enough to produce ulcers. These drugs should *not* be used to relieve sour stomach, heartburn, or similar symptoms.

Aspirin

Like the NSAIDs, aspirin can irritate the stomach lining and should *not* be used for treating symptoms associated with heartburn.

MAKING AN END RUN
Drugs for Traveler's Diarrhea

MedRANK Life Enhancement Checklist

Pills of Wisdom: Most cases of acute diarrhea are caused by viral infections and will resolve themselves *without* any treatment whatsoever. If symptoms are mild, the best approach is to take plenty of fluids, in order to prevent dehydration, and wait it out. Even mild to moderate cases of diarrhea can produce enough dehydration to make you feel tired and weak. Consequently, drinking plenty of fluids is an important part of treatment. Solutions rich in electrolytes and sugar will help you absorb water. A glass of fruit juice, to which is added a pinch of salt and a teaspoon of honey or table sugar, is a good place to start. Nondiet cola drinks that have been allowed to stand and lose their carbonation are reasonable substitutes.

More severe symptoms—especially severe cramping and watery diarrhea—may require a drug such as Lomotil or Imodium (which is available without a prescription). Kaopectate is not harmful but

may not be all that effective either. When bacterial infection is the cause, as in traveler's diarrhea, antibiotics can play an important role. Finally, if diarrhea persists for more than a few days, or if there is blood in your bowel movement, you should see your doctor for a complete evaluation.

OPTIMAL FOR PREVENTION
(HIGHLY RECOMMENDED/ BEST OF CLASS)

Cipro (ciprofloxacin)
Floxin (ofloxacin)
Noroxin (norfloxacin)

Traveler's diarrhea is a common condition, also known as *turista* when acquired in Mexico. It is caused by bacteria (enterotoxigenic *E. coli*) and usually is a self-limited illness, lasting for three to seven days.

Excellent medications are available to *prevent* traveler's diarrhea, although many physicians prefer to start treatment only *after* symptoms begin. I believe the decision should depend on *your* comfort level and *past experience.* But if you have traveled to a specific place or region over and over again, and predictably have acquired traveler's diarrhea each time, with the vacation-killing symptoms it produces, it would make sense to consider pills for prevention. If you fit this profile, my advice is, "Just take it."

Cipro (ciprofloxacin), Floxin (ofloxacin), and Noroxin (norfloxacin) are the most effective medications for prevention. State-of-the-art for preventing traveler's diarrhea, these broad-spectrum antibiotics are all dosed on a once-daily basis. You shouldn't take them for longer than three weeks and they should not be used in children. Start these pills two days before your trip and continue until two days after you return home. Pepto-Bismol also can work but is much more cumbersome to take (two tablets four times daily), changes the color of your tongue and bowel movements, and can cause an unpleasant ringing in your ears.

OPTIMAL FOR TREATMENT
(HIGHLY RECOMMENDED/ BEST OF CLASS)

Cipro (ciprofloxacin)
Floxin (ofloxacin)
Noroxin (norfloxacin)

If you get the *turista* and you feel bad enough, get help. It should be stressed that taking antibiotic pills for traveler's diarrhea is generally indicated if your symptoms are severe enough to get in the way of your daily activities. Not surpisingly, Cipro, Floxin, and Noroxin, the three antibiotics used for *prevention,* are also the best options for *treatment.* The daily dose is *doubled,* however, for treating the acute symptoms, and you should take the medications until the symptoms resolve or no longer than three days. These antibiotics should *not* be used routinely for *all* cases of mild to moderate diarrhea, but they can be very effective if you and your doctors suspect you have a severe case of traveler's diarrhea. Imodium and over-the-counter medication can also be used in conjunction with them.

RECOMMENDED
(ACCEPTABLE WITH RESERVATIONS)

Imodium (loperamide)
Diar-aid Caplets
Loperamide (generic)

These over-the-counter pills for diarrhea are safe and can be a life-saver. When required, most adults should take a 4 mg dose initially, and then 2 mg for each unformed stool, until symptoms are relieved. You should not take more than 8 mg/day of Imodium.

Lomotil (diphenoxylate HCL with atropine sulfate)

This prescription antidiarrheal drug is very effective and is recommended when quick and definitive relief of symptoms is desired. Don't take more than the prescribed dose. Lomotil should not be used in combination with monoamine oxidase inhibitors (MAOIs).

DISCOURAGED FOR INITIAL USE (BUT MAY BE REQUIRED IN SELECTED PEOPLE)

Septra (trimethoprim sulfa)

Many physicians still use Septra, which is not recommended as a first-line choice because resistance to this drug has developed in many areas.

Pepto-Bismol (bismuth subsalicylate)

If you are serious about preventing traveler's diarrhea or want rapid relief of symptoms, my recommendation is to stick with the antibiotics discussed in the "Optimal" category. In the event you are stuck overseas and can't get a prescription for antibiotics, Pepto-Bismol is a decent fallback.

Kaopectate (and similar preparations)

These OTC preparations have been used for many years for diarrhea, but there are no definitive studies confirming their value. I recommend the Imodium OTC drugs. Imodium is more effective and is available without a prescription.

CHAPTER 13

DRUGS FOR BUGS AND CRUD

Antibiotics for Common Infections

"Why do I always have to take a second course of antibiotics?" my patients have asked me over the years. "Isn't there an antibiotic I can take that will work the first time around?" The answer is yes, there are antibiotics that will cure your infection in a flash—and without the nasty side effects that have plagued these drugs for so many years. The fact is, some antibiotics are more effective against certain bacteria than others. In other cases, it's just a matter of finding an antibiotic with a side-effect profile you can tolerate—and remembering that you'll optimize the chances for curing your infection if you take all the pills, exactly as prescribed.

Antibiotics are among the most widely prescribed outpatient medications. Although many studies suggest that they may be overprescribed, when used appropriately, these agents can be life-saving. Because antibiotics have very specific indications, they should be taken only when prescribed by a physician. Overuse of antibiotics can lead to resistant bacteria and unnecessary expense. On the other hand, once an antibiotic is prescribed on your behalf, you need to comply with your doctor's instructions.

☺ *One of the main problems with antibiotics is noncompliance. How many times have you been prescribed ten days of antibiotic pills but neglected to take the entire course?*

Probably more often than you would care to admit. You are not alone. In fact, studies show that only eight out of one hundred people prescribed a ten-day course of antibiotics are still taking a pill on the tenth day of drug therapy. A Gallup survey confirms that only 45 percent of people who start on antibiotics complete the entire course. No wonder failure rates for common infections are so high. Not infrequently, the pills that are left over gather dust in a medicine cabinet, only to be used in the future for symptoms that the person perceives are being caused by a bacterial infection. Be careful. One antibiotic does not fit all conditions. Self-administration of antibiotics (taking them without a physician's approval) is discouraged because these medications need to be dosed appropriately and matched to specific infections.

☺ *Antibiotics vary widely in terms of patient-friendliness, ease of use, safety, and effectiveness.*

Today, so-called "warhorse antibiotics" such as penicillin and amoxicillin are used less widely than in the past because resistant organisms have emerged over time. In addition, penicillin, amoxicillin, and erythromycin, which require administration three to four times daily, have been replaced by new antibiotics such as Zithromax (azithromycin), Biaxin (clarithromycin), and Ceftin (cefuroxime), which require only one or two administrations daily.

☺ *Whether generic antibiotics are as good as brand-name antibiotics is a hotly debated issue. In some cases they are, and in other situations they are not.*

In general, however, I recommend *brand-name* antibiotics because they tend to provide better coverage against most bacteria, are easier to take, and have a lower risk of side effects. Studies show that patients are more likely to comply with a medication dosed on a *once-daily* basis than with one that requires three or four doses per day.

Most generic drugs used to treat infections have to be taken more than once daily for as long as seven or even ten days. Many brand-name antibiotics are available that are dosed once daily and that require shorter courses of treatment. For example, in addition to requiring fewer doses each day, Zithromax requires only five days of treatment for bronchitis, walking pneumonia, and skin infections. Even though it is taken for only five days, it provides antibiotic coverage that lasts for a full ten. Newer antibiotics also tend to have fewer side effects, which means they are less likely to produce nausea, abdominal cramping, or diarrhea.

☺ *There also are safety issues to consider. Antibiotics have the potential to cause drug interactions.*

They can interact with antihistamines, asthma medications, and drugs used for epilepsy. For example, erythromycin and Biaxin should not be taken with the antihistaminic medication Hismanal (astemizole). Life-threatening irregularities of heart rhythm are possible, or have been reported, in patients who have done so. Drug interactions between fluoroquinolone antibiotics (Cipro, Noroxin) and theophylline have also been documented. Generally speaking, you should ask your physician what antibiotic offers the simplest dosing schedule, shortest course of therapy, and best side-effect profile for your particular condition. If this antibiotic is available at an acceptable price, your likelihood of being cured the first time around will be greatly increased.

These principles also apply to the selection of antibiotic suspensions for children. Children are especially fussy when it comes to taking medications that have poor palatability. Some antibiotic suspensions, such as

Biaxin, Vantin, Pediazole, and Cefzil—among others—simply don't taste very good. They have a palatability profile that some children find unacceptable. In contrast, such medications as Amoxil (amoxicillin), Zithromax (azithromycin), and Lorabid (loracarbef) consist of flavored formulas that most children find more desirable.

☺ *Some pediatric antibiotic suspensions don't work because bacteria have become more and more resistant to antibiotics.*

One of the most common organisms causing middle ear infections in children is *Streptococcus pneumoniae*. Although once exquisitely sensitive to many different antibiotics, this bacterium has become increasingly *difficult* to treat, especially with drugs such as Amoxil (amoxicillin), Suprax (cefixime), and Ceclor (cefaclor). As a result, newer or more powerful medications, including Augmentin, Zithromax, and Lorabid, have been pressed into service in order to overcome resistant organisms.

☺ *With antibiotics, gastrointestinal symptoms (like nausea and diarrhea) and skin rashes are the most common side effects you are likely to encounter.*

You should discontinue an antibiotic at the first appearance of a rash, facial swelling, difficulty breathing, or other allergic signs. If you develop nausea, vomiting, or diarrhea when taking an antibiotic, you should inform your doctor so you can be switched to an alternative medication if necessary. Some antibiotics may cause sensitivity to sunlight. In most cases, if you miss a dose of an antibiotic, take the next dose as soon as possible. If you miss more than one dose, or if it is necessary to establish a new dosage schedule, you should contact your doctor or pharmacist.

Antifungals such as fluconazole, ketoconazole, and griseofulvin are used to treat fungal infections of the hair, skin, and nails; for *candida* infections of the vagina and thrush; and for serious conditions such as cryptococcal meningitis, a brain infection seen in patients with AIDS. As a therapeutic class, antifungal agents are associated with a high risk for producing drug interactions. Consequently, if you have been prescribed an antifungal medication, you should ask your physician about possible drug interactions. Antifungal medications are available both as oral formulations and as topical preparations.

Antiviral drugs have diverse uses, but varying degrees of toxicity. Antiviral medications for herpes infections have only mild to moderate toxicity, whereas those used to treat HIV infection and cytomegalovirus are much more toxic (see Chapter 15). Valtrex, Famvir, and Zovirax are often used to treat first attacks and recurrent outbreaks of herpes infections. They are most effective when taken at the very first sign of infection. Famvir and Valtrex have advantages over Zovirax because they are usually dosed *twice* a day, as compared to five times for Zovirax, for treating the *first* episode of a herpes infection. These drugs also are used to accelerate healing and provide pain relief for shingles outbreaks. Amantadine is available for preventing and treating respiratory symptoms associated with the flu. Because of possible side effects and inconsistent efficacy, I do *not* recommend amantadine for routine use in all patients. Generally speaking, this drug should be reserved for "high-risk" patients who have underlying heart, lung, or immunodeficiency problems. The best approach for preventing influenza infection is a *flu shot*, which is especially important in older individuals and in all people who have a debilitating chronic disease.

☺ *Vaccines can be grouped into two categories: immune serums and agents for active immunization.*

Generally speaking, an immune serum consists of immune globulins that provide protection against certain diseases, but only for a short period of time. Immune globulins provide so-called passive immunization. The protection against infection conferred by passive immunization is of rapid onset but lasts for only a few *months*. In contrast, the protection offered by *active* immunization takes longer to come on but lasts for *years*. You can refer to the MedRANK Checklists in this chapter and in Chapter 4 for information about adult and childhood vaccinations, respectively.

☺ *Some infections can be prevented by using immune serums, which contain antibodies that can protect against infections caused by bacteria as well as viruses.*

There are a number of immune serums available for routine use, including immune globulin, hepatitis B immune globulin, tetanus immune globulin, and RHo(D) immune globulin. The hepatitis B immune globulin (HBIG) is used for people who have been exposed to possible hepatitis B–containing materials. For example, accidental needle sticks, splashes, or oral ingestions of blood or saliva from people with known hepatitis usually require administration of hepatitis B immune globulin. Tetanus immune globulin (Hyper-Tet) is used for temporary protection against tetanus. This immune serum is given to people who have wounds that can cause tetanus but an uncertain history of tetanus shots. RHo immune globulin is used to prevent hemolytic disease of the newborn. It is given when an Rh-negative mother who was not previously exposed to the Rh-positive factor has an Rh-positive baby. It is also used in certain Rh-negative patients after incomplete pregnancies or transfusions. Your doctor will use a blood test to determine your Rh status and assess your suitability for RHo immune globulin.

☺ *Not surprisingly, the best approach to infection is prevention. Practicing good hygiene, using condoms, and avoiding contact with individuals known to have highly contagious conditions can reduce antibiotic use.*

In addition, flu shots, immunizations that may be required if you are traveling to exotic locations, and vaccines used to prevent ear infections, meningitis, and pneumonia have decreased our reliance on antibiotic therapy for many common conditions. But prevention-oriented measures are not perfect. Consequently, if antibiotics *are* required, ask your doctor about *one-dose, cure-here-now treatment options*. This approach emphasizes getting the job done with only one—usually rather concentrated—dose of an antibiotic, bypassing the need for a prolonged course of therapy. One-dose therapies are available for chlamydial infections (Zithromax), head lice (Vermox), *candida* vaginitis (Diflucan, Vagistat), gonorrhea (Cipro, Suprax, Zithromax), and many other infections. For more information, see the MedRANK Checklist "Antibiotics" on page 214.

COLD COMFORT PHARM
Treatments for the Common Cold

MedRANK Life Enhancement Checklist

Pills of Wisdom: Colds are a pain. They divide the world into the "haves" and "have snots." Getting one is as guaranteed as death and taxes. Sure, there's the good news: The prognosis for recovery is excellent. But then there's the bad news: The sneeze-peppered, nose-plugged, raw-throated journey to cure, more often than not, sucks the sweetness and light out of life for up to a week. And their severity is getting worse.

Who needs these neither-here-nor-there infections that do little more than get under our mucous membranes and occupy the lowest station on the Great Chain of Virological Being? What have we done to deserve this perennial, omnipresent biological irritant that seems to serve no evolutionary purpose and whose sole raison d'être is to punctuate human life with episodes of third-rate physical distress? Does the cold have no self-respect? It's "just" a cold. How common can you get?

Sure, there's the orange-juice-glass-is-half-full argument: A cold won't cause you permanent harm. But the nasal congestion, scratchy throat, minor aches, and sinus stuffiness that accompany it can make life very unpleasant for four to seven days, depending on the brand of rhinovirus that hits you and the overall sturdiness of your protoplasm. Because there are so many different kinds of cold virus and because these 110

variants are mutating at such a rapid clip, it has been very difficult to develop a vaccine against this annoying illness. Thus far, cure has proven to be elusive.

Colds are spread by the airborne transmission of virus-rich particles, and by direct mucous membrane contact with the virus from contaminated hands, other skin surfaces, and even tabletops. You can get infected with the cold virus simply by touching your eyes or nose. There are no proven methods for preventing a cold once you've been infected, no proven methods for curing it, and no proven methods that entirely eliminate all its symptoms.

But help is on the way. A "cold comfort pharm" is slowly developing that includes effective methods for reducing the severity of cold symptoms and shortening the time between sickness and health. Please consult the following MedRANK Checklist for cold remedies that work and those that don't. And remember, when all else fails, there's always chicken soup, chamomile tea, and a warm bubble bath illuminated by a scented candle to ease the pain.

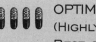 OPTIMAL
(HIGHLY RECOMMENDED/
BEST OF CLASS)

Soup (chicken, minestrone, matzoh ball, and other varieties)
It would be heresy not to include this time-honored antidote here. After all, the first priority is comfort, and "comfort food" is an

excellent place to start. Taking soup is a good way to stay hydrated and keep your mucous membranes moist.

Cold-eeze Lozenges (zinc gluconate lozenges)

Medical science says zinc lozenges (not zinc capsules) work. The Cleveland Clinic conducted one of those randomized, double-blind, placebo-controlled trials—the standard in the drug-testing business—and found that people who took zinc lozenges (as opposed to placebo) had fewer days with throat symptoms, coughing, headache, nasal congestion or drainage, and hoarseness. The time required to get rid of cold symptoms was about four and a half days for those who took the zinc lozenges, and about seven and a half days for those who didn't. That translates into three extra days of "feel good" time, which in this time-pressured world is not insignificant.

A few qualifications regarding the anti-cold "magic" of zinc should be mentioned. First, the lozenges must be taken within twenty-four hours of the onset of cold symptoms to be maximally effective. Then they have to be taken every two hours until your symptoms are gone. That's a lot of suck time. Are you willing to become a lozenge lush for the sake of cold relief?

Second, the benefits of zinc lozenges were seen when they were used in combination with the all-around pain reliever Tylenol. Finally, about 20 percent of people who used zinc lozenges reported nausea. So there's a trade-off here, and you must make the final decision.

Tylenol (acetaminophen)

What's not to like about Tylenol? It's a safe, all-purpose pain and ache reliever that alleviates muscle, joint, and head discomfort.

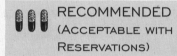

RECOMMENDED
(Acceptable with Reservations)

Atrovent Nasal Spray (ipratropium bromide)

Atrovent Nasal Spray contains ipratropium, an anticholinergic medication that can block nasal discharge. Some people don't like putting a spray canister up their nose and therefore will find no use for this approach. If you can tolerate a nasal inhaler, Atrovent, used three times daily for about four days, can be expected to reduce the nasal discharge (rhinorrhea) and sneezing associated with the common cold. It has little effect on nasal congestion per se. On the downside, an irritating nasal dryness and headache are seen more frequently in people using the nasal spray. This medication is available by prescription only.

Echinacea

The effectiveness of echinacea is hotly debated. A steady flow of scientific studies has been coming in from Germany, where clinical trials suggest that echinacea can speed up recovery from colds and the flu. Unfortunately, these studies have evaluated the effectiveness of injected echinacea. Whether American preparations designed for oral ingestion produce the same results is simply not known. It's a coin toss, so don't expect dramatic results.

DISCOURAGED FOR INITIAL USE
(BUT MAY BE REQUIRED IN
SELECTED PEOPLE)

Antihistamines/decongestants
Don't expect a miracle. These OTC medications can reduce the severity of some cold symptoms, but only if they are taken within the first couple of days after the illness has started. Their main downside is dry mouth.

Vitamin C
Despite the initial hype, study after study suggests that vitamin C (at high or low doses) neither prevents a cold nor decreases the severity of symptoms.

Steam inhalation
Studies show this is of no value.

Antiseptic mouthwash
Studies show this is of no value.

 AVOID IF POSSIBLE
(NOT RECOMMENDED)

Antibiotics
If you think—or your doctor says—that you are suffering from a cold, don't look to antibiotics for relief. Common colds are caused by viruses, against which antibiotics are completely ineffective. What's more, widespread overuse of antibiotics can lead to resistant bacteria, which can make future infections much more difficult to treat. Remember, too, that antibiotics can alter the growth of "normal bacteria" in a way that predisposes women to vaginal infections. And besides, the side effects of many antibiotics are far worse than the symptoms of a cold.

A doctor or a patient who uses antibiotics for the common cold does a service for no one. But colds can trigger bacterial infections in some people. If you are one of those individuals in whom a cold frequently triggers a bacterial infection of the sinus or middle ear, then antibiotics may be required—but only if bacteria, and not the cold virus, are suspected of being the principal offender.

ANTIBIOTICS
One-Dose, Cure-Here-Now Pills and Other Short-Duration Treatments for Common Infections

 MedRANK Life Enhancement Checklist

Pills of Wisdom: This MedRANK Checklist brings together the most effective one-dose or short-duration cures that have been identified for common infections. If you are diagnosed as having one of these infections and you are prescribed a course of antibiotics that is *longer* than the ones presented here, you might ask your physician whether you are suitable for a one-dose or short-course option. Your compliance will usually be better, and the results ought to be at least as good.

NONSPECIFIC BACTERIAL VAGINOSIS
Flagyl (metronidazole) 2 g by mouth, once

TRICHOMONIASIS
Flagyl (metronidazole) 2 g by mouth, once (contraindicated during first trimester of pregnancy)

CANDIDA VAGINITIS
Diflucan (fluconazole) 150 mg by mouth, once
OR
Vagistat (tioconazole) 6.5% vaginal ointment

GONORRHEA
Rocephin (ceftriaxone) 125 mg intramuscular shot
OR
Zithromax (azithromycin) 2 g by mouth, once

OR
Suprax (cefixime) 400 mg by mouth, once
OR
Cipro (ciprofloxacin) 500 mg by mouth, once
OR
Floxin (ofloxacin) 400 mg by mouth, once

CHANCROID
Zithromax (azithromycin) 1 g by mouth, once

CHLAMYDIA INFECTION
(UNCOMPLICATED, AS IN CERVICITIS, URETHRITIS)
Zithromax (azithromycin) 1 g by mouth, once

SKIN INFECTION
(CELLULITIS, AS IN STAPHYLOCOCCUS AUREUS, STREPTOCOCCUS)
Zithromax (azithromycin) for five days of treatment

EAR INFECTION
(OTITIS MEDIA IN CHILDREN)
Rocephin (ceftriaxone) 50 mg/kg intramuscular shot, once
OR
Zithromax oral suspension, for five days of treatment

URINARY TRACT INFECTION
(UNCOMPLICATED)
Septra (trimethoprim/sulfamethoxazole)

4 double-strength tablets, by mouth (high relapse rate, 35%)
OR
Septra (trimethoprim/sulfamethoxazole) 1 double-strength tablet, twice daily for three days (relapse rate reduced to 15%)

WHIPWORM INFECTION
(TRICHURIS TRICHIURA)
Zentel (albendazole) 400 mg by mouth, once

PINWORM INFECTION
(ENTEROBIUS VERMICULARIS)
Vermox (mebendazole) 100 mg by mouth; repeat after 2 weeks

HOOKWORM
(NECATOR AMERICANUS)
Zentel (albendazole) 400 mg by mouth
OR
Vermox (mebendazole) 100 mg, by mouth

SCABIES/MITES
(SARCOPTES SCABIEI)
Permethrin (5%) massage from head to soles; wash off after 8–14 hours

HEAD LICE
(PEDICULUS HUMANUS CORPORIS)
Mectizan (ivermectin) one dose of 200ug/kg taken by mouth

BODY LICE
(PEDICULUS HUMANUS CORPORIS)
Pyrethrin (with piperonyl butoxide) apply lotion for 10 minutes, then bathe and repeat

CORTICOSTEROIDS
(ASTHMA, ALLERGIC REACTIONS)
A short (5–7 day) tapering of steroids is as effective in most cases as longer tapering courses

ANTIBIOTICS FOR "WALKING" PNEUMONIA

  MedRANK Life Prolongation and Enhancement Checklist

Pills of Wisdom: "Walking" pneumonia is a bacterial infection in the lung that is acquired in a community setting. It is usually of mild to moderate severity and is most often seen in younger (less than 60 years of age), previously healthy adults. As a rule, this infection is treated out of the hospital, especially when it occurs in young adults. Of course, older people with this condition may need to be hospitalized, although sometimes they can be given antibiotic treatment at home.

The critical issue is finding an antibiotic that kills all the *likely* bugs that cause walking pneumonia. In the overwhelming number of cases, a doctor simply can't tell which specific bug you're infected with, so the antibiotic is chosen on an *empirical* basis, which means the one that has the greatest *odds* of covering *all* the likely possibilities.

The point is, if your physician treats you with a drug that works against *all* the common offenders, the chance of cure the first time around is greatly increased, and the likelihood that you'll need to be retreated with another drug or that you'll get worse is significantly decreased.

In previously healthy people, there are four likely bacterial culprits. The good news is, we know who they are: *S. pneumoniae, H. influenzae, M. catarrhalis,* and *Mycoplasma* (and sometimes *Chlamydia*). The principal offender is *S. pneumoniae.* The bad news is, only three antibiotics—Zithromax, Levaquin, and Biaxin—will predictably cover all four of these bacteria. The other bad news is that there is a growing bacterial resistance to *S. pneumoniae.* The MedRANK Checklist takes these and other factors into account when evaluating antibiotics used for this infection.

OPTIMAL FOR PEOPLE UNDER 60
(HIGHLY RECOMMENDED/ BEST OF CLASS)

Zithromax (azithromycin)

Convenient. Comfortable. Consistent. Safe. Curative. In my view, this "less is more" antibiotic is the top-of-the-line choice for walking pneumonia, in young and middle-aged adults, that is mild enough to be treated out of the hospital.

Its strong points include a compliance-enhancing, five-day course of once-daily medication, and no risk of significant drug-drug interactions. It covers all the likely bacteria that cause walking pneumonia in most people. The gastrointestinal symptoms associated with so many antibiotics are seen in less than 5 percent of people who take the five-day course of therapy. And the likelihood of producing vaginal yeast infections is less than 2 percent. In short, it's patient-friendly.

An important point of information: Although Zithromax is taken for a total of only five days, it's as if you are still actually *taking* the medication on the sixth through tenth days. That's because the antibiotic stays in the body's tissues at the site of infection (in the lung), wiping out the bacteria until the job is done. At about $40 for a course of therapy, Zithromax is a steal.

Biaxin (clarithromycin)

This drug shares with Zithromax excellent activity against the four likely bugs that cause pneumonia in outpatients. It is widely used with excellent results. Its principal downside, compared with Zithromax, is that it has to be taken twice daily for ten days, and that it can produce a steely "gunmetal" taste in the mouth. At $58–$60, it costs a bit more than Zithromax.

OPTIMAL FOR PEOPLE 60 OR OLDER
(HIGHLY RECOMMENDED/ BEST OF CLASS)

ONE-DRUG THERAPY

Levaquin (levofloxacin)

This new once-daily fluoroquinolone is effective against *Streptococcus pneumoniae, Moraxella catarrhalis, Hemophilus influenzae,* and *Mycoplasma pneumoniae.* In addition, it is active against Legionella, an "atypical" organism that can be deadly in the elderly. Its convenient dosing schedule and extensive spectrum of coverage, including gram-negative bacteria, make Levaquin an excellent one-drug choice for outpatient treatment of the elderly patient with pneumonia.

This antibiotic covers all the common bacteria that cause "walking pneumonia." One potential problem, however, is that it has a much broader spectrum of coverage than is usually necessary for this condition, which can increase the risk of producing resistance bacteria. Selective use is recommended, such as in the elderly.

TWO-DRUG THERAPY

> **Ceftin (cefuroxime)** *plus*
> **Zithromax (azithromycin),** *or*
> **Biaxin (clarithromycin),** *or*
> **Erythromycin**

If you are 60 or older and you develop a bacterial pneumonia, the chances are very good that you will be hospitalized for a few days of intravenous antibiotics. But *some* very healthy seniors who develop pneumonia can be treated at home with antibiotics.

If a doctor chooses to treat an older individual out of the hospital, many experts agree that *two* different antibiotics should be taken as part of the medication program. Two antibiotics are required as an "insurance" policy because additional bacteria that are *not* covered by Zithromax or Biaxin alone can cause pneumonia in this age group. The two-drug program that is most reliable includes a combination of Ceftin *plus* either Biaxin, Zithromax, or erythromycin.

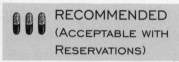 **RECOMMENDED** (ACCEPTABLE WITH RESERVATIONS)

Erythromycin

I have serious reservations about this warhorse drug, especially now that pharmaceutical science has produced equally effective, safer, and better-tolerated—albeit more costly—options. I believe that Zithromax should replace erythromycin as the drug of choice for walking pneumonia. Largely because it's dirt cheap, however, many HMOs and managed care plans advocate erythromycin as the first drug that should be used for walking pneumonia. Other experts also cite the value of this antibiotic as an "out of the gate" choice.

But erythromycin is one of the least convenient and comfortable antibiotics that physicians prescribe. It requires three to four doses per day, and 20–25 percent of people who take it get moderate to severe gastrointestinal discomfort, which can include cramping, nausea, and diarrhea. In addition, it does not cover one of the important bugs (*H. influenzae*) that can cause walking pneumonia, especially in smokers and people with other lung conditions. Erythromycin causes serious drug interactions, most important with such antihistamines as Seldane and Hismanal, and therefore it should never be taken in combination with them.

On balance, erythromycin raises concerns about convenience, comfort, (potential) safety, and coverage. Consequently, I discourage initial use of it for walking pneumonia, although it may be appropriate and provide effective therapy in selected patients. My advice: Stick with the Optimal choices, Zithromax and Biaxin.

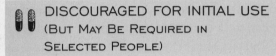

DISCOURAGED FOR INITIAL USE
(BUT MAY BE REQUIRED IN SELECTED PEOPLE)

Amoxil (amoxicillin)

The inconvenient, three-times-per-day dosing and the failure to cover *Mycoplasma*—a not-infrequent cause of walking pneumonia—explain why amoxicillin is not at the top of the comfort, effectiveness, and consistency list. Increasing resistance of this antibiotic to *S. pneumoniae* also is of concern.

Augmentin (amoxicillin-clavulanate)

Same concerns as with Amoxil for *Mycoplasma*. Twice-daily dosing is an improvement, but this drug produces diarrhea in up to 15 percent of those who take it.

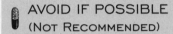

AVOID IF POSSIBLE
(NOT RECOMMENDED)

Cipro (ciprofloxacin)

This drug is effective for many conditions, especially serious kidney infections, but it should not be used routinely for most cases of walking pneumonia because it is only moderately effective against *S. pneumoniae* and is not indicated for *Mycoplasma*.

Ceclor (cefaclor)

Too many bacterial strains are becoming resistant to this antibiotic.

Penicillin

This antibiotic *used* to be the drug of choice for treating pneumonia. Now, however, it simply doesn't cover enough of the bugs predictably enough to have much use as empirical treatment.

ANTIBIOTICS FOR UNCOMPLICATED SINUS INFECTIONS*

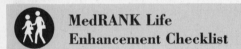

MedRANK Life Enhancement Checklist

Pills of Wisdom: Millions of Americans suffer from recurrent sinus infections. When a sinus infection is caused by bacteria—and is serious enough to cause symptoms such as thick, discolored nasal discharge, headache, tenderness over the sinus areas of the face or forehead, and/or fever—antibiotics are usually necessary. It should be pointed out, however, that not all sinus discomfort and symptoms are caused by bacterial infections that require antibiotics. Some sinus problems are caused by viruses or allergies and will *not* benefit from antibiotics. It is up to your doctor to determine if antibiotics, which should never be overused, are indicated in your particular case.

This list ranks antibiotic options for what is called acute or uncomplicated sinusitis: a sinus infec-

* In addition to antibiotics, most cases of acute, uncomplicated sinusitis will also benefit from an oral decongestant and three to five days of a topical decongestant administered into the nasal passage. If allergic symptoms have triggered your sinus infection, an oral antihistamine may be very helpful. (Please see the MedRANK Checklist "Antihistamines for Allergies" on page 156.)

tion that has come on fairly suddenly—perhaps after a cold, allergic episode, air travel, or other triggering event. Such acute infections often are easy to cure with a single course of antibiotics. They are much different from chronic sinus infections, or a series of stubborn infections that recur frequently and never seem to go away completely. If your sinus infections seem to dovetail one into the next, you may have what is considered a chronic or "subacute" condition. Chronic, ongoing sinus infections are much more difficult to treat and usually will require a referral to an ear, nose, and throat specialist.

Even simple, acute sinus infections can be stubborn and difficult to cure. They sometimes require *two* courses of antibiotics, especially if the patient is not 100 percent compliant with the medication. The important point is to take the *full course* of antibiotics, and any other medications, exactly as prescribed. In addition, if you have any conditions that can trigger a sinus infection—nasal congestion from allergies, in particular—be sure these are addressed by your physician. This MedRANK Checklist ranks medications that are useful for acute, bacterial sinus infections.

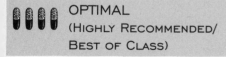

OPTIMAL
(HIGHLY RECOMMENDED/
BEST OF CLASS)

Biaxin (clarithromycin)
This drug is FDA-indicated for acute, uncomplicated bacterial infections of the sinus. It has excellent activity against the likely bacterial strains that are known to cause such infections.

Its principal downside, as compared with Zithromax, is the fact that it has to be taken twice daily for ten days, and that it can produce a steely "gunmetal" taste in the mouth. *Caution:* Biaxin should not be taken in combination with the antihistamines Seldane and Hismanal.

Septra (trimethoprim/sulfamethoxazole)
This inexpensive, relatively effective, twice-daily antibiotic is widely used for treating sinus infections. Its main advantage is cost.

Zithromax (azithromycin)
What is unique about this antibiotic is that, for all practical purposes, you get a full ten days of antibiotic coverage by taking it for only five days. Convenience-wise, this puts Zithromax in a class of its own. Although it does *not* carry an official FDA indication for treating bacterial sinus infections, it is widely and successfully used as an "off-label" treatment for this condition.

For most infections, the typical course of therapy with Zithromax is once-a-day for five days. Some physicians, however, are uncomfortable giving this drug only five days for a condition that probably requires a full ten days of bug-drug contact.

But I feel that the short course and once-daily dosing—strong compliance-enhancing features—are strong positives for Zithromax, especially for a sinus infection, when it is so critical to complete a full course of pills. The fact is, even though Zithromax is taken for a total of only five days, it's as if the patient were actually still taking it on the sixth through tenth days, because the antibiotic stays in the body's tissues—in this case, in the sinus cavity—fighting the infection until the job is done.

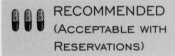

RECOMMENDED
(Acceptable with Reservations)

Augmentin (amoxicillin-clavulanate)

Now that this gold-standard and FDA-approved antibiotic for treating sinus infections is available as a twice-daily pill (as opposed to the old three-dose-per-day variety), it's more attractive. But it still requires twenty doses over ten days, which isn't ideal, and 10–15 percent of people will get diarrhea, a side effect that can make them bail out before the entire course is completed. Augmentin is particularly useful in people whose stubborn, resistant sinusitis evolves into a chronic problem.

Ceftin (cefuroxime)

This FDA-approved drug is usually reserved for treatment of stubborn, resistant sinusitis that has evolved into a chronic problem. It is safe and effective, and it is more expensive than Biaxin, Zithromax, Septra, and Augmentin.

DISCOURAGED FOR INITIAL USE
(But May Be Required in Selected People)

Amoxil (amoxicillin)

Too much resistance has developed. Therefore, it is not a first-choice medication.

Cefzil (cefprozil)

Other, equally effective drugs are available.

Vantin (cefpodoxime)

Other, equally effective drugs are available. Palatability may be a problem in children.

AVOID IF POSSIBLE
(Not Recommended)

Cipro (ciprofloxacin)

This drug is effective for many conditions, especially serious kidney infections, but should not be used routinely for bacterial sinus infections.

Ceclor (cefaclor)

Too many bacterial strains are becoming resistant to this antibiotic.

Penicillin

Penicillin simply doesn't cover enough of the bugs predictably enough to have much use in sinus infections.

ANTIBIOTICS FOR CHLAMYDIA INFECTIONS

 MedRANK Life Enhancement Checklist

 Pills of Wisdom: Sexually transmitted diseases and complications caused by chlamydia infection are responsible for about $3 billion in health care costs annually. Chlamydial infection of the cervix (and urethra) can be a "silent" condition without many symptoms, even as the disease progresses and leads to such complications as scarring of the tubes, infertility, and tubal pregnancy. Consequently, detecting this disease in its "quieter" stages is a high priority. Just as critical is selecting an antibiotic that will work the *first* time around.

No antibiotic can measure up to this standard every time, but some come very close, especially those drugs that require only one dose to achieve a cure. Zithromax, the optimal drug for treating uncomplicated chlamydial infection of the cervix, satisfies this important criterion.

 OPTIMAL
(HIGHLY RECOMMENDED/ BEST OF CLASS)

Zithromax (azithromycin)

There is no serious competition for Zithromax when it comes to treating chlamydial infection of the cervix. You take 1 gram (either as a liquid or pills), and in 94 percent of cases it's a done deal—the infection is eradicated. This is the only single-dose therapy approved by the Centers for Disease Control and Prevention (CDC). Be sure your sexual partner(s) is (are) treated, that you or your partner use condoms for protection, and that you abstain from intercourse for about one week after treatment.

RECOMMENDED
(ACCEPTABLE WITH RESERVATIONS)

Doxycyline

Prior to Zithromax, this used to be gold-standard therapy. Although very effective against chlamydia in the test tube, in the real world a sizable percentage of people just didn't comply with the seven-day, fourteen-pill regimen. With a condition like chlamydia, which can spread to many other people, there's no sense in taking chances. My vote goes to the one-dose, cure-now approach using Zithromax.

 DISCOURAGED FOR INITIAL USE
(BUT MAY BE REQUIRED IN SELECTED PEOPLE)

Erythromycin

The dosage is four pills a day for seven days. It's even more difficult to take than doxycycline, and the gastrointestinal side effects don't help.

Floxin (ofloxacin)

The dosage is twice-daily therapy for seven days. It's not to be used in pregnant women or in individuals less than 18 years of age.

 AVOID IF POSSIBLE
(NOT RECOMMENDED)

Tetracycline

The dosage is four pills per day for ten days—the risk of noncompliance is simply too great.

PILLS FOR VAGINAL CANDIDIASIS
("Yeast Infection")

 MedRANK Life Enhancement Checklist

 Pills of Wisdom: One oral tablet and many ointments and vaginal tablets are approved by the FDA for treating *Candida* (fungal) infection of the vagina. These infections produce thick, cheesy discharges. As every woman knows, some of these ointments, creams, and suppositories are uncomfortable to use and, therefore, encourage premature discontinuation of therapy. The key to success in treating candida infections is to use something that is convenient, safe, and comfortable. All the approved medications listed in this MedRANK Checklist produce cure rates that are about equivalent, as long as the patient *complies* with the medication program. Finally, intercourse should be avoided for three to five days after treatment has started.

OPTIMAL
(Highly Recommended/ Best of Class)

Diflucan (fluconazole)
One 150 mg oral tablet does the job. It doesn't get more convenient than that. The downside is that about 15 percent of patients develop some gastrointestinal distress that may include nausea, abdominal pain, or diarrhea.

Vagistat (tioconazole)
One application of 4.6 g of intravaginal ointment does the job. It's another attractive, one-dose therapy. But Vagistat is almost twice as expensive as Diflucan.

Mycelex-G (clotrimazole)
Use one vaginal tablet once. It's a matter of preference—tablet versus cream.

 RECOMMENDED
(Acceptable with Reservations)

Terazol-3 (terconazole)
Use one suppository at bedtime for three days. It's also available as intravaginal cream, to be used for three days.

Monistat-3 (miconazole)
Use one suppository at bedtime for three days.

Femstat (butoconazole)
Use this intravaginal cream at bedtime for three days.

 DISCOURAGED FOR INITIAL USE
(But May Be Required in Selected People)

Terazol-7 (terconazole)
Use this intravaginal cream at bedtime for seven days.

Monistat-7 (miconazole)
Use this intravaginal cream at bedtime for seven days.

Mycelex-7 (clotrimazole)
Use this vaginal tablet or cream at bedtime for seven days.

Gyne-Lotrimin (clotrimazole)

Use this vaginal tablet or cream at bedtime for seven days.

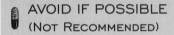

Nystatin (generic)

Use one vaginal tablet at bedtime for fourteen days.

BACTERIAL INFECTIONS OF THE VAGINA

MedRANK Life Enhancement Checklist

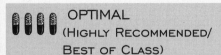

Pills of Wisdom: As opposed to candida infections, bacterial infections of the vagina involve bugs such as *Trichomonas* ("Trich"), *Gardnerella vaginalis*, bacteroides, *Mobiluncus*, *Mycoplasma*, and other organisms. These bacterial infections are frequently called *nonspecific bacterial vaginosis* (NBV), since a mixed bag of infecting bacteria is involved. The bad news is that these infections can cause more problems than initially suspected: Having bacterial vaginosis early in pregnancy increases by *fivefold* the risk of premature labor and later miscarriage. The good news is, effective medications are available for treatment, although some are easier to take than others.

OPTIMAL
(HIGHLY RECOMMENDED/
BEST OF CLASS)

Flagyl (metronidazole) (one-dose regimen)

Although the CDC recommends using Flagyl at 500 mg twice daily for seven days, studies show that cure rates are just as good with a *one-dose* approach, in which 2 grams of Flagyl are taken (by mouth) once. Flagyl should be avoided during the first trimester (twelve weeks) of pregnancy. If Flagyl is going to be used later in pregnancy, it is probably preferable to use the seven-day regimen. (See "Recommended.") This medication can cause nausea, upset stomach, headache, cramping, furry tongue, and vomiting. It can make you feel spaced out. It's not the most pleasant pill to take, but a single dose is preferable to a dosage over several days.

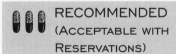

RECOMMENDED
(ACCEPTABLE WITH
RESERVATIONS)

Flagyl (metronidazole) (seven-day regimen)

Although the CDC recommends using Flagyl at 500 mg twice daily for seven days, studies show that cure rates for mild to moderate infections are just as good using a one-dose approach, in which 2 g of Flagyl are taken (by mouth) once. For more serious infections, it is reasonable to be on the longer course, but the one-dose approach is always worth a try. Please see "Optimal" for Flagyl side effects.

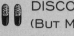 **DISCOURAGED FOR INITIAL USE**
(BUT MAY BE REQUIRED IN
SELECTED PEOPLE)

Cleocin (clindamycin)

Clindamycin can be used either as a seven-day course of oral tablets or as a 2 percent vaginal cream for seven days. Flagyl is clearly a more convenient option.

Gyne-Lotrimin (clotrimazole)

Vaginal tablets are sometimes used for four-teen days if the infection is diagnosed during pregnancy. The problem is, the cure rates are very low (about 20 percent), and the woman usually needs to be treated with Flagyl after moving into the later stages of pregnancy.

 AVOID IF POSSIBLE
(NOT RECOMMENDED)

ALL OTHERS

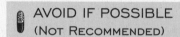 **PILLS FOR STREP THROAT, TONSILLITIS, AND PHARYNGITIS**
(Bad Sore Throat, "White Spots on My Tonsils," "Tonsil Infection")

 MedRANK Life Enhancement Checklist

Pills of Wisdom: The treatment for this very common condition is in a state of flux. Although it is usually referred to as "strep throat," it actually can be caused by a number of other bacterial strains as well. Penicillin has been the gold-standard treatment for strep throat. The problem is that, although many of the newer antibiotics will cure the infection and kill the bacteria causing it, only penicillin has actually been *proven* to *prevent* rheumatic fever, the dreaded complication of inadequately treated strep throat. (On the other hand, although newer antibiotics have not been shown to prevent rheumatic fever, there is no reason to think they will be less effective in this regard.) As a result, many doctors still stick to the old "less convenient" penicillin. Regardless of which antibiotic is prescribed on your behalf, the bottom line is that you must complete the entire course of therapy, even if your symptoms are gone before all your pills have been taken.

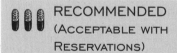 **OPTIMAL**
(HIGHLY RECOMMENDED/
BEST OF CLASS)

Benzathine penicillin G (intramuscular shot)

It may be a pain, but this one-shot cure for strep throat is a sure thing and eliminates the risk of noncompliance.

Penicillin V

This penicillin approach also works, but it does require taking a pill four times a day for ten days. If this is your (or your physician's) preference, be *sure* you take all forty pills.

RECOMMENDED
(ACCEPTABLE WITH
RESERVATIONS)

Erythromycin

If you are allergic to penicillin, erythromycin is recommended by the American Heart Association for prophylaxis against rheumatic fever. *Caution:* Erythromycin causes troublesome gastrointestinal symptoms in about 20 percent of people who take it. Moreover, the multiple daily doses are not optimally convenient.

Zithromax (azithromycin)

A five-day course of therapy with this antibiotic is the next-simplest thing to a one-shot penicillin cure.

Biaxin (clarithromycin)

The ten days of therapy with twenty pills make this drug more convenient than penicillin.

Vantin (cefpodoxime)

Once-daily treatment makes this an attractive option.

 DISCOURAGED FOR INITIAL USE (BUT MAY BE REQUIRED IN SELECTED PEOPLE)

Ceftin (cefuroxime)
Lorabid (loracarbef)

Ten days of treatment, twenty pills, and expensive, relatively speaking. These drugs are as effective as the options in the "Recommended" category.

 AVOID IF POSSIBLE (NOT RECOMMENDED)

ALL OTHERS

ANTIVIRAL PILLS FOR GENITAL HERPES INFECTION*
("Herpes," "Vaginal Herpes," "Genital Blisters," "Blister Herpes")

 MedRANK Life Enhancement Checklist

Pills of Wisdom: An estimated 20 million American men and women suffer from the sexually transmissible genital herpes infection. The impact of this disease should not be underestimated. In addition to pain and discomfort, it can produce symptoms of fatigue, upper respiratory discomfort, and muscle burning. Herpes also increases the risk of cervical cancer, and pregnant women are advised not to have a vaginal delivery *if* labor begins while they are having an *acute* outbreak of their infection. Consequently,

we have powerful incentives to prevent transmission of this disease with safe sexual practices, and to reduce recurrence rates (flare-ups) in high-risk individuals, so that fewer people will be exposed to viral transmission.

Although there is currently no *cure* for genital herpes, antiviral medications can significantly reduce the length and severity of a first attack. Equally important, these pills can dramatically reduce the recurrence rates (outbreaks of genital blisters) in people who suffer from several episodes per year. Zovirax, the first drug approved for this indication, has to be taken five times a day to treat a first attack. Newer drugs such as Valtrex require only twice-daily dosing

---

* There is no proof that these medications prevent shedding, or transmission of the herpes virus from one sexual partner to another. Consequently, practicing safe sex using a condom barrier method is mandatory, whether medications are being taken or not. Do not share these medications with anyone, including sexual partners.

and are just as effective. The problem with all antiviral drugs for herpes is that they are quite expensive (about $100–$125 for a course of therapy).

All of the medications in this MedRANK Checklist will be equally effective *if* you take them exactly as prescribed. Accordingly, it is convenience and comfort factors that distinguish between more and less desirable pills.

 OPTIMAL FOR TREATMENT
OF FIRST ATTACKS
AND RECURRENCES
(Highly Recommended/
Best of Class)

Valtrex (valacyclovir)

Approved by the FDA for treatment of genital herpes, Valtrex is easier to take and is as effective as the old standard, Zovirax. Valtrex is the optimal pill for herpes for the simple reasons of convenience and compliance. Among people with their *first* attack of herpes, a *twice*-daily dosing regimen for ten days with Valtrex was as effective as a *five*-times-per-day regimen with Zovirax. Valtrex has not been extensively studied for long-term prevention (see "Optimal for Long-Term Prevention"), and therefore its use should be restricted to treating first attacks or acute flare-ups as they occur. This drug is quite comfortable for most people to take, although gastrointestinal upset, headache, and rash can occur.

 OPTIMAL FOR LONG-TERM
PREVENTION OF
RECURRENT ATTACKS
(Highly Recommended/
Best of Class)

Zovirax (acyclovir)

For people who suffer more than six flare-ups (or outbreaks) of their genital herpes infection, *prevention* for six to twelve months is usually advised. For *prevention* purposes, Zovirax is dosed on a *twice-daily* basis, which is quite tolerable. The drug has been shown to be effective (more than 90 percent reduction in flare-ups) for a period of up to three years. It is the drug of choice for long-term prevention.

Famvir (famciclovir)

With a twice-daily dosing schedule, this drug is effective for treating *recurrent* attacks.

 RECOMMENDED FOR
TREATMENT OF FIRST ATTACKS
(Acceptable with
Reservations)

Zovirax (acyclovir)

Zovirax *was* the gold standard for treating first attacks of herpes. The problem is that it is usually given five times per day—a dosing schedule that most people find inconvenient. A three-times-per-day approach also has been shown to be effective. Because Valtrex and Famvir have the advantage of twice-daily dosing, however, most patients will prefer them over Zovirax.

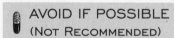 DISCOURAGED FOR INITIAL USE
(But May Be Required in
Selected People)

All Others

 AVOID IF POSSIBLE
(Not Recommended)

All Others

PILLS FOR SHINGLES (HERPES ZOSTER)
Pills for Chronic Nerve Pain (Postherpetic Neuralgia)

 ## MedRANK Life Enhancement Checklist

Pills of Wisdom: Shingles is a common, potentially painful infection that involves inflammation, blisters, skin eruptions, burning pain, and electric shock–like sensations on the surface of the skin. The condition is caused by the reactivation of a dormant virus that was originally introduced into the nerves by an earlier bout of varicella-zoster (chicken pox) infection. The older you are, the greater your risk of getting a shingles outbreak, which is also much more common in HIV-infected patients, individuals with cancer, and children with leukemia.

The pain associated with a shingles eruption tends to go away within a week or two. Middle-aged adults (people under 50) may be able to tolerate a first attack with no medications whatsoever, whereas *older* individuals frequently have *severe* attacks that require antiviral pills and anti-inflammatory medications. These pills can reduce the *length* and *severity* of symptoms. Attacks can be recurrent, but the most troublesome complication of shingles is the chronic, recurrent nerve pain and irritating skin sensations—what is called *postherpetic neuralgia*—which can last for a year, or even longer, following an acute outbreak.

Although postherpetic neuralgia is difficult to treat—and can be especially severe in the elderly—the medications discussed in this MedRANK Checklist offer the best options for dealing with this problem.

 ## OPTIMAL
(HIGHLY RECOMMENDED/ BEST OF CLASS)

ANTIVIRAL MEDICATIONS

Famvir (famciclovir)

Because their shingles attacks are prolonged and painful, people 50 or older should probably receive treatment with antiviral medications, which can reduce the severity and length of the attacks. Famvir is given three times per day for seven days and should be started *as soon as the diagnosis is made.* In the case of recurrent outbreaks, it should be started as soon as the typical rash appears.

In addition to Famvir—or any of the other antiviral drugs listed here—the corticosteroid *prednisone* should be started at once and gradually discontinued over twenty-one days. Although these medications do *not* completely eliminate postherpetic neuralgia, they help clear up the skin lesions and reduce the duration of nerve pain by about two months.

Valtrex (valacyclovir)

This effective antiviral drug is dosed three times per day. See "Famvir" for timing and indications.

CORTICOSTEROIDS

Prednisone

In older patients, especially those with more severe symptoms, this once-daily corticosteroid pill will improve symptoms and reduce pain over the short term. It doesn't completely prevent postherpetic neuralgia.

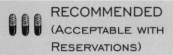

RECOMMENDED
(ACCEPTABLE WITH RESERVATIONS)

ANTIVIRAL MEDICATIONS

Zovirax (acyclovir)

This antiviral drug is effective, but patients have to take five doses per day for seven days, as opposed to three doses per day for Famvir and Valtrex.

PAIN RELIEVERS

NSAIDs (ibuprofen)

Of questionable benefit.

Vicodin (hydrocodone)

May be of some benefit.

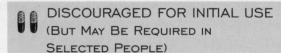

DISCOURAGED FOR INITIAL USE
(BUT MAY BE REQUIRED IN SELECTED PEOPLE)

ANTIDEPRESSANT MEDICATIONS

Elavil (amitriptyline)

For people who have persistent, troublesome, and incapacitating pain that doesn't respond to mild pain relievers, this antidepressant, at very low doses, has been shown to work.

Norpramin (desipramine)

Same as for Elavil.

Capsaicin cream

This cream may relieve pain, but no definitive studies have been done to demonstrate its effects conclusively.

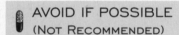

AVOID IF POSSIBLE
(NOT RECOMMENDED)

ALL OTHERS

PILLS FOR UNCOMPLICATED URINARY TRACT INFECTIONS IN WOMEN
(Bladder Infection, Cystitis, Urethritis, UTI, Urinary Infection)

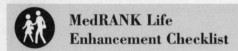

MedRANK Life Enhancement Checklist

Pills of Wisdom: Treating patients with simple urinary tract infections (bladder infections or cystitis) is getting easier all the time. Rather than ten days, women can be treated with only three days of antibiotics in most circumstances. Longer courses of antibiotics are needed only if the shorter course of therapy fails.

Typical symptoms of bladder infection include burning, increased frequency of urination, and the sensation of needing to urinate. When the infection is more serious and involves the kidney, fourteen days of antibiotics are required—no shortcuts permitted. In simple cases, antibiotics are chosen on an empirical basis—that is, drugs that are likely to eliminate all the bugs known to cause this kind of infection are used first. But when the infection is more serious and involves the kidney, or when it occurs in someone who is pregnant, bacterial cultures of the urine should be taken and antibiotics modified (if necessary) according to the results.

Women who suffer more than one episode of urinary tract infection in a year should be considered for *preventive* therapy, which usually consists of an every-*other*-day dose of an inexpensive antibiotic such as Septra. When these infections follow sexual intercourse (so-called "honeymoon cystitis"), diligent attention to one-dose treatments in the postcoital period is very effective. If urinary tract infections are recurrent in a postmenopausal woman, estrogen cream (0.5 mg of estriol cream once each night for two weeks, followed by two applications per week for eight months) can reduce repeated infections and antibiotic use.

Finally, it should be stressed that symptoms of urinary infection—burning and discomfort—can also represent infection with a sexually transmissible disease such as chlamydia, which is effectively treated with a different class of antibiotics. (See the MedRANK Checklist "Antibiotics for Chlamydia Infections" on page 221.)

OPTIMAL
(HIGHLY RECOMMENDED/ BEST OF CLASS)

Bactrim (trimothoprim/ sulfamethoxazole)
Septra (trimethoprim/sulfamethoxazole)

This drug is cheap, effective, and safe. Almost every doctor will agree that it is the logical pill to try first in a woman with an uncomplicated bladder infection. With one-dose treatment, the success rate is only about 60–65 percent. But when this twice-daily pill is given for *three* days, the cure rate jumps to 85 percent or better. That's the time period for treatment I recommend. If you fail the three-day course, you'll need a urine culture and a full ten days of treatment with this or another antibiotic.

Monurol

This one-dose treatment for urinary tract infection is effective and convenient.

SPECIAL CONSIDERATION FOR RECURRENT INFECTIONS IN POSTMENOPAUSAL WOMEN

Vaginal estrogen cream

Vaginal estrogen cream is not a primary medication used to treat urinary tract infections, but it can be very effective in preventing recurrent infections in postmenopausal women. Using 0.5 mg of estriol cream once each night for two weeks, followed by two applications per week for eight months, can reduce repeat episodes by about 50 percent. It is not to be used during pregnancy.

RECOMMENDED
(ACCEPTABLE WITH RESERVATIONS)

QUINOLONE ANTIBIOTICS

Trovan (trovafloxacin)
Cipro (ciprofloxacin)
Floxin (ofloxacin)
Noroxin (norfloxacin)

These antibiotics are every bit as effective as, and perhaps even more effective than, Septra-like drugs for more serious urinary tract infections. For an uncomplicated bladder infection, however, they are a bit pricey compared with Septra, which does the job in about 90 percent of cases. They also should be used in short courses, usually a three-day period, although one-dose treatments have also been shown to be effective. These drugs should not be used during pregnancy.

CEPHALOSPORINS

Ceftin (cefuroxime)
Lorabid (loracarbef)
Vantin (cefpodoxime)

These cephalosporin antibiotics are excellent drugs for complicated urinary tract infections that involve the kidney.

 DISCOURAGED FOR INITIAL USE
(BUT MAY BE REQUIRED IN SELECTED PEOPLE)

Augmentin (amoxicillin-clavulanate)

Augmentin is a good drug for urinary tract infections. It does an excellent job at eliminating the appropriate bacteria, and it is especially useful for more serious kidney infections. Its effectiveness for short courses is not as well studied as for the quinolone antibiotics and Septra. Its drawbacks are its cost and its gastrointestinal side effects.

Doxycycline

This antibiotic is sometimes used for treating simple urinary tract infections. How effective it is for short three-day courses is not known, and therefore preference is given to the antibiotics in the "Optimal" and "Recommended" categories.

Nitrofurantoin

This drug is effective, but better, safer options are available.

 AVOID IF POSSIBLE
(NOT RECOMMENDED)

Amoxil (amoxicillin)

Too many bacterial strains involved in bladder infections have become resistant to amoxicillin, so this drug is no longer recommended for bladder infections.

ANTIBIOTICS FOR BACTERIAL BRONCHITIS
(Bronchitis, "The Crud," "Lung Infection," "Chest Cold")

 MedRANK Life Enhancement Checklist

Pills of Wisdom: Bacterial bronchitis is a bacterial infection of the bronchial air passages in someone who is known to have chronic obstructive pulmonary disease (COPD). This includes individuals with chronic bronchitis, emphysema, and other forms of lung disease. The majority are smokers or have been exposed to secondhand smoke. Chronic bronchitis, the most common condition, is characterized by a chronic cough that is productive of abnormal quantities of yellow-colored sputum.

Flare-ups of these chronic lung conditions are often caused by a bacterial infection. When this is the case, antibiotic treatment will usually help accelerate recovery and restore breathing status. It should be stressed that the precise value of antibiotics for these flare-ups is not established, although most doctors agree that these pills are worth a try in *most* patients with *significant* symptoms. Because the value of antibiotics in these cases is so controversial, for many doctors cost is the main factor driving pill selection.

Younger adults and adolescents frequently suffer from what is called *acute bronchitis*. Usually this illness is caused by a virus or other organism against which antibiotics are *ineffective*. People with fever and severe symptoms—coughing, wheezing, and sputum—should see their doctors to be sure they don't have pneumonia. (See the MedRANK Checklist "Antibiotics for 'Walking' Pneumonia" on page 215.)

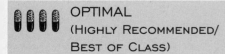 OPTIMAL
(HIGHLY RECOMMENDED/
BEST OF CLASS)

Zithromax (azithromycin)

Convenient. Comfortable. Consistent. Safe. Curative. In my view, this "less is more" antibiotic is the best choice for people with chronic lung conditions who get flare-ups of bronchitis caused by bacterial infection. Its strong points include a compliance-enhancing, five-day course of once-daily doses. It has no risk of significant drug-drug interactions, which is important because people with lung problems are frequently taking other medications. It eliminates all the likely bacteria that cause bronchitis flare-ups in people with chronic lung diseae. The gastrointestinal symptoms associated with many antibiotics are seen in less than 5 percent of people who take a five-day course of therapy. And the likelihood of producing a vaginal yeast infection is less than 2 percent. In short, Zithromax is patient-friendly. From a convenience and comfort perspective, it is impossible to beat. But if the cost is a problem, consider Septra or Vibramycin in the "Recommended" category.

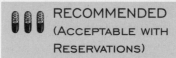 RECOMMENDED
(ACCEPTABLE WITH
RESERVATIONS)

Biaxin (clarithromycin)

This drug shares with Zithromax excellent activity against the likely bugs that cause bronchitis flare-ups in patients with chronic lung disease. It is widely and successfully used, with excellent results. Its principal downside, as compared to Zithromax, is the fact that it has to be taken twice daily for ten days and that it can produce a steely "gunmetal" taste in the mouth. It can produce drug interactions, so a bit more caution is required. At $58–$60, it's a touch more expensive than the Optimal drug Zithromax.

Trovan (trovafloxacin)
Levaquin (levofloxacin)

These once-daily antibiotics require seven days of treatment and cover all the likely bacteria that cause flare-ups of bronchitis. Its spectrum of coverage is a bit broad for routine bronchitis, and therefore its use as an initial drug is questionable.

Vibramycin (doxycycline)

This drug also covers the appropriate bugs that cause acute bronchitis flare-ups. It's very attractively priced among the twice-daily antibiotics that are indicated for this condition.

Septra (trimethoprim/sulfa)

Septra is an effective twice-daily medication when taken for ten days. It has many of the same advantages as doxycycline, including an attractive price (less than $15).

Ceftin (cefuroxime)

A very effective but rather expensive drug ($80–$100 for a course of therapy) for this condition. Other drugs (Biaxin, Zithromax, Septra, Vibramycin) do the job with equal or better convenience for fewer dollars.

 ## DISCOURAGED FOR INITIAL USE (BUT MAY BE REQUIRED IN SELECTED PEOPLE)

Augmentin (amoxicillin-clavulanate)

This antibiotic is effective. However, it is more expensive than some other effective pills (Septra, Vibramycin) that require twenty doses over ten days. This isn't ideal, and 10–15 percent of people will get diarrhea, a side effect that can make some people bail out before the course is completed. It's in the "Discouraged" category because of its price and side effects.

Amoxil (amoxicillin)

Its inconvenient three-times-per-day dosing and its failure to effectively eliminate all bacterial strains causing bronchitis explain why amoxicillin is not at the top of the comfort and consistency list. Increasing resistance of this antibiotic to *S. pneumoniae* (one of the principal bacterial offenders in this condition) is also a concern.

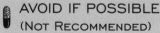 ## AVOID IF POSSIBLE (NOT RECOMMENDED)

Tetracycline

Tetracycline has the same effectiveness as Vibramycin (see "Recommended"), but it has to be taken four times daily, which is a liability as far as convenience and compliance are concerned.

Erythromycin

Erythromycin doesn't eliminate all the bacteria (*H. influenzae*) causing bacterial bronchitis in people with chronic lung disease.

Ceclor (cefaclor)

Better drugs are available than Ceclor. Bacteria such as *S. pneumoniae* are becoming increasingly resistant to it.

Penicillin

It's not effective in bronchitis because too many bacteria are resistant to it.

QUINOLONE ANTIBIOTICS

Floxin (ofloxacin)
Cipro (ciprofloxacin)
Maxaquin (lomefloxacin)

These rather costly ($60–$80) antibiotics work fairly well for bronchitis, but they are difficult to justify as first-out-of-the-gate choices because less expensive options provide greater coverage at much lower cost. An exception is Levaquin (see "Recommended").

VACCINATIONS THAT PROLONG LIFE AND PREVENT SERIOUS OR FATAL DISEASES IN ADULTS*

  MedRANK Life Prolongation and Enhancement Checklist

Pills of Wisdom: Children are not the only people who require vaccinations for disease prevention. Adults can benefit from vaccinations too. Yet many adults fail to take advantage of prevention-oriented shots that can reduce their risk of serious illnesses such as influenza and pneumonia. Most adult vaccinations are targeted at specific groups of people who are most likely to benefit. This MedRANK Checklist identifies adult immunizations than can help you or members of your family.

IMMUNIZATION CHECKLIST FOR ADULTS

Influenza vaccine (flu shots)

Who should get a flu shot? My philosophy has always been, if you're not sure if you qualify, just get one. Flu shots are cheap and safe, and even if you're not a high-risk (weakened or debilitated) patient, the flu can put even the most fit person on their back. If you are 65 or older, though, or if you have a chronic lung or heart problem, diabetes, kidney problems, asthma, or just about any other debilitating condition, you should get a flu shot by all means. Doctors, nurses, home health care providers, and people providing essential community services should be vaccinated. If you are traveling to the Tropics at any time of year or to the Southern Hemisphere between April and September, you should be vaccinated. The vaccine is considered safe for pregnant women.

Even a "touch" of influenza in a person with a significantly weakened immune system can turn into a strong handshake with pneumonia or even death. The slope is slippery. HIV-infected individuals, who may already be warding off respiratory conditions, such as *Pneumocystis carinii* pneumonia (PCP), need all the protection they can get, and flu shots are a good, harmless place to start.

Influenza outbreaks in the United States usually begin in December and peak in January and February. A flu shot will start protecting you about ten days after the injection and will last for up to six months, so the best time to get a flu shot is probably between mid-October and mid-November. Some studies suggest that cancer patients on chemotherapy may benefit from two flu shots.

Pneumovax 23

A polyvalent pneumococcal vaccine effective against the twenty-three most common strains of *S. pneumoniae* bacteria that cause pneumonia. Pneumonia is nobody's friend these days, least of all the elderly, people with

* See the MedRANK Checklist "Preventing and Treating Infections While Traveling" on page 234 for additional vaccinations required under special circumstances.

chronic lung or heart problems, or HIV-infected individuals. About one-third of all people between the ages of 50 and 64 have indications for the Pneumovax vaccine. (Being 65 or older is an automatic indication.) Unfortunately, *only 25 percent* of eligible people actually *get* vaccinated. Protection against pneumonia is neither perfect nor forever, but lowering risk against it is a priority. One shot lasts about six years, maybe longer.

Varicella vaccine (against chicken pox)

Although this vaccine is directed *primarily* at infants and children, it is approved for use in "susceptible" adults and adolescents, because when adults get chicken pox, it can be quite severe. The vaccine is recommended for health care workers, people with immune-deficiency diseases, people working in day-care centers or schools, nonpregnant women of childbearing age (to reduce risk for congenital varicella), and international travelers.

PREVENTING AND TREATING INFECTIONS WHILE TRAVELING*
(Traveler's Diarrhea, Turista, Hepatitis A, Malaria, Polio, and Others)

  MedRANK Life Prolongation and Enhancement Checklist

Pills of Wisdom: If you are planning to travel to countries where diseases such as Traveler's Diarrhea, malaria, and hepatitis are known to be endemic, you will want to contact the Centers for Disease Control (CDC) by telephone (404-332-4559) or fax (404-332-4565) for information relating to legal requirements, epidemiological conditions, and preventive measures that are appropriate for a given location at a given time. The following prudent recommendations will also make your travels safer and more comfortable.

Traveler's Diarrhea

This common condition, also known as *turista* when acquired in Mexico, is caused by a bacterium (enterotoxigenic *E. coli*) and is usually self-limited, lasting for three to seven days. Although excellent medications are available to *prevent* traveler's diarrhea, many physicians prefer to start treatment only *after* the symptoms begin. I believe the decision should depend on your comfort level and past experience. In other words, if you have traveled to a specific place or region several times and repeatedly have acquired traveler's diarrhea during your visits, it would make sense to consider a pill for prevention. If you fit this profile, my advice is, just take it. The most effective medications for prevention are Cipro (ciprofloxacin), Floxin (ofloxacin), and Noroxin (norfloxacin). They are state-of-the-art for preventing traveler's diarrhea and the vacation-killing symptoms it produces. These

* As a rule, more than one vaccination can be given at the same time. Pregnant women and people with immunologically compromised disease should not receive live virus vaccines. Measles vaccine, however, is recommended for HIV-infected people and pregnant women who cannot avoid exposure.

broad-spectrum antibiotics are all dosed on a once-daily basis, and you shouldn't take them for longer than three weeks. Start taking them two days before your trip begins and continue until two days after you return home.

Pepto-Bismol can also work but is much more cumbersome to take (two tablets four times daily), changes the color of your tongue and bowel movements, and can cause an unpleasant ringing in your ears.

If you *haven't* taken preventive pills and develop traveler's diarrhea during or just after your trip, you'll want treatment, especially if the symptoms are distressing enough to interfere with your daily routine (which is usually the case). Not surprisingly, the same three drugs are also the best treatment options.

The daily dose is *doubled*, however, for *treating* acute symptoms, and you should take the medications until the symptoms resolve, and no longer than three days. It should be stressed that taking antibiotic pills for traveler's diarrhea is generally indicated if your symptoms are severe enough to get in the way of your daily activities. Imodium, an over-the-counter medication, can be used in conjunction with Cipro, Floxin, or Noroxin to relieve diarrhea symptoms.

Finally, many physicians still use Septra or Bactrim, but they are *not* recommended as first-line choices because resistance to them has developed in many areas.

Malaria

If you are going to a region known to have chloroquine-resistant malaria, Lariam (mefloquine) 250 mg once a week is the drug of choice. (Chloroquine resistance is quite common and has been reported wherever malaria occurs, except for Central America west of the Panama Canal Zone, Haiti, Mexico, the Dominican Republic, and the Middle East.) If you are traveling to a chloroquine-sensitive area, the preventive pill of choice is Aralen (chloroquine) 300 mg once a week. Call the CDC for more information.

Hepatitis A

If you are planning a trip to an area where hygiene is known to be sorely lacking—and especially if you will be traveling off the beaten path—you will want to get vaccinated against hepatitis A at least 15 to 21 days before you start. The two recommended hepatitis A vaccines are Havrix and Vaqta. They are given as a single dose to adults and as two doses, one month apart, to children. This is followed by a booster dose in six to twelve weeks.

Hepatitis B

Vaccination against hepatitis B is *not* routinely recommended, except for medical and related personnel who may be handling body fluids, or people who expect to have sexual contact, receive medical or dental care, or stay for six months or more in Southeast Asia or sub-Saharan Africa.

Yellow Fever

If you are traveling to rural areas of yellow-fever-endemic zones, which includes most of tropical South America and most of Africa between 15 degrees north and south latitude, you should get yellow fever vaccine about ten days prior to your trip. Boosters are given every ten years.

Polio

If you have not been previously immunized against polio and are planning travel to developing or tropical countries outside the Western Hemisphere, you should receive a primary series of enhanced inactivated polio vaccine (eIPV). If you require immediate protection (within four weeks), a single dose of eIPV or trivalent (live) oral polio vaccine (OPV) is recommended. Be aware that OPV can (rarely) cause vaccine-induced polio (in one case per million vaccinations).

Japanese Encephalitis

This potentially fatal disease seen in rural Asia is transmitted by mosquitoes. A vaccination (JE-Vax) should be strongly considered if you plan to travel extensively in rural rice-growing areas that would bring you in contact with mosquitoes. Despite its name, the condition rarely occurs on the main islands of Japan.

Cholera

Tourists have a very low risk of acquiring cholera. The vaccine that is currently licensed in the United States is marginally effective and not recommended.

CHAPTER 14

■

COCKTAILS FOR LIFE

Cancer Medications

Over the years, the questions I have been asked about medications used to treat cancer have been very predictable and, almost without exception, very appropriate. People want to know the benefits of these pills as well their downside—the risks of hair loss, depression, fatigue, and other toxic side effects. Who can blame them? More than with other classes of medications, the decision to use these powerful drugs must be an educated one. "What are the chances chemotherapy will cure my cancer?" patients anxiously inquire. "And how bad will the side effects be? Are these drugs worth it?" Usually, the answer is yes. As you might expect, however, every case is different.

☼ *The good news is that many chemotherapy regimens, in combination with other treatment options—usually surgery or radiation therapy—can cure or significantly prolong life in people who have been diagnosed with cancer.*

Among those malignancies that respond to chemotherapy, significant strides have been made for breast cancer, lymphoma, and leukemia, among others. You can consult the MedRANK Checklist "Cancer Chemotherapy Regimens" on page 242 for an evaluation of the effectiveness of various regimens for specific cancers.

Drugs used to treat cancer—so-called chemotherapy medications—work by a variety of different mechanisms. Some chemotherapeutic agents can actually cure disease, as in the case of Hodgkin's lymphoma, whereas other anticancer medications are used to produce remissions (temporary elimination of the signs and symptoms of cancer). These drugs must always be prescribed by a physician, preferably an oncologist who is familiar with their indications, side effects, and approved protocols. I believe they should be prescribed by an oncologist, a cancer specialist, or hematologist, because the field is evolving very quickly, and cancer specialists are more likely to keep abreast of the latest advances.

☺ *The anti-breast cancer drug tamoxifen (Nolvadex) has been shown to reduce the rates of recurrence and death from the disease among a wide range of women. Despite its potential benefits, the drug is prescribed for far too few patients.*

The finding that tamoxifen has the capacity not only to prevent recurrence of breast cancer but that it can prevent this malignancy in women at high risk for the disease has important implications for women of all ages. Contrary to what many doctors had believed, tamoxifen benefits breast cancer patients of all ages, not just those who have gone through menopause, and the drug is effective whether the cancer was localized to the breast or had spread to lymph nodes in the armpit. The drug is also effective whether the cancer was removed surgically (lumpectomy or mastectomy) or treated with radiation or chemotherapy drugs. A new finding is that the drug is also effective in women whose tumors were negative for estrogen receptors.

The benefits of treating women with breast cancer with tamoxifen outweigh any risk in endometrial cancer, which is often curable if caught early. It also carries a small risk of causing potentially fatal clots to the lung. Over a period of ten years, however, it is estimated that tamoxifen can prevent 80 deaths due to breast cancer per 1000 women taking tamoxifen for a period of five years, but may cause 2 deaths per 1000 women due to uterine cancer and one death from blood clots in the lung.

What is clear is that tamoxifen is underprescribed in women with breast cancer, and could save an additional 20,000 lives worldwide if prescribed for more women. If you or a family member has or has had breast cancer, it is important to inquire of your suitability as a candidate for this medication. The overwhelming majority of women with breast cancer will benefit from this drug.

Finally, whether tamoxifen's benefits outweigh the risks for *protecting* high-risk women against breast cancer remains uncertain. The National Cancer Institute stopped a study on the preventative effects of the drug, more than a year early, after initial results showed it reduced the incidence of first time breast cancer by more than 45 percent. Given these impressive results, tamoxifen's benefits will likely extend to younger women with breast cancer, as well as those at high risk who are likely to benefit from prevention.

☺ *Although anticancer drugs can be highly effective, as a group of medications, their side effects are more troublesome and potentially serious than those seen in most other therapeutic classes.*

If you require chemotherapy, you will want to know what's coming down the road and make decisions that balance the benefits against the pitfalls. The problem is that although development efforts are directed toward finding medications that work only on cancer cells, most drugs now used to treat malignancies also cause significant toxicity in *normal* tissues.

This toxicity can cause a wide range of side effects, including fatigue, decreased energy levels, low blood counts, hair loss and skin changes, and nausea and vomiting. Fortunately, most of these side effects are transient in nature and will normalize after the chemotherapy regimen has been completed. You will want to review the MedRANK Checklist "Side Effects and Complications of Chemotherapy" on page 248 to learn what side effects and problems you can expect with specific anticancer drugs.

If you or a family member requires chemotherapy, the following caveats are worth remembering. First, for the management of most malignant diseases, combinations of cancer drugs are generally superior to single drug therapy. This means that you will take a specific combination of medications according to a predetermined sequence or dosing schedule. It is important that you follow this dosing schedule precisely as outlined by your prescribing physician. Always ask for detailed instructions and a written appointment schedule. Combinations of cancer drugs usually lead to higher response rates and longer remissions. The reason for this is that many of these medications work by different mechanisms. Because cancer cells may acquire resistance to a single agent, combination therapy is frequently effective in cases where a single drug has failed to produce a remission or cure. Moreover, increased responsiveness to combination therapy may permit the dosage of many individual medications to be reduced and therefore decrease their toxic side effects.

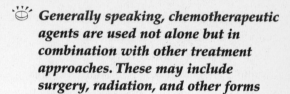 ***Generally speaking, chemotherapeutic agents are used not alone but in combination with other treatment approaches. These may include surgery, radiation, and other forms of drug therapy.***

Although attempts have been made to reduce the adverse side effects of anticancer medications, the fact is, patients who require chemotherapy must prepare themselves for *moderate to severe impairments in their quality of life during the program.* Some regimens will require visits to the doctor's office or hospital to receive medications that are administered intravenously. In some cases, hospitalization may even be required during the initial course of therapy.

Virtually all anticancer agents require laboratory monitoring to ensure that the white blood cell, red blood cell, and platelet counts do not fall into a range that can lead to serious complications, such as bleeding, infection, or anemia.

As a rule, your physician will order these tests at precise points following the administration of your medication, and depending upon your blood counts, he or she may modify the dosage for your next treatment cycle. Because chemotherapy agents can lower your body's ability to fight infection, you should be aware of any signs of infection, including fever, sore throat, rashes, or shaking chills, all of which suggest the need for further evaluation. Because many of these medications can produce fetal abnormalities, birth control measures are usually recommended during treatment. You should always contact your doctor if you suspect pregnancy while receiving a course of chemotherapy.

Special precautions are required if you accidentally miss a dose. As a rule, you should take the next dose as soon as possible, as long as no more than one to two hours has elapsed. On the other hand, if several hours have passed or it is time for the next dose, do not double the dose in order to catch up, unless you are advised by your doctor to do so. If you missed more than one dose, it may be necessary to establish a new dosage schedule, in which case you should contact your doctor immediately.

☺ *Chemotherapy programs differ in length—some last as short as six weeks, and others as long as six months or more. Probably the most difficult part of maintaining a regimen is coping with the nonlife-threatening but uncomfortable quality-of-life-impairing side effects, such as nausea, vomiting, fatigue, decreased energy, and hair loss.*

Fortunately, excellent medications are available that will reduce gastrointestinal symptoms such as nausea and vomiting. If these symptoms are intolerable or get in the way of your normal daily activities, you should ask your physician to prescribe an antinausea medication, some of which are extremely effective. (See the MedRANK Checklist "Taking the Edge Off" on page 250.)

Managing fatigue and decreased energy is more difficult. Because these symptoms are caused by both the direct toxic effects of the medications, as well as by decreased blood counts, you may have to wait until your course of chemotherapy is over before you recover energy level.

☺ *Many physicians suggest temporary treatment with an antidepressant to improve outlook on life and energy level. I recommend this approach when necessary.*

Because many anticancer medications can produce depression, it is reasonable to consider antidepressant therapy in conjunction with them. Fortunately, the hair loss caused by anticancer drugs is almost always temporary, and once your chemotherapy program is complete, your hair will grow back. During periods of hair loss, you may wish to use a turban, wig, or other cosmetic approach.

☺ *Drinking plenty of liquids, getting exercise as tolerated, and maintaining social activities and strong family relationships will help you negotiate many of the problems and pitfalls associated with anticancer therapy.*

Chemotherapy support groups are also useful for sharing fears, anxieties, and other quality-of-life issues. Your physician or hospital can usually direct you to these support groups, as well as to other sources of information.

☺ *Pain relief is of paramount importance in people who have cancer. It should be emphasized that drugs are the cornerstone of pain management for the cancer patient.*

When appropriate, aspirin, acetaminophen, or nonsteroidal anti-inflammatory drugs (NSAIDs) are the initial agents of choice. As required, they should be supplemented by narcotic medications such as codeine or hydrocodone. In more severe cases, morphine, methadone, and fentanyl are appropriate. These medications should be given on an around-the-clock basis, with additional doses available on an as-needed basis. You should be aware that tolerance and dependence are predictable consequences of using potent high-dose narcotic analgesics, but this should not preclude the use of adequate doses to achieve acceptable pain relief. As emphasized, antidepressants and other medications may also be useful in combination with opioid (narcotic) medications.

☺ *Unfortunately, pain management is woefully inadequate for many patients with cancer. To minimize this problem, be sure that you provide your physician with an accurate, complete history of your pain patterns, including severity and time of day.*

Fortunately, pain medications are relatively inexpensive, they usually work fairly quickly, and they entail acceptable risks. Except for medications that affect blood-clotting factors, such as aspirin and NSAIDs, most pain medications can be given safely in combination with a chemotherapy program.

☺ *Although the specific pain regimen will always have to be tailored to the individual patient, a useful protocol has been developed by the World Health Organization. (See the MedRANK Checklist "The Three-Step Approach to Cancer Pain Management" on page 252.)*

Initially, aspirin, acetaminophen, or an NSAID is instituted, followed by the addition of an opioid such as codeine or hydrocodone (often as a fixed combination pill because of synergistic effects). These potent agents should be started at the *outset* in patients with *moderate to severe* pain due to their malignancy. Patient-controlled analgesia, using programmable pumps to deliver drugs intravenously, subcutaneously, or by other routes, are especially useful to treat pain that breaks through an established drug regimen. Furthermore, psychosocial support and other medications may be useful as adjuncts to opioid medications. For severe, refractory pain syndromes, radiation therapy, nerve blocks, or surgical procedures should be considered.

CANCER CHEMOTHERAPY REGIMENS

  MedRANK Life Prolongation and Enhancement Checklist

Pills of Wisdom: The following combinations of medications are considered by many experts and panels to provide the best results against specific tumors and cancers. They are grouped according to the following categories: (1) chemotherapy drugs that are potentially curative for specific types of cancer; (2) those in which moderate to reasonable results can be expected; and (3) those for which only minimal or less-than-satisfactory results can be anticipated. Other chemotherapy combinations *not* mentioned in the table may also be used as alternatives.

Chemotherapy regimens have become increasingly complex and sophisticated—and also more effective. In fact, new combinations of drugs—sometimes as many as five or six different medications—have been shown to have synergistic effects against tumors. Usually, the decision to endure a course of chemotherapy for a potentially *curable* cancer is not a difficult one to make. Living is a powerful incentive, and most people will seize the opportunity to take a life-saving course of anticancer drugs—let's say for Hodgkin's disease or lymphoma, or as adjuvant therapy for breast cancer—despite the significant side effects. The decision to prolong life by a few weeks or months in those with terminal cancer is a much more difficult one and should be individualized for the patient.

Considering the complexity and toxicity of chemotherapy regimens, identifying which one is most appropriate for you is beyond the scope of this book. Moreover, because these drugs are highly toxic —and because the treatment protocols for specific

cancers are constantly evolving—you *always* should see a cancer specialist (oncologist) or be referred to a cancer center for optimal treatment.

Remember, for some cancers (leukemia and lymphoma) chemotherapy is the primary approach, whereas in other cancers (breast, ovary, lung), chemotherapy is used as an "adjunct" to other treatment strategies, including surgery and/or radiation therapy. Sometimes, chemotherapy drugs are used prior to surgery to improve overall results. In still other cases, cancer therapy is palliative—in other words, there is little impact on long-term survival, but the medications can "shrink" the tumor and make people feel much better as a result.

Although selecting the appropriate chemotherapy program is ultimately the responsibility of your doctor, you *will* want to ask a number of important questions before beginning an intensive treatment program. Some of the questions you will want to ask include:

- What can I realistically expect in the way of results?
- What are the bottom-line benefits of the chemotherapy regimen being proposed for my specific type and stage of cancer?
- Will this chemotherapy, alone or in combination with other modalities, *cure* my cancer, or is it intended to induce a *remission* for a length of time, after which I can expect a recurrence?
- *If a remission can be expected:* How long is the remission likely to last?
- *If the regimen is not curative:* How long will chemotherapy prolong my life?
- *If the regimen is potentially curative:* What percentage of patients taking this chemotherapy program *are* cured of their disease? How many people

survive ten years? How many survive two or five years? What factors explain the different survival rates?

- How well does chemotherapy work against my particular *kind* of tumor?

You also will want to know how long your survival is likely to be if you decide *not* to use chemotherapy. Some stages of prostate cancer and lymphomas do *not* benefit *dramatically* from chemotherapy, and many people prefer to avoid the risks and discomfort of anticancer drugs. This may be an option in your case, and you should have the pros and cons explained to you.

Although some of the technical and scientific issues are likely to be beyond your comprehension, you certainly should ask why a particular chemotherapy combination is being selected for your case. If more than one option is available, ask which has produced the best results in people with your particular type of cancer, and whether there are significant differences in their side effects or toxicity. The side effects associated with anticancer drugs vary according to the type of medication, but they can include nausea, vomiting, diarrhea, hair loss, anemia, low platelet counts, low white blood cell counts, increased risk of infection, skin rashes, and allergic reactions.

ANTICANCER DRUGS WITH BEST RESULTS

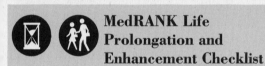 **MedRANK Life Prolongation and Enhancement Checklist**

BRAIN: MEDULLOBLASTOMA

Vincristine *plus* carmustine *with or without* mechlorethamine *with or without* methotrexate
OR
Mechlorethamine *plus* vincristine *plus* procarbazine *plus* prednisone (MOPP)
OR
Vincristine *plus* cisplatin *with or without* cyclophosphamide

BRAIN: PRIMARY CENTRAL NERVOUS SYSTEM LYMPHOMA

Methotrexate *with or without* cytarabine
OR

Cyclophosphamide *plus* doxorubicin *plus* vincristine *plus* prednisone (CHOP)

BREAST

In combination with surgery and radiation:
Cyclophosphamide *plus* methotrexate *plus* fluorouracil (CMF)
OR
Cyclophosphamide *plus* doxorubicin *with or without* fluorouracil (AC or CAF)
OR
Tamoxifen (when indicated, for estrogen-sensitive tumors)

For widespread disease, i.e., metastatic:
Cyclophosphamide *plus* methotrexate *plus* fluorouracil (CMF)
OR
Cyclophosphamide *plus* doxorubicin *with*

or without fluorouracil for receptor-negative and/or hormone-refractory tumors
AND
Tamoxifen for receptor-positive and/or hormone-sensitive tumors

CHORIOCARCINOMA

Methotrexate *with or without* leucovorin
OR
Dactinomycin

EMBRYONAL RHABDOMYOSARCOMA

Vincristine *plus* dactinomycin *with or without* cyclophosphamide
OR
Vincristine *plus* ifosfamide with mesna *plus* etoposide

EWING'S SARCOMA

Cyclophosphamide (*or* ifosfamide with mesna) *plus* doxorubicin *plus* vincristine (CAV) *with or without* dactinomycin

LEUKEMIA: ACUTE LYMPHOCYTIC LEUKEMIA (ALL)

To promote (induce) remission:
Vincristine *plus* prednisone *plus* asparaginase *with or without* daunorubicin

Maintenance therapy:
Methotrexate *plus* mercaptopurine

Patients with bad prognosis:
Bone marrow transplant

LEUKEMIA: ACUTE MYELOID LEUKEMIA (AML)

To promote (induce) remission:
Cytarabine *plus* either daunorubicin *or* idarubicin

Postinduction:
High-dose cytarabine *with or without* other drugs such as etoposide
OR
Bone marrow transplant

LEUKEMIA: CHRONIC LYMPHOCYTIC LEUKEMIA (CLL)

Chlorambucil *with or without* prednisone
OR
Fludarabine

LEUKEMIA: CHRONIC MYELOID LEUKEMIA (CML)

Chronic phase of illness:
Bone marrow transplant
OR
Interferon alfa
OR
Hydroxyurea

BLAST CRISIS

Lymphoid type:
Vincristine *plus* prednisone *plus* L-asparaginase *plus* intrathecal methotrexate (*with or without* maintenance with methotrexate *plus* 6-mercaptopurine)

Myeloid type:
High-dose cytarabine plus daunorubicin

LEUKEMIA: HAIRY CELL LEUKEMIA

Pentostatin
OR
Cladribine

LUNG: SMALL CELL (OAT CELL)

Cisplatin *plus* etoposide (PE)

OR
Cyclophosphamide *plus* doxorubicin *plus* vincristine (CAV)
OR
PE alternated with CAV
OR
Cyclophosphamide *plus* etoposide *plus* cisplatin (CEP)
OR
Doxorubicin *plus* cyclophosphamide *plus* etoposide (ACE)

LYMPHOMA: HODGKIN'S

Early stages curable with radiation:
Doxorubicin *plus* bleomycin *plus* vinblastine *plus* dacarbazine (ABVD)
OR
ABVD alternated with MOPP
OR
Mechlorethamine *plus* vincristine *plus* procarbazine (*with or without* prednisone) *plus* doxorubicin *plus* bleomycin *plus* vinblastine (MOP[P]–ABV)

LYMPHOMA: NON-HODGKIN'S, BURKITT'S LYMPHOMA

Cyclophosphamide *plus* vincristine *plus* methotrexate
OR
Cyclophosphamide *plus* high-dose cytarabine *with or without* methotrexate with leucovorin
OR
Intrathecal methotrexate *or* cytarabine

LYMPHOMA: DIFFUSE LARGE-CELL

Cyclophosphamide *plus* doxorubicin *plus* vincristine *plus* prednisone (CHOP)

LYMPHOMA: FOLLICULAR

Cyclophosphamide
OR
Chlorambucil

MYCOSIS FUNGOIDES

PUVA (psoralen plus ultraviolet A), mechlorethamine (topical) interferon alfa, electron beam radiotherapy, methotrexate

OVARIAN

Cisplatin (*or* carboplatin) *plus* paclitaxel
OR
Cisplatin (*or* carboplatin) *plus* cyclophosphamide (CP) *with or without* doxorubicin (CAP)

RETINOBLASTOMA (EYE)

Doxorubicin *plus* cyclophosphamide *with or without* cisplatin *with or without* etoposide *with or without* vincristine

TESTICULAR

Cisplatin *plus* etoposide *with or without* bleomycin (PEB)

WILMS' TUMOR

Dactinomycin *plus* vincristine *with or without* doxorubicin *with or without* cyclophosphamide

POTENTIALLY LIFE-PROLONGING CHEMOTHERAPY REGIMENS

BLADDER

Methotrexate *plus* vinblastine *plus* doxorubicin *plus* cisplatin (MVAC)
OR
Cisplatin *plus* methotrexate *plus* vinblastine (CMV)

BRAIN: ANAPLASTIC ASTROCYTOMA

Procarbazine *plus* lomustine *plus* vincristine

BRAIN: ANAPLASTIC OLIGODENDROGLIOMA

Procarbazine *plus* lomustine *plus* vincristine

COLORECTAL

Adjuvant therapy for colon cancer:
Fluorouracil *plus* levamisole
OR
Fluorouracil *plus* leucovorin

Therapy for metastatic spread:
Fluorouracil *plus* leucovorin

ESOPHAGEAL HEAD AND NECK: SQUAMOUS CELL

Cisplatin *plus* fluorouracil
OR
Methotrexate

KAPOSI'S SARCOMA (AIDS RELATED)

Etoposide
OR
Interferon alfa
OR
Vinblastine
OR
Doxorubicin *plus* bleomycin *plus* vincristine *or* vinblastine (ABV)

MULTIPLE MYELOMA

Melphalan (*or* cyclophosphamide) *plus* prednisone
OR
Melphalan *plus* carmustine *plus* cyclophosphamide *plus* prednisone *plus* vincristine
OR
Dexamethasone *plus* doxorubicin *plus* vincristine (VAD)
OR
Vincristine *plus* carmustine *plus* doxorubicin *plus* prednisone (VBAP)

NEUROBLASTOMA

Doxorubicin *plus* cyclophosphamide *plus* cisplatin *plus* teniposide *or* etoposide
OR
Doxorubicin *plus* cyclophosphamide
OR
Cisplatin *plus* cyclophosphamide

OSTEOGENIC SARCOMA

Doxorubicin *plus* cisplatin *with or without* etoposide *with or without* ifosfamide

SARCOMA: SOFT TISSUE, ADULT

Doxorubicin *with or without* dacarbazine *with or without* cyclophosphamide *with or without* ifosfamide with mesna

MINIMALLY EFFECTIVE CHEMOTHERAPY REGIMENS

BRAIN: GLIOBLASTOMA

Carmustine
OR
Lomustine

CANCER OF THE CERVIX

Cisplatin
OR
Ifosfamide *with* mesna
OR
Bleomycin *plus* ifosfamide *with* mesna *plus* cisplatin

UTERINE (ENDOMETRIAL)

Megestrol *or* another progestin
OR
Doxorubicin *plus* cisplatin *with or without* cyclophosphamide

STOMACH

Fluorouracil *with or without* leucovorin

ISLET CELL: PANCREAS

Streptozocin *plus* doxorubicin

LIVER

Doxorubicin
OR
Fluorouracil

LUNG: NON–SMALL CELL

Cisplatin plus etoposide
OR
Cisplatin *plus* vinblastine *with or without* mitomycin
OR
Cisplatin *plus* vinorelbine

MELANOMA

Interferon alfa
OR
Dacarbazine

KIDNEY

Aldesleukin
OR
Interferon alfa

SIDE EFFECTS AND COMPLICATIONS OF CHEMOTHERAPY

 MedRANK Side Effects and Drug Toxicity Checklist

Pills of Warning: Anticancer drugs are among the most toxic medications used to treat human diseases. Any decision regarding the use of them must take into account their possible side effects and toxicity. You must be watchful for side effects so that medication adjustments—dosage changes, drug substitutions, treatment for side effects—can be made if necessary. This MedRANK Checklist helps identify anticancer medications that may be causing problems.

INFLAMMATION OF THE MOUTH

(MUCOUS MEMBRANE INFLAMMATION, MOUTH ULCERS, SORENESS)

Adriamycin
Methotrexate
Doxorubicin
Interleukin-2
Mercaptopurine
Mithramycin
Nitrosoureas
Procarbazine
Vinblastine
Vincristine
5-fluorouracil
Busulfan
Bleomycin
Actinomycin-D
Cyclophosphamide
Daunorubicin

HAIR LOSS

(ALOPECIA)

Amsacrine
Bleomycin
Cyclophosphamide
Cytarabine
Dactinomycin
Daunorubicin
Dacarbazine
Doxorubucin
Etoposide
5-Fluorouracil
Hydroxyurea
Ifosfamide
Interleukin-2
Methotrexate
Nitrosoureas
Procarbazine
Vinblastine
Vincristine

BLOOD PROBLEMS

(LOW WHITE BLOOD CELL COUNTS AND LOW PLATELET COUNTS. ANTI-CANCER DRUGS THAT ARE MOST LIKELY TO CAUSE THIS PROBLEM ARE LISTED FIRST, AND THOSE DRUGS LEAST LIKELY TO ARE LISTED LAST)

Nitrogen mustard
Anthracycline
Antifolates
Antipyridines
Nitrosoureas
Busulfan
Carboplatin
Dacarbazine
Antipurines
Podophyllotoxins
Cisplatin
Hydroxyureas
Mitomycin
Procarbazine
Rozoxane

SKIN PIGMENTATION CHANGES

(DARKENING OF THE SKIN)

Bleomycin
Cyclophosphamide
Doxorubicin
5-Fluorouracil
Ifosfamide
Thiotepa
Methotrexate
Hydroxyurea
Methotrexate

ALLERGIC REACTIONS
(HYPERSENSITIVITY)

L-Asparaginase
Paclitaxel
Docetaxel
Elliptinium
Teniposide
Cisplatin
Procarbazine
Carboplatin
Melphalan
Mechlorethamine
Diaziquone
Etoposide
Cytarabine
Mitomycin

EYE PROBLEMS
(BLURRED VISION, INFLAM-
MATION, GLAUCOMA, BLIND-
NESS, DRYNESS OF THE
EYES, OR NERVE DAMAGE)

Busulfan
Chlorambucil
Cisplatin
Cyclophosphamide
Nitrogen mustard
Nitrosoureas
Doxorubicin
Mithramycin
Mitomycin C
Cytosine arabinoside
5-Fluorouracil
Methotrexate
Tamoxifen
Vinblastine
Vincristine
Cyclosporine

Mitotane
Paclitaxel

HEART DAMAGE
(DECREASING FORCE
OF HEART MUSCLE
CONTRACTIONS)

Adriamycin
Doxorubicin
Idarubicin
Epirubicin
Daunorubicin
Cyclophosphamide
Mitomycin C
Etoposide
Melphalan
Vincristine
Bleomycin
Cisplatin

LUNG PROBLEMS

Bleomycin
Peplomycin
Liblomycin
Mitomycin C
Doxorubicin
Vincristine
Vinblastine
Vindesine
Busulfan
Cyclophosphamide
Ifosfamide
Melphalan
Chlorambucil
Methotrexate
Azathioprine
Cytarabine
Fludarabine

NAUSEA AND VOMITING
(DRUGS LISTED FIRST HAVE
THE GREATEST POTENTIAL
FOR CAUSING NAUSEA AND
VOMITING; DRUGS LISTED
LAST HAVE THE LEAST)

Cisplatin
Dacarbazine
Dactinomycin
Cyclophosphamide
Lomustine
Carboplatin
Doxorubicin
Daunorubicin
Cytarabine
Procarbazine
Etoposide
Mitomycin
Methotrexate
Fluorouracil
Hydroxyurea
Bleomycin
Vinblastine
Vincristine
Chlorambucil

NEUROLOGICAL PROBLEMS
(CONFUSION, INFLAMMATION
OF BRAIN TISSUE, SEIZURES,
SLEEPINESS, CENTRAL NER-
VOUS SYSTEM PROBLEMS)

Asparaginase
Carmustine
Cisplatin
Corticosteroids
Cytarabine
Fludarabine
5-Fluorouracil

Etoposide
Ifosfamide
Interferon
Interleukin-2
Methotrexate
Procarbazine
Retinoic acid
Tamoxifen
Thiotepa
Vincristine

NERVE OR MUSCLE PROBLEMS

(NERVE PAIN, MUSCLE ACHES, MUSCLE WEAKNESS)

Cisplatin
Corticosteroids
Cytarabine

Docetaxel
Etoposide
Paclitaxel
Procarbazine
Suramin
Vincristine
Vinorelbine

CANCER-CAUSING MEDICATIONS

(CHEMOTHERAPY DRUGS THAT ARE CARCINOGENIC OR ARE ASSOCIATED WITH AN INCREASED RISK OF A "SECOND" MALIGNANCY SUCH AS LEUKEMIA)

Busulfan
Carmustine

Chlorambucil
Chlornaphazine
Cisplatin
Cyclophosphamide
Dacarbazine
Ifosfamide
Lomustine
Melphalan
Nitrogen mustard
Mitomycin C
Procarbazine
Semustine
Thiotepa
Treosulphan
Uracil mustard

TAKING THE EDGE OFF
Pills for Nausea and Vomiting

 MedRANK Life Enhancement Checklist

 Pills of Wisdom: Nausea and vomiting are among the most uncomfortable side effects seen with chemotherapy drugs. This checklist identifies medications that are best able to suppress these distressing symptoms.

OPTIMAL
(HIGHLY RECOMMENDED/ BEST OF CLASS)

Zofran (ondansetron)

This is a very effective medication for people who are taking chemotherapy drugs that pro-duce *severe* nausea and vomiting. The most common side effect is headache. When the going gets very rough with respect to nausea and vomiting and nothing else seems to work, this drug will provide the best results. It can be taken by mouth or given intravenously. Its side effects are quite tolerable, and its effectiveness is improved by using it in conjunction with Decadron (a steroid medication, dexamethasone).

Kytril (granisetron)

Similar to Zofran.

RECOMMENDED
(ACCEPTABLE WITH RESERVATIONS)

Compazine (prochlorperazine)

Compazine has a long and respectable track record as an effective treatment for mild to moderate nausea associated with chemotherapy. It can produce muscle cramps and uncomfortable, involuntary movements of the arms and legs. When it does not provide adequate relief—which may be the case in people who take cisplatin, a drug known to produce severe nausea—you will need to use more potent antinausea drugs such as Zofran and Kytril (see "Optimal").

Torecan (thiethylperazine)

Similar to Compazine.

Benadryl (diphenhydramine)

When Compazine or Torecan produces involuntary muscle movements of the arms and legs, Benadryl can be used to prevent or treat these side effects.

DISCOURAGED FOR INITIAL USE
(BUT MAY BE REQUIRED IN SELECTED PEOPLE)

Ativan (lorazepam)

This benzodiazepine may be useful as an add-on to drugs listed in the more favorable categories. It can produce drowsiness.

Marinol (dronabinol)

Dronabinol is the principal psychoactive substance present in *Cannabis sativa L* (marijuana). It is used to suppress nausea and vomiting in patients who are not responding to conventional treatment with the Optimal and Recommended drugs. It is also approved for use as an appetite stimulant in AIDS patients with severe weight loss. This drug may produce uncomfortable sensations (dysphoric reactions) in some people. Use only if necessary.

THE THREE-STEP APPROACH TO CANCER PAIN MANAGEMENT

 MedRANK Life Enhancement Checklist

 Pills of Wisdom: Cancer pain is usually caused when tumors invade vital body organs or spread to bone or other tissues. This approach to pain management follows the three-step guidelines issued by the World Health Organization.

For patients with advanced stages of cancer and severe pain, many medications are administered by vein, through patient-activated infusion pumps, or by other drug delivery systems. Radiation and chemotherapy treatments also play an important part in pain management and are used in conjunction with "pain medications." Other drugs (like stool softeners) may be used to treat side effects (such as constipation) caused by pain relievers. Many of these approaches are beyond the scope of this book and should be implemented by a cancer specialist. However, regardless of what pill or regimen is used, people with cancer-related pain should *always demand* an acceptable and comfort-making pain-relieving program.

OPTIMAL
(HIGHLY RECOMMENDED/
BEST OF CLASS)

STEP 1: MILD PAIN

First consider:
Tylenol
OR
Extra-Strength Tylenol

If not effective, consider these alternatives:
Aleve
OR
Motrin
OR
Advil
OR
other NSAID

If pain increases or is persistent, go to Step 2.

STEP 2: MODERATE PAIN

First consider:
Tylenol #3
OR
Codeine *plus* an NSAID

If not effective, consider alternatives:
Vicodin
OR
Percodan (Percocet, Tylox, etc.) *plus* an NSAID

If pain increases or is persistent, go to Step 3.

STEP 3: SEVERE PAIN

First consider:
Percodan *plus* an NSAID

If not effective, consider these alternatives:
Morphine
OR
Dilaudid *plus* an NSAID

CHAPTER 15

—

MEDICATIONS
FOR HIV INFECTION

The Arsenal

No one is ready to say there is a *cure* for HIV infection quite yet: *cure* would mean the complete, permanent, and irreversible eradication of HIV from the blood and all other human tissues in the infected person. But the prognosis is improving month by month. Remarkable progress has been made in blocking replication of the human immunodeficiency virus (HIV) and in managing the serious infections that complicate this disease. Without question, medications have played the pivotal role in prolonging life and improving the quality of life in HIV-infected individuals. (Please see the MedRANK Checklist "Life-Prolonging Pills for HIV Infection" on page 255.) Because strategies for combining, sequencing, and timing drug therapy are changing rapidly, expert-based care is mandatory. Hence, if you, a friend, or a family member is infected with HIV, you will get the best results by seeing a physician who has had a broad range of experience treating this condition.

☺ *Antiviral agents such as didanosine, zidovudine, and protease inhibitors are now used in combination cocktails very early in the course of HIV infection.*
It should be stressed that these medication regimens have not yet been proven to cure HIV infection, but they do improve *survival* and reduce the symptoms associated with viral infection. Zidovudine (AZT) inhibits the growth of the HIV virus in HIV-positive patients and may also delay the onset of acquired immunodeficiency syndrome (AIDS). The protease inhibitors, a new class of medications that are now used as part of the treatment "cocktail," have been shown to decrease the progression of AIDS.

☺ *Clinical studies have found that combining protease inhibitors with medications such as AZT can reduce the amount of virus in the patient's blood to undetectable levels.*

To benefit maximally from AZT therapy, patients should be identified as early as possible in the course of HIV infection. Current treatment recommendations include the use of protease inhibitors in conjunction with other antiretroviral agents. At precisely what point in the natural history of HIV infection triple therapy is useful remains to be determined from additional clinical trials.

☺ *The second arm of drug therapy in HIV-infected patients is protecting them against infection.*

People infected with this virus develop many unusual so-called "opportunistic" infections because of their compromised immune status. These infections, more often than not, are the fatal blow in people with AIDS. Protease inhibitors plus zidovudine (AZT) and other nu-cleoside analogs—ddI, ddC, d4T, and 3TC—help prevent these infections by inhibiting the growth of the virus. This helps the body to maintain a more active immune response. Generally speaking, these medications are prescribed according to the patient's CD4 cell counts. They should never be shared with anyone else.

☺ *At certain stages, patients with HIV infection and low CD4 lymphocyte counts will require prophylaxis against opportunistic infections.*

Medications used for this purpose include trimethoprim-sulfamethoxazole, azithromycin, fluconazole, and many other drugs. Antibiotics and antiviral agents should always be taken with physician supervision. As a group, antiviral medications are associated with a number of drug interactions and side effects. You can identify the best pills for preventing infection by consulting the Med-RANK Checklist "Pill Combinations for HIV Infection" on page 257.

LIFE-PROLONGING PILLS FOR HIV INFECTION*

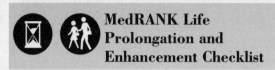

MedRANK Life Prolongation and Enhancement Checklist

Pills of Wisdom: The advances against HIV infection have been startling. When currently available medications are used in strategic, synergistic combinations, at high enough doses and for long enough periods of time, people infected with HIV can recover their much-needed infection-fighting CD4 T-cell counts; they can decrease their virus load to the point that HIV is no longer even detectable in their bloodstream; they can decrease their susceptibility to opportunistic infections; and they can prolong the *quality* and *quantity* of their life. Though it is not a cure as yet, from the perspective of most physicians as well as their patients, it is progress indeed.

OPTIMAL
(HIGHLY RECOMMENDED/ BEST OF CLASS)

NUCLEOSIDE ANALOGS
These are the original drugs used to fight HIV infection. Called reverse transcriptase inhibitors, they disrupt the early stages of viral replication. They are no longer used *alone* but are still used in *combination* with each other and with the *protease inhibitors* in order to provide a more potent attack strategy against HIV infection.

Retrovir (AZT, zidovudine)
This time-tested nucleoside analog is somewhat successful at inhibiting one of the critical steps in HIV replication. It can temporarily decrease the level of viral particles circulating in the blood, increase the levels of CD4 T-cells (which the body needs to fight infection), and decrease the number of infections that can overwhelm a body debilitated by a poorly functioning immune system.

But this drug needs *help.* Like the other nucleoside analogs, therapy with AZT *alone* is no longer the treatment of choice. As this book goes to press, a triple-drug "cocktail" therapy that includes AZT plus another nucleoside analog (like ddI, ddC, or d4T) and a protease inhibitor (like Crixivan) appears to be the most desirable (potent) antiretroviral combination.

Over time, HIV becomes *resistant* to AZT, and new drugs to replace AZT are brought into the "cocktail." The drug has many side effects, including anemia, low white blood cell counts, vomiting, headache, fatigue, muscle wasting, and liver problems.

Videx (didanosine, ddI)
This drug, commonly referred to as ddI, is often used along with AZT to increase the power of the anti-HIV "cocktail," or as a replacement for AZT in people who cannot tolerate AZT or in whom HIV resistance to AZT has developed.

* For recommendations regarding combinations of these medications, please see the MedRANK Checklist "Pill Combinations for HIV Infection" on page 257.

ddI can produce all the benefits of AZT—and resistance to it can also develop. The main side effects are pain in nerves of the skin and soft tissues, inflammation of the pancreas, and gastrointestinal symptoms.

Hivid (ddC, zalcitibane)

Giving ddC along with AZT is more effective than giving AZT alone. (These drugs are no longer used by themselves as *single* therapy.) It appears to be at least as effective as ddI. The main side effect is pain in the nerves of the skin and soft tissues.

Zerit (stavudine, d4T)

This drug is active against most strains of HIV that have become resistant to AZT. It is used in patients with advanced HIV infection who cannot tolerate AZT or fail to show good results with it. d4T is more effective than AZT alone in preventing progression of disease in people who have been on AZT for at least six months and shown resistance to it. The main side effect is pain in the peripheral nerves of skin and soft tissue.

Epivir (lamivudine, 3TC)

When this drug is used alone, resistance develops rapidly. However, in combination with AZT, 3TC improves survival, as compared with AZT alone. Among the nucleoside analogs, this one probably has the best side-effect profile and therefore appears to be the best tolerated among the nucleoside analogs.

Protease Inhibitors

For HIV to infect new cells, large protein molecules must be broken down into smaller components, which are then assembled into "complete" virus particles. The protease inhibitors *prevent* the breaking-down of these large proteins, which in essence puts a glitch into the viral-particle assembly line. The use of protease inhibitors, in combination with two nucleoside analogs early in the course of HIV infection, has produced dramatic improvement in HIV-infected people and has prolonged survival. Protease inhibitors must be used in *combination* with the nucleoside analogs.

Norvir (ritinovir)

This is a very effective drug against HIV, and resistance develops slowly. In patients who have not previously received treatment for HIV, this drug raised the CD4 (fighter) T-cell counts more than AZT alone did. In patients with advanced HIV infection (AIDS) who were treated with other medications previously, it has been shown to *prolong* life.

The side-effect profile of this drug is rough. Nausea, diarrhea, vomiting, funny sensations around the mouth, altered taste, and tingling sensations in the limbs are common. It also can be involved in many drug-drug interactions.

Crixivan (indinovir)

This very potent drug, in one study, lowered HIV particles in the blood to *undetectable* levels in 90 percent of previously treated patients within six months of treatment, when used in combination with AZT and lamivudine. When used in combination with AZT and ddI in previously untreated patients, indinovir lowered HIV blood levels to undectable levels in about 60 percent of patients. Even when used alone for up to a year, indinovir has eliminated HIV from the blood in 40 to 60 percent of patients.

The drug is well-tolerated, although kidney stones occur in 2 to 3 percent of people who take it. To prevent this complication, people who take this drug should drink at least one and a half quarts of water each day, and the pills should be taken with water one or two hours after a meal.

Invirase (saquinavir)

This appears to be the *least effective* of the protease inhibitors. Resistance develops when saquinavir is used alone, and HIV strains that have become resistant to this drug are usually susceptible to the other two protease inhibitors (ritinovir and indinovir). It is the best tolerated drug in this class. Many drug-drug interactions are possible.

PILL COMBINATIONS FOR HIV INFECTION

MedRANK Life Prolongation Checklist

Pills of Wisdom: Advances in AIDS therapy have been moving at a fairly blistering pace. This MedRANK Checklist presents the anti-HIV "cocktails" (or drug combinations) that were optimal as this book went to press. They are made on the basis of the most current clinical trials, with the understanding that many drug evaluations in HIV patients are even now in progress and have not yet been reported at scientific meetings or in the medical journals. The results of these trials will certainly lead to changes in current guidelines.

At this writing, these cocktails are potent enough to eliminate all detectable traces of HIV from the blood, at least for a year, or two, or maybe more—no one is quite certain. The fact that HIV is undetectable in the blood does not mean it is not there. A coterie of surviving virus particles—hard-core retroviral guerrillas—may have taken refuge, gone "underblood," in some other body tissue, like the brain, testicles, or lymph glands. When patients in whom the virus has been bludgeoned into nondetection eventually go *off*

their medications, we will see whether an HIV strike force re-emerges to start the infectious cycle all over again.

Even in the face of this uncertainty, some pills appear to be better than others. Based on what we know now, some drugs are felt to be more potent (effective) than others, and some are much more user-friendly. When all these factors are taken into account, optimal starting regimens to counter HIV infection can be devised.

Specific information about each of these individual medications can be found in "Life-Prolonging Pills for HIV Infection" on page 255. Regardless of which multipill cocktail your physician selects, the bottom line is to attack HIV infection *early, hard, and as definitively as possible with a "multiflank" strategy* that includes, for now, *three* drugs—one protease inhibitor and two nucleoside analogs.

Which two nucleoside analogs (among AZT, ddI, ddC, and so on) provide the best and most durable combination for use with a protease inhibitor is simply not known. AZT, however, has the longest track record, and lamivudine seems to be the best tolerated. As for the protease inhibitors, indinavir and ritonavir are the most effective, although ritonavir has a higher risk for drug interactions and appears to be less well tolerated than indinavir.

How effective are these cocktails? *Time* magazine's "Man of the Year," Dr. David Ho, along with other researchers at the University of Alabama, has discovered that immediately after the HIV virus infects the body, it engages in a fierce battle with the immune system. This insight has prompted speculation that delivering aggressive, full-throttle antiviral drugs early on may sufficiently favor the body's infection-fighting warriors (lymphocytes, macrophages, and other virus-inhibiting cells) to tip the balance and battle in the patient's favor—perhaps (no one knows for sure) permanently, or at least for many more years than we could have imagined only a short time ago.

The precise timing for unleashing this multipill warhead is also a matter of debate, so recommendations may change rapidly in this regard. The trend is to treat with all *three* drugs when the CD4 count is less than 500, although some clinicians have proposed treating people *as soon as infection is confirmed*, regardless of the CD4 count.

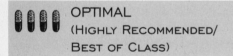

OPTIMAL
(Highly Recommended/ Best of Class)

All of these combinations use AZT as the "anchor" nucleoside analog and either indinavir or ritonavir as the protease inhibitor of choice.

Zidovudine (AZT) *plus* Lamivudine (3TC) *plus* Indinavir

OR

Zidovudine (AZT) *plus* ddI *plus* Indinavir

OR

Zidovudine (AZT) *plus* Lamivudine (3TC) *plus* Ritinovir

OR

Zidovudine (AZT) *plus* ddC *plus* Ritinovir

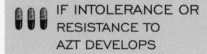

IF INTOLERANCE OR RESISTANCE TO AZT DEVELOPS

If the patient becomes *intolerant* of AZT or if AZT resistance develops—and the disease progresses—the physician will usually replace AZT with another nucleoside analog or, on occasion, continue AZT and add another nucleoside. These drug regimens require careful monitoring by the physician for side effects and effectiveness, including blood counts.

ddI *plus* Lamivudine (3TC) *plus* Indinavir

OR

ddI *plus* Lamivudine (3TC) *plus* Ritinovir

OR

AZT *plus* ddC *plus* Lamivudine (3TC) *plus* Ritinovir

OR

Stavudine *plus* Lamivudine (3TC) *plus* Ritinovir

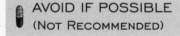

AVOID IF POSSIBLE
(Not Recommended)

Single drug therapy. Optimizing life prolongation in HIV infection appears to require, at a minimum, *three*-drug therapy for initial treatment. Starting anti-HIV therapy "gradually" with one drug is associated with inferior outcomes.

PILLS FOR PREVENTING INFECTIONS IN HIV-INFECTED INDIVIDUALS

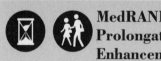 **MedRANK Life Prolongation and Enhancement Checklist**

Pills of Wisdom: There are two basic approaches to medication-based treatment of people infected with the HIV virus. The first approach is a head-on, *anti-HIV*, full-gun assault that moves hard and fast against the HIV virus. This strategy attacks the enemy head-on. The best pills—and the most potent cocktails—for accomplishing this goal are presented in the two MedRANK Checklists in this chapter.

But the HIV virus is only *part* of the problem. If primary antiretroviral treatment is *not* successful, the virus undergoes frenzied replication, producing billions of copies of itself each day, a cycle that gradually overwhelms the body's infection-fighting cells. The devastation is measured by the decline in CD4+ T-cell counts in the blood. This deterioration permits other enemies—*bacteria, non-HIV viruses such as CMV and herpes zoster, parasites, fungal organisms,* and *tuberculosis*—to take advantage of the weakened, overworked immune system, set up an infection, and deal a debilitating blow to the patient with AIDS.

Hence, the second basic approach to treating patients with AIDS is to prevent infection by these "opportunists." The key is to be proactive. *An ounce of medication is worth a pound of prevention, and a pound of prevention is worth a ton of cure.* Initiation of prevention and/or suppression therapy for these infections, to a great extent, is based on the CD4 counts. In other cases, suppression therapy is automatic, especially in people who have had a first infection and need continuing, low-dose medication to keep the offending organism from recurring.

This MedRANK Checklist identifies the most important prevention-oriented pills and vaccinations. The risk of drug interactions is especially high with pills used to treat AIDS-related conditions. Consequently, a meticulous review, with your physician or pharmacist, of potential incompatibilities is a *must* before you add another pill to your infection-preventing cocktail.

 OPTIMAL
ALL HIV-INFECTED PEOPLE NEED THESE VACCINES

Influenza vaccine (flu shots)

By all means get one—maybe two. A touch of influenza in a person with a significantly weakened immune system can turn into a strong handshake with pneumonia or even death. The slope is slippery. HIV-infected individuals, who may already be warding off respiratory conditions, such as *Pneumocystis carinii pneumonia* (PCP), need all the protection they can get, and flu shots are a good, harmless place to start.

Outbreaks of influenza in the United States usually begin in December and peak in January and February. A flu shot will start protecting you about ten days after the injection and will last for up to six months. People in the middle to advanced stages of HIV infection may have a less-than-optimal response—in terms of producing protective antibodies—but they should be vaccinated anyway. Some studies suggest that cancer patients on chemotherapy may benefit from *two* flu shots. The best time to get a flu shot is probably between mid-October and mid-November.

Pneumovax 23

A polyvalent pneumococcal vaccine effective against twenty-three of the most common strains of *S. pneumoniae* bacteria that cause pneumonia.

Pneumonia is nobody's friend these days, least of all the person with AIDS. One vaccination is a good start, but the protection is neither perfect nor forever. Preventing a bout of pneumonia is a priority, so people with AIDS who have had one Pneumovax shot should consider having a second shot after six years.

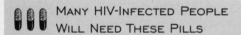

MANY HIV-INFECTED PEOPLE WILL NEED THESE PILLS

Septra DS Tabs (trimethoprim sulfa)

Chronic preventive therapy against PCP. If your CD4 count falls below 200, you will want to take trimethoprim sulfa DS tablets, one a day, for prevention against PCP. There are other approaches, including Dapsone, but none is as convenient or cost-effective as trimethoprim sulfa.

Zovirax (acyclovir)

Chronic suppressive therapy for genital herpes infection. For HIV-infected patients who suffer more than six outbreaks of genital herpes within a year—as well as those who have fewer but particularly severe recurrent attacks —chronic suppressive therapy for at least six to twelve months is usually advised. For *prevention* or suppression purposes, Zovirax is the optimal drug. When dosed on a twice-daily basis, it is very safe and quite tolerable. The

drug has been shown to be effective (more than 90 percent reduction in flare-ups) for up to three years. It is the drug of choice for long-term prevention in patients with HIV infection.

Diflucan (fluconazole)

This drug provides chronic suppressive therapy against cryptococcosis. If you are at high risk for or have had this fungal infection, protection against a recurrence is best accomplished with suppressive therapy, that is, using drugs to keep the infecting offenders at bay and prevent a full-blown infection. Diflucan 200 mg, taken once daily, is the most user-friendly approach for people at risk for cryptococcosis. This antifungal medication also can prevent thrush (candida) infections of the mouth.

Mycostatin (nystatin)

Chronic suppressive therapy against recurrence of oral candida fungal infection of the mouth. The use of nystatin tablets, three to five times daily, can prevent recurrent thrush infections of the mouth. This medication may not be necessary in people already taking the antifungal drug Diflucan, since it also protects against thrush.

Sporanox (itraconazole)

Chronic suppressive therapy against histoplasmosis. Histoplasmosis is another fungal infection that can be devastating. Suppressive therapy with itraconazole is currently the most reasonable approach. Side effects include nausea, stomachache, rash, and headache.

Zithromax (azithromycin)

For prevention against disseminated mycobacterium avium complex (MAC) infection.

If your CD4 count falls below 75—some experts say below 50—you will want to prevent against MAC infection. MAC is life-threatening, the terminal infection in up to 20 percent of patients with AIDS. Two other medications, Biaxin and Rifabutin, also are used for this purpose, but Zithromax requires only fifty-two doses per year (one dose by mouth each week), is the most reasonably priced option, and is as well-tolerated as the other pills. Zithromax plus Rifabutin produces more effective prevention than either drug alone, but Rifabutin is expensive and has many side effects.

Cytovene (fanciclovir)
For suppression of cytomegalovirus (CMV) infection. CMV can cause a debilitating infection involving the eye (retina), colon, or esophagus. A relapse can be delayed with ganciclovir, an oral medication that is given on a daily basis. It can lower white blood cell counts, especially when used with AZT.

Pyrimethamine and sulfadiazine
For suppression of toxoplasmosis infection. These two medications are the drugs of choice for preventing a recurrence of toxoplasmosis, which can cause serious infections of the brain.

Isoniazid (INH)
For prevention against tuberculosis. People with HIV infection should get a skin test called PPD to see whether they have been exposed to tuberculosis. If this skin test is positive, preventive therapy with INH will be required.

CHAPTER 16

■

BONES AND MOANS

Medications for Osteoporosis and Arthritis

"I've tried everything, and the pain is no better than it was a year ago. First my doctor tried Motrin. That irritated my stomach. Then he put me on Meclomen, and I developed terrible diarrhea." This is how patients with disabling arthritis usually begin their saga. Then the pill plot gets thicker: "The codeine made me nauseated. The Vicodin worked, but it made me constipated, and he took me off it because he said he didn't want me to get too dependent on it. I asked for Voltaren, but he said that could cause liver problems. He didn't want to give me Feldene because he said I was too old. Now I'm in constant pain, I'm not on anything, and I'm at my wit's end. Isn't there something new for arthritis?" The answer is, yes and no.

Perhaps more than any other group, people who suffer from arthritis are stuck between a rock and a hard place. Many are elderly and have the free time to participate in social and family activities. Yet they become progressively debilitated by degenerating—and in the case of rheumatoid arthritis, inflamed—bones and joints, which produce enough pain to make life miserable and curtail their normal functioning.

☺ *As far as arthritis is concerned, the goal is to strike a comfortable balance between pain relief and side effects.*

Complicating the "to medicate or not to medicate" dilemma is the fact that elderly people as a group are much more susceptible to the side effects and risks of pain-relieving drugs such as NSAIDs, methotrexate, steroids, narcotics, aspirin, and gold therapy. The drugs that can reduce inflammation, relieve pain, or prevent bone wasting have the potential downside of drug-related problems. For the physician and the older patient, this problem presents a treacherous decision tree—or pharmacological roulette wheel.

☺ *The best approach is to use medications only when necessary to maintain or restore physical function, and to use them in conjunction with a graduated, supervised exercise program that will improve muscle strength and minimize damage to injured joints.*

Finally, weight loss—when indicated—is an excellent way to reduce mechanical stress and prevent joint deterioration. When obesity co-exists with arthritis, weight loss should be considered a critical component of the overall treatment program. (For more information on pain relief, see Chapter 17.)

☺ *Osteoarthritis. The most common cause of bone and joint pain in the United States is osteoarthritis (OA). A disease of bone trauma and aging, osteoarthritis produces significant discomfort in 10 to 20 percent of people over age 65.*

It accounts for almost one-third of all office visits to primary care physicians, and it is the most common cause of physical disability in the elderly. The symptoms—which can include chronic pain in the knees, hips, fingers, thumbs, neck, and lower spine—are the result of damaged cartilage. What causes osteoarthritis? Although the simplistic "wear and tear" hypothesis is no longer in fashion, exactly what causes cartilage to fray, shred, and crack over time is not known. But once major defects appear in the cartilage, it cannot repair itself, and the disease progresses with age. Many of the problems—and much of the pain—associated with osteoarthritis are the result of excessive bone growth and spurs that intrude into the joint space, as well as "remodeling" changes that cause pain with joint movement.

☺ *At present, there is no confirmed cure for osteoarthritis, but medications can offer relief of the symptoms.*

There is, however, widespread public and scientific interest in a recently proposed "miracle" cure for this disease. In this approach, pills that contain key components of damaged cartilage are said to halt cartilage deterioration—and promote cartilage regeneration. Confirmation of this breakthrough will require more extensive study.

☺ *For the time being, the best approach for relieving pain in people who do not have inflamed joints is the use of analgesics (pain relievers). Because OA is a chronic condition, it makes sense to use a pill that is relatively inexpensive and safe.*

Tylenol (acetaminophen) is the most reasonable option because of its safety. It doesn't produce the stomach ulcers seen with chronic aspirin or NSAID use, although it has a *small* risk of kidney problems if it is used at very *high* doses for *many* years. Although many people use aspirin, the risk of causing stomach ulcers is worrisome, especially at the higher doses required to treat arthritis. Moreover, even "coated" preparations of aspirin, such as Ecotrin, can cause ulcers, a finding that reduces the overall attractiveness of this medicine-cabinet staple as an anti-arthritic pain reliever. *My advice:* Tylenol over aspirin.

☺ *Although NSAIDs are widely prescribed for OA, there is no convincing proof that they provide any more relief —for people with mild arthritis—than pure analgesics such as Tylenol.*

People respond differently to medications, and treatment should always be individualized. Generally, however, I recommend that you begin with Tylenol, and if this does not adequately relieve your pain, you and your doctor may raise the ante and try an NSAID next.

Rheumatoid Arthritis. Rheumatoid arthritis (RA) is a much different disease from osteoarthritis. It is a common, very painful, and physically debilitating condition that produces tremendous inflammation in joint tissue. In fact, the inflammation is so intense— and the potential for joint destruction is so great—that a formidable arsenal of medications has been pressed into service to combat this condition. The best sequence for RA pills and information on controversies regarding treatment are presented in the MedRANK Checklist "Pills for Rheumatoid Arthritis" on page 271.

Anyone who has ever had RA knows about steroids. Except for estrogen-containing medications, the adrenal cortical steroids (otherwise known as glucocorticoids) are probably the most widely used synthetic hormones. These medications, of which prednisone is the most common, have potent anti-inflammatory properties, and as a result they are used to treat a number of conditions, including RA.

Proceed cautiously with these pills, and use them only if necessary to provide relief from severe pain. Their main side effects include impaired wound healing, enlargement of fat pad areas in the body (obesity in the midsection), acne, and gastrointestinal problems. Individuals who have been on long-term corticosteroid therapy must avoid sudden withdrawal from it. In addition, because of the wide range of potential side effects that can result from chronic therapy with corticosteroids, they should be used only when absolutely indicated.

☺ *If at all possible, you should be prescribed the lowest daily dose of corticosteroids that will provide a level of symptomatic relief compatible with an acceptable quality of life.*

The severity of side effects associated with low-dose, *short-term* steroid therapy is controversial. But most physicians and pharmacists feel that the positive effects that steroids have on inflammatory conditions outweigh the risks of using them on a short-term basis. Long-term administration of steroid therapy is another matter altogether, and most experts recommend using the *lowest* dose possible. An area of particular concern is the effect of these medications on bone mass. It is widely known that chronic use of steroid medications can cause osteoporosis in older individuals, which can lead to bone fractures. Even low-dose corticosteroid therapy (doses of greater than 10 mg per day) can cause a significant decrease in bone mineral density.

☻ *Osteoporosis, or Bone Wasting. Thin bones put people on thin ice, and the bone-wasting disease called osteoporosis, which commonly affects elderly women, places people at increased risk for back and hip fractures.*

Fortunately, this is one condition in which an ounce of prevention is worth a ton of cure—and medications are the linchpin of health maintenance. The best pills for preventing bone wasting are estrogen, Fosamax, calcium, and vitamin D. The various pills are rated and compared in the MedRANK Checklist "Pills for Osteoporosis" below. Here you will find a pill-by-pill comparison of available medications and approaches to designing pill "cocktails" for slowing the process of bone demineralization over time.

☻ *Exercise is an important part of this prevention program.*

In addition, older patients, who are prone to osteoporosis, benefit from calcium supplementation and/or vitamin supplements that contain vitamin D. In fact, many physicians prescribe calcium supplementation for healthy postmenopausal women on an ongoing basis. One gram of elemental calcium is the recommended dosage. Some studies suggest that calcium supplementation continued over thirty years of postmenopausal life may lead to a cumulative benefit of a 10 percent reduction in bone loss. This result, it has been estimated, could reduce the risk of bone fractures by as much as 50 percent. On the other hand, excessive amounts of calcium can produce constipation, kidney disease, and other side effects. Consequently, your calcium intake should be monitored by your family physician.

PILLS FOR OSTEOPOROSIS

MedRANK Life Prolongation and Enhancement Checklist

☻ **Pills of Wisdom:** All postmenopausal women should be considered candidates for drug therapy to prevent osteoporosis. In simple terms, osteoporosis is characterized by a gradual thinning of bones, a process that predisposes the person to bone fractures and other skeletal deformities. The risk of fracturing a bone—especially in the hip—increases with age, doubling every ten years for women in their post-

menopausal years, and peaking between 85 and 90 years of age. Protecting women against bone wasting is an important health priority because fractures cause not only discomfort but disability, are associated with depression, and can shorten life expectancy.

Fortunately, many medications have been shown to slow osteoporosis during the postmenopausal years. Some of these pills (estrogen) are more or less *essential*, whereas others (slow fluoride) are not. Where the evidence for life prolongation with some pills (estrogen) is overwhelming, the evidence for others (Fosamax) is not. What is clear is that women must have answers to the following questions:

- When should I start taking medications to prevent osteoporosis?
- How long do I have to take them in order to achieve permanent benefits?
- What are the risks of taking them over the long term?

This MedRANK Checklist identifies medications that have been *proven* to strengthen bones over time, increase stature, and reduce the risk of broken bones—especially hip fractures—in postmenopausal women. As you review this information, please note that recommendations for medications—in particular, for estrogen pills—will vary depending upon whether the woman has a uterus or has had a hysterectomy (surgical removal of the uterus).

Estrogen, in particular, is the most widely used and potentially effective medication for preventing and improving osteoporosis. But taking estrogen for the purpose of long-term hormonal replacement therapy (HRT) is an *individualized* decision that you *and* your doctor must make. It must always take into account the following issues and concerns: (1) your previous history of heart disease, breast cancer, cancer of the uterus, or other uterine conditions; (2) your willingness to tolerate postmenopausal breakthrough bleeding; (3) the degree of osteoporosis; and (4) the beneficial effects estrogen has on your postmenopausal symptoms and cardiovascular health.

OPTIMAL
(HIGHLY RECOMMENDED/ BEST OF CLASS)

ESTROGEN REPLACEMENT THERAPY*

Before you start, consider these points: Estrogen replacement therapy is a highly recommended life-prolonging strategy that should be strongly *considered* in *all* postmenopausal women who do not have current medical conditions (including breast cancer, cancer of the uterus, and blood clots), or a history of them, that would make estrogen therapy potentially unsafe.

The benefits of estrogen are maximized if a woman begins taking it *immediately* at the onset of menopause and continues to take it for at least *seven* years. It appears that older women (up until age 75) who start estrogen replacement and continue it for at least two years also benefit. But the really substantial benefits, in terms of decreasing the risk of broken bones, require at least *five to seven years of treatment.* Discontinuing estrogen is followed by an accelerated rate of bone wasting equivalent to that in untreated women. So, long-term compliance is a must.

There are other reasons—especially its life-prolonging effects related to heart disease—for taking estrogen and that make it a bulwark of prevention against the deterioration that accompanies aging.

Your risk for developing complications related to osteoporosis can be assessed using a noninvasive test called bone densimetry, which measures how much calcium your bones have. This test may help to decide whether you are a strong or weak candidate for estrogen, at least as far as the bone issue is concerned.

Warnings: "Unopposed estrogen" (Premarin, Estrace)—that is, estrogen taken alone,

---

* For more information about the benefits, risks, options, and side effects associated with estrogen replacement therapy, see Chapter 19.

without progesterone (Provera)—is not advised for most women *with* a uterus. This group should have *progesterone added to the estrogen* in order to *decrease* the risk of uterine cancer. (See "Estrogen Replacement Regimen for Women Who Have a Uterus" below.) Continuous combined therapy with Prempro is the best choice.

In addition, women who have a history of breast cancer, cervical cancer, endometriosis, abnormal Pap smears, uterine fibroids, blood clots, migraine, liver disease, or elevated triglyceride levels may not be ideal candidates for estrogen and, therefore, should weigh the relative risks and benefits carefully with their physicians.

Estrogen Replacement Regimen for Women Who Do Not Have a Uterus

Premarin 0.625 mg (conjugated estrogens) each day

OR

Estrace 1 mg (estradiol) each day

This is the preferred regimen for women who do not have a uterus.

Estrogen Replacement Regimen for Women Who Have Their Uterus

Prempro (preferred approach)

OR

Premarin 0.625 mg *plus* Provera 2.5 mg each day

OR

Estrace 1 mg *plus* Provera 2.5 mg each day

The cyclic combined estrogen and progestin regimen is also effective, but compliance is not as good. (See the "Recommended" category.) The use of progesterone along with estrogen is complicated by breakthrough bleeding, which many women find disturbing. The frequency of this side effect is reduced with the *continuous-combined* approach, and as many as 80 percent of women have no bleeding after one year of hormone replacement. Prempro combines estrogen and progesterone into a single pill.

Calcium Nutritional Supplements

Calcium nutritional supplements are advised for postmenopausal women, inasmuch as studies suggest that elderly women who take calcium and vitamin D have a lower risk of breaking a hip than those who do not. In addition, most of the other medications—estrogen, Fosamax, etc.—that are recommended to prevent osteoporosis have been evaluated in women who were also taking calcium supplementation.

How much calcium do you need to take? A panel of experts from the National Institutes of Health recommends 1,000 mg per day for women 25 to 50 years old, and 1,250 mg per day for women 51 to 65 years old who are taking estrogen. If you are more than 65 years old, this panel recommends a daily intake of 1,500 mg of calcium.

The average diet provides less than 800 mg per day, which means that to ensure adequate calcium intake, women over 50 should take one 500–600 mg calcium tablet per day, and women over 65 should take *two* of these tablets per day.

Calcium Carbonate

Caltrate 600

Os-Cal 500

Tums 500

Calcium carbonate regimens are optimal because they are the simplest and most convenient to take. These supplements are usually well tolerated, although gastrointestinal symptoms such as constipation and bloating are sometimes seen.

Calcium Citrate

Citracal

Citracal + D

These tablets are equally convenient. See "Calcium carbonate" for additional details.

Vitamin D Supplementation

Vitamin D

I recommend vitamin D (a daily dose of 400 International Units) along with calcium supplementation to prevent and treat bone wasting caused by osteoporosis.

Biphosphanates

Fosamax (atredonate)

This drug, which promotes bone formation—and, in turn, counters bone wasting—is approved by the FDA for both prevention and treatment of osteoporosis. Unlike estrogen, it is not used *routinely* in postmenopausal women for prevention but is reserved as treatment for people who, on the basis of tests confirming the presence of osteoporosis, are deemed to be at high risk for breaking bones and suffering other complications of this disease, like diminishing stature.

To achieve best results, this drug should be taken as part of a regimen that also includes estrogen and calcium supplements. Taken once daily on an empty stomach, it is well-tolerated, except for occasional gastrointestinal side effects. If you have been on one of the other biphosphanates—Didronel (etidronate) or Aredia (pamidronate)—which are *not* approved by the FDA for treatment of osteoporosis, you should strongly consider asking your doctor to *switch* you to Fosamax.

Warning: A potentially serious condition, ulcerative esophagitis—in which the coating of the esophagus becomes eroded—has been reported in women who took this medication while lying down. It is a very rare complication, but nevertheless you should take Fosamax in the morning with a glass of water, then wait a few minutes in an upright position before eating or drinking anything else.

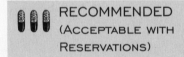

RECOMMENDED (Acceptable with Reservations)

Evista (Raloxifene)

Raloxifene was approved by the FDA in December of 1997 and marked the introduction of a new class of hormones known as selective estrogen reception modulators (SERM). Approved for the prevention of bone wasting (osteoporosis), Evista has been the subject of intense investigation by the pharmaceutical industry because it has the capacity to stimulate estrogen receptors in some tissues, while blocking the effects of estrogen stimulation in other tissues. In this regard, Evista has estrogen-like effects on bones and cholesterol levels, but does not appear to stimulate, and may even act as an "antiestrogen" in, breast and uterine tissues.

Currently, this drug is approved for prevention of bone wasting in postmenopausal women, and is very effective for this indication. The usual dose is 60 mg daily without regard to meals, and supplemental vitamin D and calcium is recommended if dietary intake is inadequate. The daily cost of the drug is about $1.90, which is about five times the cost of Premarin.

The decision to use Evista versus standard estrogen therapy (Premarin) must be individualized. However, before you jump on the Evista bandwagon, you should be aware of the following comparisons between Evista and the traditional conjugated estrogens. First, although Evista shows promise, long-term outcomes are not known—studies are presently underway to settle some of these issues. Hormone replacement with estrogen has been around for many years and has been shown to be safe and effective—and much less expensive.

The proven benefits of estrogen replacement, including prevention of osteoporosis, heart disease, and possibly Alzheimer's disease, are in stark contrast to the unknown effect of Evista on these diseases. Estrogen has also been shown to prevent heart disease after coronary artery bypass surgery. Even in the case of bone wasting, the increase in bone mineral density with Evista was not as impressive as it is for 0.625 mg of Premarin. And while we expect Evista to protect against breast cancer (like another SERM, tamoxifen), this is not yet proven.

Second, the potential disadvantages of Evista should be mentioned. This drug worsens postmenopausal symptoms such as hot flashes, vaginal dryness, and decreased sexual desire.

Evista should be seen as an alternative to estrogen for the prevention of osteoporosis. It should be viewed as an option for women afraid or unable to take estrogen or concerned about protecting their bones and breasts, but it should not be seen as an alternative to estrogen yet.

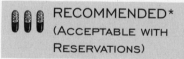

RECOMMENDED*
(ACCEPTABLE WITH RESERVATIONS)

ESTROGEN REPLACEMENT THERAPY

The Cyclical-Combined Regimen for Women Who Still Have Their Uterus

Premarin 0.625 mg each day is taken on Days 1 through 25. On Days 13 through 25, a low-dose progestogen is taken.
The cyclic-combined estrogen progestin approach to hormone replacement therapy is less

---

* These "cyclic-combined estrogen and progestin" regimens are just as effective and safe as the continuous-combined regimen discussed in the "Optimal" category. They are downgraded to the "Recommended" category only for convenience reasons (including medication compliance and more breakthrough bleeding).

convenient than the continuous-combined approach described in the "Optimal" category. Women who have breakthrough bleeding on this cyclic regimen can be switched to the continuous regimen in order to eliminate this troublesome symptom.

The use of progesterone along with estrogen is complicated by breakthrough bleeding, which many women find disturbing. The frequency of this side effect is reduced with the continuous-combined approach, and as many as 80 percent of women have no bleeding after one year of hormone replacement.

For additional information related to estrogen therapy, please see the "Optimal" category.

Miacalcin Nasal Spray (calcitonin)

This FDA-approved nasal spray consists of the hormone calcitonin, which prevents the thinning of bone. It is a safe approach to preventing bone loss, but the effectivness of Miacalcin does not appear to be in the league of either estrogen or Fosamax. An adequate intake of vitamin D and calcium is required for this medication to achieve the best possible results.

DISCOURAGED FOR INITIAL USE
(BUT MAY BE REQUIRED IN SELECTED PEOPLE)

Slow fluoride (slow-release fluoride)

This medication is not yet approved in the United States. Many experts are still concerned about its safety, although it clearly has a very beneficial effect on bone strength. Some individuals will require slow fluoride as part of their treatment regimen. At this point in time, the combination of estrogen replacement, Fosamax, and Miacalcin—in conjunction with calcium therapy—offers the optimal approach in severe cases.

AVOID IF POSSIBLE
(NOT RECOMMENDED)

Didronel (etridonate)
Aredia (pamidronate)

Not approved for treatment of osteoporosis. If you are taking these medications for treatment of bone wasting, you should strongly consider being switched to Fosamax. (See "Optimal" category.)

PILLS FOR RHEUMATOID ARTHRITIS*

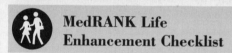

MedRANK Life Enhancement Checklist

Pills of Wisdom: Rheumatoid arthritis (RA) is a common, painful, and debilitating disease that, almost without exception, requires medications for acute flare-ups and long-term maintenance. Many different pills and approaches have been pressed into service to combat the pain, chronic suffering, and disabilities associated with this disease.

Unfortunately, nearly all the medications that appear to work can produce serious side effects. For example, aspirin and nonsteroidal anti-inflammatory medications (NSAIDs) can cause bleeding ulcers and kidney problems; corticosteroids can produce bone wasting, obesity, and skin fragility; methotrexate can produce liver and lung toxicity; and gold and penicillamine can be toxic to the kidneys.

The main area of debate surrounding the treatment of RA is how long to use the so-called "first-line" drugs and exactly when to add the "second-line" drugs (which tend to be more toxic) to the "cocktail" of medications. Many arthritis experts are leaning toward adding the second-line drugs much *earlier* because of speculation that they might actually slow down progression of the disease. The thinking is that the more aggressive cocktails may decrease the rate of bone, joint, and cartilage destruction. No one knows for sure if this approach will really retard joint destruction, but many doctors are giving it a try.

Currently, if you or a family member has RA, you can expect a sequence of drug therapy that begins with aspirin, an NSAID, or a low-dose corticosteroid medication (considered the "first-line" of therapy), which will then be followed by the second-line or "disease-modifying" drugs—so called because they may actually affect the *progression* of joint destruction.

The important point is that the addition or sequencing of these drugs will depend on your physician and will differ from patient to patient. Some doctors will be more aggressive and use the second-line drugs right away. Naturally, if you're not getting better with the initial medications, and your disease is progressing rapidly, it makes sense for your doctor to raise the ante and try the more aggressive drugs. With few established guidelines for the second-line drugs, a case-by-case, "let's see how you do on this drug" approach may be the best you can expect for now.

Generally speaking, low-dose methotrexate is the most commonly used second-line drug and is considered by most rheumatologists (physicians who specialize in joint and tissue diseases) to be the second-line drug of choice, especially for severe RA. It works quickly, is relatively safe if you are carefully monitored, and it reduces joint inflammation.

If the disease is relatively mild, hydroxychloroquine (Plaquenil), a drug that is also used for malaria, is frequently used in place of methotrexate. You should be aware that relapse rates for people with RA are high, regardless of which therapy is used—which is another way of saying that medications for this condition are woefully inadequate, in part because of their ineffectiveness in many people, and in part because of their toxic effects. Anyone embarking on

---

* Most of the medications used to treat rheumatoid arthritis are quite toxic. Consequently, it is recommended that the pills in this MedRANK Checklist be prescribed by arthritis specialists (rheumatologists) who are experienced in treating this condition.

medical treatment for RA will have to muster all the patience they can and be prepared for continued laboratory monitoring and less-than-perfect results.

Finally, as is the case with heart disease and AIDS, there is an increasing movement to use full-throttle "cocktail" therapy with three of the disease-modifying pills—methotrexate, hydroxychloroquine, and sulfasalazine—especially in people who have responded poorly to one drug only.

OPTIMAL
(HIGHLY RECOMMENDED/ BEST OF CLASS)

NSAIDS (NONSTEROIDAL ANTI-INFLAMMATORY DRUGS)

Naprosyn (naproxen)
Motrin (ibuprofen)
Relafen (nabumetone)
Daypro (oxaprozin)
Ansaid (fluriprofen)
Aleve (naproxen)
Many others

These drugs are the best place to *start*, with the understanding that they can cause many problems, especially in older people. But almost without exception, the pain and disability that characterize RA are so severe that NSAIDs will be pressed into service, despite their downsides.

Is it possible to recommend one NSAID over another? Yes and no. First, it should be made clear that no one has ever shown definitively that one NSAID is any more effective than another, or that the safety profile of one NSAID, used at its effective dose, will be safer or produce fewer side effects than any other NSAID used at its effective dose. Nevertheless,

some NSAIDs appear to cause more side effects than others, and therefore they are relegated to "Avoid If Possible" status.

From a practical standpoint, this means if one NSAID isn't working or is producing troubling side effects, your physician will switch you to another NSAID that you *can* tolerate and that will produce the relief you need. Expect this kind of trial-and-error approach to pain and inflammation management. It comes with the territory when using NSAIDs.

Warning: NSAIDs do pose a significant safety risk, especially in high-risk individuals —the elderly, and people with stomach or peptic ulcers, kidney disease, RA, diabetes, heart disease, nasal polyps, high blood pressure, bleeding disorders, and persons taking multiple medications. NSAIDs can erode the stomach lining. If you are over 70 or have previously had an ulcer or bleeding from your gastrointestinal tract, you probably should be on a medication called Cytotec (misoprostol), in order to reduce the risk of developing ulcers.

Cytotec will have no effect on the RA; it is a preventive medication against developing gastrointestinal side effects from NSAIDs. Most older people with RA fall into this high-risk category and, therefore, will require Cytotec treatment. Accordingly, people who use NSAIDs for RA should be followed very carefully by their physician. They should report any stomach or abdominal pains, darkening in the color of the stool, bleeding problems, breathing problems, and changes in urinary habits.

The bottom line is that for many, but not all, patients with RA, NSAIDs are effective pain relievers and joint-function improvers. However, many people will *not* get better with NSAIDs and will need to be started on more aggressive, second-line drugs. This is the rule, rather than the exception, so expect a "cocktail" approach—two or three drugs in combination—if you do not show immediate improvement with NSAIDs.

Among the NSAIDs, Relafen and Daypro have the advantage of once-daily dosing, and therefore are recommended for people who require NSAIDs for longer courses (weeks) of treatment and for those who have to manage multiple medications.

Rheumatrex (methotrexate)

If your joint disease takes an aggressive turn, and you are not responding all that well to NSAIDs, methotrexate is the next logical step. Its toxic effects appear to be lessened when it is given in low doses on a *once-weekly* basis. In most patients its benefits will outweigh its risks. People with RA are more likely to continue methotrexate than they are any of the other second-line drugs. But it can cause problems, including nausea, abdominal pain, diarrhea, and vomiting. Liver failure can occur in a very small percentage of patients, especially the very old and those who have been on the drug for long periods.

Plaquenil (hydroxychloroquine)

This drug, which is also used to treat malaria, is used for people with slowly progressive RA. It is less toxic than most of the other drugs used for RA and therefore is favored as an early second-line agent.

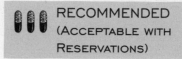

RECOMMENDED
(ACCEPTABLE WITH RESERVATIONS)

CORTICOSTEROIDS

Prednisone

Steroids, as they are usually called, reduce inflammation, swelling, and joint pain in people with RA. Their use is somewhat controversial, because they also have some very undesirable side effects when used for prolonged periods.

The way to maximize the benefits of steroids and reduce the toxic side effects is to have your doctor prescribe them at the lowest dose possible (5 to 10 mg per day). They are especially useful in older people, as an alternative to the even more toxic second-line drugs, and in younger people to help control flare-ups. Side effects include weight gain, bone wasting, cataracts, risk of infection, elevated blood pressure, ulcers, bleeding, and skin changes.

Azulfidine (sulfasalazine)

This drug has shown increasing promise for treatment of RA. In one study, when used in combination with methotrexate and hydroxychloroquine in patients who had shown a poor response to other medications, people with severe RA showed significant improvement.

Zostrix (capsaicin)

This drug is made from a substance found in hot peppers. Many people have found that continued use of this cream can improve joint pain.

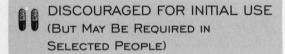

DISCOURAGED FOR INITIAL USE (BUT MAY BE REQUIRED IN SELECTED PEOPLE)

Aspirin

Aspirin was one of the original treatments for RA. I no longer recommend it because multiple daily doses are required, which can be very inconvenient for RA sufferers, who frequently have to take many other pills. In addition, the dose of aspirin required to reduce inflammation is high enough to cause stomach irritation and other gastrointestinal complications in a significant percentage of people. NSAIDs are preferred over aspirin.

Depen (penicillamine)

Depen is not as effective as the second-line drugs in "Optimal" and "Recommended." This medication can cause a rash, itching, altered taste sensations, and blood count problems.

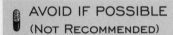

AVOID IF POSSIBLE (NOT RECOMMENDED)

Sandimmune (cyclosporine)

This drug should be avoided if possible. It can cause serious kidney problems and have toxic effects on the liver as well. Its use is experimental and should be reserved for people in whom all else has failed.

Myochrysine (gold sodium thiomalate)

Gold by injection should be avoided because of its toxic effects on the kidneys. Gold taken by mouth (orally) appears to be less toxic but is also less effective than the drugs mentioned in the "Optimal" and "Recommended" categories.

Imuran (azathioprine)

This cancer chemotherapy drug can affect the immune system and cause liver problems. It may predispose people to getting a type of cancer called lymphoma.

Chlorambucil

This chemotherapy drug can compromise the immune system and lead to an increased risk of infections and certain cancers.

Cyclophosphamide

This chemotherapy drug can compromise the immune system and lead to an increased risk of infections and certain cancers.

Meclomen (meclofenamate)

This NSAID is much more likely to produce severe diarrhea than other drugs in this class, and therefore should be avoided.

Feldene (piroxicam)

This is one of the best pain relievers and anti-inflammatory drugs among the NSAIDs. It has been embroiled in controversy over its relative risk for causing gastrointestinal bleeding in elderly people with chronic arthritis. No long-term study has convincingly proven that piroxicam does produce a higher risk of bleeding. Some studies suggest it does, others say no. Geriatric experts tend to avoid this NSAID. Its use as a first-line drug was more attractive a few years ago, when it was the only once-daily NSAID available. Now that other options (Daypro and Relafen), with equal convenience, are approved, Feldene's advantages are less convincing.

CHAPTER 17

—

NO PAIN IS YOUR GAIN

Medications for Pain Relief

"My back still hurts, doc" is the common refrain. "Can't you give me something stronger?" There is almost always something stronger for pain relief—but stronger may not be better in a particular case. With increased potency and effectiveness comes the risk of such troubling side effects as sleepiness, constipation, heartburn, nausea, vomiting, and—last but not least—the risks of physical dependence and drug withdrawal symptoms.

In people who have advanced cancer and are suffering from excruciating, chronic pain syndromes, these risks are well worth it for the relief they provide. Senior citizens with disabling arthritis also may be suitable candidates for long-term therapy with narcotic analgesics. In addition, for people who have had surgical procedures or trauma, the value of short-term treatment with potent pain relievers is well-documented. On the other hand, caution is required whenever you find yourself taking any kind of pain reliever for a

long period of time, especially for conditions that are less well defined. Chronic pain can be a sign of depression, in which case an entirely different class of medications will be required.

When choosing a pain reliever (analgesic), you should keep three things in mind. First, be sure your doctor has explained the cause of your pain. This is important so you don't fall into the trap of masking the pain caused by a potentially serious medical problem that has not yet been diagnosed. Second, be sure that the strength of the medication is matched to the degree of pain you are experiencing. If a drug feels too strong, ask your physician for something milder. On the other hand, if it isn't even touching your pain, you may need to be reevaluated—maybe your condition is more severe than initially suspected—or considered for treatment with a more potent drug. Finally, many pain syndromes respond much better to nonanalgesic medications that are specifically targeted at remedying the underlying cause of the pain. For example, nitrates, calcium channel blockers, and beta-blockers are useful for relieving the chest pain (angina) caused by narrowed arteries in the heart; Imitrex (sumatriptan) is the best approach to relieving migraine headaches; and antiviral drugs such as Famvir, Zovirax, and Valtrex are essential for treating the pain of genital herpes and shingles.

☺ *An enormous choice of pain relievers is available to you and your physician. The overarching principle for optimizing their use is to start with pills that are "weak and safe," then graduate— slowly, and only if necessary—to analgesics that are "potent and problematic."*

For a drug-by-drug comparison and pill-for-disease matchup, you will want to consult the MedRANK Checklist "Pills for Mild, Moderate, and Severe Pain" on page 278.

☺ *For most minor aches and pains, Tylenol (acetaminophen) is probably the safest and most convenient pain reliever available. It has few drug interactions, and as long as it isn't used in people who are heavy drinkers or have liver problems, it is very safe.*

Aspirin is also effective, but it has a much *greater* risk for drug interactions. Important interactions can occur between aspirin and the following medications: antacids, steroids, Axid, ACE inhibitors, oral anticoagulants (Coumadin), heparin, diuretics, methotrexate, probenicid, oral sulfonyureas (Glucotrol XL,

Amaryl, Micronase), insulin, valproic acid, and NSAIDs. In addition, at doses required to produce pain relief, aspirin can produce heartburn, stomach ulcers, kidney problems, and ringing in the ears, especially in the elderly.

☺ *If Tylenol doesn't do the job and inflammation is the most likely cause of your pain, it makes sense to "graduate" to a nonsteroidal anti-inflammatory drug (NSAID).*

NSAIDs are widely used and highly effective for treating pain syndromes associated with headache, athletic injuries, menstrual cramps, and viral syndromes. These medications reduce inflammation—pain, redness, and swelling—by inhibiting the production of chemicals, called prostaglandins, that can produce tissue irritation and inflammation. A number of prescription and nonprescription formulations are available, including ibuprofen, ketoprofen, naproxen, and many others.

☺ *NSAIDs are also associated with a number of drug-related side effects. The most important forms of toxicity that you should be aware of include worsening of kidney disease, stomach ulcers, and drug interactions.*

The elderly appear to be at increased risk for these side effects, especially stomach ulcers and gastrointestinal bleeding. As a result, if you or a family member is over the age of 65, you should use NSAIDs with great care and under a physician's supervision. Lower doses may still produce acceptable results while reducing the risk of drug-related problems. (See the MedRANK Checklist "NSAIDs for Osteo-arthritis and Other Painful Diseases" on page 287.)

If you are considering self-administering an NSAID, you should take the following precautions. First of all, these medications should not be consumed in excessive doses. Studies show that the risk of bleeding from the gastrointestinal tract is increased with larger doses of the medication. Consequently, you should take as little of the medication as is required to produce beneficial effects, and never exceed the recommended dosages that appear on the package insert. If you have a previous history of gastric ulcer, peptic ulcer, or gastrointestinal bleeding from any cause, you should consult a physician before taking one of these medications. In addition, if you have a history of heart disease, congestive heart failure, or diabetes, you are at greater risk for experiencing side effects caused by these drugs.

If you have ever been told that you have any kind of kidney disease, you may be especially vulnerable. Unfortunately, kidney problems may occur very quickly and with relatively low doses of the medications, including over-the-counter sources. Generally speaking, you should avoid taking high doses of aspirin or alcoholic beverages while taking NSAIDs. Finally, because there are significant differences among drugs in this therapeutic class, brand interchange is not recommended.

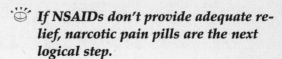 **If NSAIDs don't provide adequate relief, narcotic pain pills are the next logical step.**

Narcotic pain medications are useful for relieving moderate to severe pain syndromes. A number of different formulations are available, but, in general, all of these drugs can cause sleepiness, confusion, and withdrawal syndromes. You can develop tolerance to and/or physical dependence on narcotic pain relievers. This can occur after months or even days of continuous therapy. Tolerance is manifested by the need for increasing dosages in order to maintain pain relief. In addition, long-term use may lead to addiction.

Early signs of addiction include ineffective pain relief and reliance on high-dosage formulations.

Because narcotic pain relievers can make you sleepy, cautious use is required, especially when combined with other medications affecting mental alertness, as well as alcohol and antihistamines. In particular, the narcotic meperidine should never be used in combination with a monoamine oxidase inhibitor (MAOI).

Pain relief must be individualized. Collaboration between you and your doctor is essential. The MedRANK Checklist in this chapter can help guide you to the best and safest pain relievers available for pain syndromes from which you or your family members may suffer.

PILLS FOR MILD, MODERATE, AND SEVERE PAIN*

 MedRANK Life Enhancement Checklist

Pills of Wisdom: Methods for relieving pain associated with medical conditions, surgical procedures, and injuries are very controversial. Many physicians, fearing that their patients will become *addicted* to narcotic medications, prescribe pills that provide *inadequate* relief, whereas other practitioners prescribe very potent medications with a high potential for physical dependence, for conditions with only mild to moderate pain.

There are no simple answers because people can respond very differently to similar pain stimuli. A medication may produce dramatic pain relief for one person, but be perceived as inadequate by another. As a result, your physician may have to experiment and try different pills within the same class—or try another class of drugs altogether—in order to get the relief you want.

Whether you use OTC or prescription pain medications, be sure you know the *cause* of your pain. Because pain is something you experience for a reason, you will always want to be sure it is not an indication of a serious illness—a heart attack, a ruptured abdominal artery, cancer, pneumonia, a kidney stone —that requires immediate medical attention to correct the underlying problem. You don't want to mask a serious condition by taking a pain medication. If your chronic pain is a sign of underlying depression, then you will get better results from antidepressant medications than with pain relievers per se.

In other words, you always should be told what is causing your pain. Ask your doctor these questions: "What organ or part of my body is the pain coming from? How long is the pain likely to last? How long should I take pain medications? How can I gradually reduce my dependence on pain medications?" Once the source of pain is identified, you can relieve it with medications that are appropriate for your condition.

Don't be a victim of *undertreatment*. As long as the cause of your pain is well defined, you are entitled to be comfortable. Unfortunately, studies show that up to 40 percent of cancer patients, even those with advanced disease and painful symptoms, are woefully *undertreated* for pain control. The World Health Organization has established a very explicit three-step set of guidelines that should be followed when treating patients with advanced cancer for pain. (See the MedRANK Checklist "Pain Medications for Common Medical Conditions" on page 282 for a summary of these recommendations.)

Everyone agrees that the choice of a pain medication must be customized for the patient and their condition. Some people with a particular illness may have higher pain thresholds than others with exactly the same condition. The choice of drugs must account for these variations. Moreover, some very painful conditions—migraine headaches, the nerve pain of shingles or diabetes, angina, and muscle spasms—are more effectively treated with drugs that are *not* traditionally considered pain relievers. For example, migraine headache responds to Imitrex, the nerve pain of diabetes can be relieved with Elavil, and chest pain caused by angina is treated with nitroglycerine, calcium channel blockers, and beta-blockers.

This MedRANK Checklist includes both narcotic

---

* Treating moderate to severe pain with medications must always be individualized and should take place under a physician's supervision.

and non-narcotic medications that can be taken by mouth to relieve pain. It should be stressed that as a group of medications, pain relievers have the potential to produce many serious and even life-threatening side effects. For example, a drug as seemingly benign as aspirin can cause acid indigestion and, in more severe cases, bleeding into the gastrointestinal tract. The commonly used nonsteroid anti-inflammatory drugs (NSAIDs) can cause similar problems, as well as confusion, sedation, kidney problems, and many drug interactions. Narcotic drugs, such as Tylenol #3, Vicodin, Percodan, morphine, Dilaudid, and others, can cause confusion, sleepiness, drowsiness, nausea, constipation, and respiratory problems, as well as physical dependence, albeit in varying degrees depending on their potency. In summary, caution is the watchword when these drugs are used, especially in the elderly, in people with asthma and other lung conditions, in those with liver disease and ulcers, and in those with many other problems.

Chronic pain is an extremely challenging problem that frequently requires a team approach and cautious use of medications from different drug classes. The discussion of this problem is beyond the scope of this book.

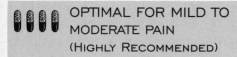

OPTIMAL FOR MILD TO MODERATE PAIN
(Highly Recommended)

Tylenol (acetaminophen)
This is the relatively safe, all-purpose gold-standard pain reliever for five-and-dime aches, pains, and garden-variety discomforts. It is a well-tolerated over-the-counter (OTC) pain reliever that is appropriate for mild pain syndromes. It has very little anti-inflammatory effect and, therefore, may not be as effective as NSAIDs in such conditions as sprains, arthritis, and gout. It's a relatively safe drug, but it

shouldn't be taken in excessive doses over the long term, especially by people who are heavy drinkers or have liver problems or kidney disease. It does not cause stomach ulcers. Overall, this good, all-purpose pain reliever has an excellent safety profile.

Aspirin (acetylsalicylic acid)
Recommended with qualifications. Aspirin is a relatively weak pain reliever when compared with NSAIDs in analgesic doses, but it is comparable in efficacy to Tylenol. It is more likely to cause gastrointestinal ulcers and burning than Tylenol and should not be given to children with influenza, chicken pox, or flulike syndromes.

Aspirin use requires special caution in the *elderly*. It has many potential drug interactions and can worsen asthma in susceptible individuals and cause excessive bleeding. Although particularly effective when given at low doses for prevention of heart disease and related conditions, it takes a backseat to Tylenol as an all-purpose pain reliever in most situations.

NSAIDs

Motrin (ibuprofen)
Advil (ibuprofen)
Naprosyn (naproxen)
Relafen (nabumetone)
Daypro (oxaprozin)
Ansaid (fluriprofen)
Aleve (naproxen)

Caution: Effective, but many adverse effects. The relative potency of these various NSAIDs is still a matter of debate, but the bottom line is that they are very effective pain relievers for a number of conditions. They do pose a significant safety risk, especially for high-risk individuals, like the elderly or people with stomach or peptic ulcers, kidney disease, diabetes, heart disease, nasal polyps, high blood pressure, bleeding disorders, or persons taking multiple medications.

NSAIDs are tailored for *younger, healthy adults* who require relief only from time to time, for mild to moderate pain syndromes (like headache, premenstrual discomfort, strains, and aches). Among the many excellent options, I recommend Aleve as a first choice. This doesn't mean it should be used right out of the gate. Try Tylenol first. If it fails to provide adequate relief, taking an NSAID for a short period will provide significant benefits at low risk.

Older patients who depend on NSAIDs for relief of chronic pain are at much greater risk for adverse side effects and complications. They should be followed very carefully by their physician. They should report any stomach or abdominal pains, darkening in the color of the stool, bleeding problems, breathing problems, and changes in urinary habits.

Among the NSAIDs, Relafen and Daypro have the advantage of once-daily dosing and therefore are recommended for people who require NSAIDs for *longer* courses (weeks) of treatment.

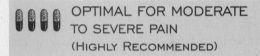

OPTIMAL FOR MODERATE TO SEVERE PAIN
(HIGHLY RECOMMENDED)

Vicodin (hydrocodone/acetaminophen)
Lortab (hydrocodone/acetaminophen)
Very effective. Relatively safe. More potent and less constipating than codeine. This is my first choice for relief of pain of moderate severity. Hydrocodone is a reliable drug, and studies have shown it to be more effective than Tylenol #3 for muscle- and bone-associated pain. It is less constipating than codeine (from which it is derived), and elixirs are available for children. You can become sleepy, nauseated, or dizzy with this pill. It is a narcotic, so physical dependence can occur, although this is rare.

Ultram (tramodol)
Because this drug is still relatively new, the jury is still out, but it has promising aspects. It is a centrally acting analgesic, which means it works in the brain to decrease pain sensations. It is indicated for moderate to severe pain. Its side effects—dizziness, nausea, constipation, headache—become more prominent with extended use.

Tylenol #3 (acetaminophen with codeine)
Commonly prescribed, but frequently doesn't produce enough pain relief. A second-best drug. Although widely used, Tylenol #3 is not a particularly potent pain reliever, at least compared with hydrocodone. Moreover, codeine can be quite constipating and produce an unsettled feeling in the stomach.

Percocet
Tylox
Percodan
Roxicet
Roxiprin
These drugs contain oxycodone, combined with either aspirin or Tylenol. They are more likely to cause dependence than either Vicodin or Tylenol #3, and they have a greater

tendency to cause drowsiness and nausea. They should be reserved for situations in which pain is quite severe and has been unresponsive to Vicodin plus NSAIDs.

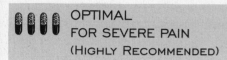

OPTIMAL
FOR SEVERE PAIN
(Highly Recommended)

Dilaudid (hydromorphone)

This high-potency narcotic pain reliever is short-acting. Because of its euphoric effects, it is particularly useful in cancer patients with severe pain. It is not recommended for indiscriminate or widespread use because it causes extreme euphoria. It is highly prized by narcotic abusers as a substitute for heroin. This drug should not be used in children, in people with severe asthma, or in individuals with fluid in their lungs due to congestive heart failure.

Morphine sulfate

This drug should be reserved for individuals with severe pain, especially caused by cancer, and for individuals with severe, incapacitating pain for which all other medication options have been exhausted. It has many precautions and drug interactions. Be sure to tell your physician about any other medications you are taking.

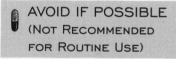

AVOID IF POSSIBLE
(Not Recommended
for Routine Use)

Indocin (indomethacin)

This NSAID is more likely to cause central nervous system symptoms—hallucinations, dizziness, and the like—and gastrointestinal distress than many of the other NSAIDs.

Generally speaking, it is *not* a first-line choice, except perhaps for gout (although safer drugs such as colchicine and other NSAIDs are available for this very painful condition) and rare inflammatory conditions of the sac lining, the exterior of the heart.

Codeine

The fact is, codeine is not all that effective as a pain reliever and has unpleasant side effects. If it is to be used for mild to moderate pain, it is more effective when combined with Tylenol.

Talwin (pentazocine)

This drug can produce "psychological" side effects, among them disorientation, episodes of panic, and hallucinations. It should not be used routinely, least of all by the elderly.

Meclomen (meclofenamate)

This NSAID is much more likely to produce severe diarrhea than other drugs in this class and therefore should be avoided.

Feldene (piroxicam)

This is one of the best pain relievers and anti-inflammatory drugs among the NSAIDs. It has been embroiled in controversy over its relative risk for causing gastrointestinal bleeding in elderly people with chronic arthritis. Its use as a first-line drug was more attractive a few years ago, when it was the only once-daily NSAID available. Now that other options (Daypro and Relafen), with equal convenience, are approved, Feldene's advantages are less convincing.

Darvon (propoxyphene)
Darvocet

These drugs have a more severe toxicity profile than drugs in the "Optimal" category.

They are not advised for routine use, especially in older persons.

Demerol (meperidine)

This drug requires very frequent dosing (every 2 hours) and high dosages to produce adequate pain relief in severe situations. It also places patients at risk for serious drug interactions, especially with the MAOI class of antidepressants.

Methadone

This drug is not recommended for pain relief. It is used in drug rehabilitation programs.

Levo-Dromoran (levorphanol)

This drug is very potent, and its effects last for long periods of time (15–20 hours). It should not be used in the elderly.

Stadol (butorphanol nasal spray)

This narcotic is sometimes used for migraine headaches. Sleepiness, dizziness, and confusion are seen in too many patients to recommend this drug as a first-line choice for treatment of pain.

PAIN MEDICATIONS FOR COMMON MEDICAL CONDITIONS*

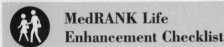 **MedRANK Life Enhancement Checklist**

Pills of Wisdom: As emphasized in the MedRANK Checklist "Pills for Mild, Moderate, and Severe Pain" on page 278, the choice of a pain medication must be customized for the individual patient. This MedRANK Checklist ranks pain medications according to the common medical conditions and injuries for which they are the most appropriate and effective. Remember, this ranking is limited to pain-relieving pills only. For many of these conditions, nondrug approaches (ACE bandages, ice, elevation), as well as prevention-oriented medications, may reduce pain. These are discussed in other chapters.

ACHES AND PAINS

(BONE, JOINT, AND MUSCLE ACHES FROM OVERUSE, INJURY, OR FLU SYNDROME)

MINOR PAIN

First consider:
Tylenol
OR
Extra-Strength Tylenol

If not effective, consider:
Aleve
OR
Motrin
OR
Advil

---

* Please see MedRANK Checklist "Pills for Mild, Moderate, and Severe Pain" on page 278 for a discussion of specific pain-relieving pills and their potencies.

OR
other NSAID

MODERATE PAIN

First consider:
Aleve
OR
Motrin
OR
Advil
OR
other NSAID

If not effective, consider:
Tylenol #3 (acetaminophen with codeine)

Tips:
Use ice for the first 12 hours to reduce swelling.

ARTHRITIS
(DEGENERATIVE OR OSTEOARTHRITIS)

MILD PAIN

First consider:
Extra-Strength Tylenol

If not effective, consider:
Extra-Strength Tylenol *plus* intermittent use of Tylenol #3

MODERATE TO SEVERE PAIN

First consider:
Extra-Strength Tylenol
OR
Ultram

If not effective, consider:
Relafen
OR
Daypro
OR
Naprosyn
OR
other NSAID

SEVERE PAIN

First consider:
Vicodin
OR
Ultram

If not effective, consider:
Vicodin *plus* NSAIDs

CANCER PAIN

Cancer pain usually is caused when a tumor invades vital body organs or spreads to bone or other tissues. These recommendations follow the three-step guidelines issued by the World Health Organization. *Please note:* Making patients with advanced stages of cancer and severe pain more comfortable may also include other medications, many of which are administered by vein, patient-activated infusion pumps, or other drug-delivery systems.

Radiation and chemotherapy treatments also play an important part of pain management and are used in conjunction with pain medications. Other drugs (stool softeners) may be used to treat side effects (such as constipation). Many of these approaches are beyond the scope of this book and should be implemented by a cancer specialist. However, regardless of what pill or pain-relieving regimen is used, always demand an acceptable and comfortable one.

MILD PAIN (STEP 1)

First consider:
Tylenol
OR
Extra-Strength Tylenol

If not effective, consider:
Aleve
OR
Motrin
OR
Advil
OR
other NSAID

MODERATE PAIN (STEP 2)

First consider:
Tylenol #3
OR
Codeine *plus* NSAID

If not effective, consider:
Vicodin
OR
Percodan (Percocet, Tylox, etc.) *plus* NSAID

SEVERE PAIN (STEP 3)

First consider:
Percodan *plus* NSAID

If not effective, consider:
Morphine
OR
Dilaudid *plus* NSAID

MENSTRUAL CRAMPS

First consider:
Extra-Strength Tylenol

If not effective, consider:
Aleve
OR
Motrin
OR
Advil
OR
other NSAID. Tylenol #3 may be used for "breakthrough" pain.

BROKEN BONES

Broken bones (also known as fractures) require rest, immobilization, and elevation (sometimes with an ice pack), along with pills for pain relief.

MILD PAIN

First consider:
Extra-Strength Tylenol

If not effective, consider:
Aleve
OR
Motrin
OR
Advil
OR
other NSAID. Tylenol #3 may be used for "breakthrough" pain.

MODERATE PAIN

First consider:
Vicodin *plus* NSAID

If not effective, consider:
Ultram

SEVERE PAIN

First consider:
Percodan

DENTAL PROCEDURES

MILD TO MODERATE PAIN

First consider:
Extra-Strength Tylenol
OR
Tylenol #3

If not effective, consider:
Vicodin

SEVERE PAIN

First consider:
Vicodin

If not effective, consider:
Percodan
OR
Percocet

SURGICAL PROCEDURES

MILD PAIN

First consider:
Extra-Strength Tylenol

If not effective, consider:
Naproxen
OR
other NSAID

OR
Vicodin

MODERATE TO SEVERE PAIN

First consider:
Vicodin *plus* naproxen
OR
Motrin
OR
other NSAID

If not effective, consider:
Percodan
OR
Percocet *plus* NSAID

GOUT (ACUTE ATTACK)

First consider:
Naproxen
OR
Colchicine

If not effective, consider:
Indocin

HEADACHES

MIGRAINE (SEE CHAPTER 11)

First consider:
Extra-Strength Tylenol
OR
NSAID (Aleve, Anaprox, Naprosyn, others)

If not effective, consider:
Imitrex
OR
Vicodin, if necessary

TENSION HEADACHE

First consider:
Extra-Strength Tylenol

If not effective, consider:
NSAID (Aleve, Anaprox, Naprosyn, others)

LOW BACK PAIN

MILD TO MODERATE SPASMS

First consider:
Extra-Strength Tylenol

If not effective, consider:
NSAID (Aleve, Anaprox, Naprosyn, other).
May be used in combination with a muscle
relaxant such as Robaxin.

SEVERE SPASMS

First consider:
Vicodin *plus* naproxen. May be combined
with a muscle relaxant such as Robaxin.

If not effective, consider:
Percodan *plus* naproxen. May be used in com-
bination with a muscle relaxant such as
Robaxin.

MUSCLE STRAINS AND SPRAINS

MILD TO MODERATE PAIN

First consider:
Extra-Strength Tylenol

If not effective, consider:
NSAID (Aleve, Anaprox, Naprosyn, other).
May be used in combination with a muscle
relaxant such as Robaxin.

SEVERE PAIN

First consider:
Vicodin

If not effective, consider:
Vicodin *plus* NSAID. May be combined with
a muscle relaxant such as Robaxin.

NERVE PAIN

SHINGLES

First consider:
If you are less than 50 years of age, you
should consider mild analgesics such as an
NSAID or Extra-Strength Tylenol.

If you are 50 or older, consider:
Antiviral medications Valtrex or Famvir, in
combination with prednisone (a corticosteroid)

GENITAL HERPES

First consider:
Extra-Strength Tylenol *plus* Famvir
OR
Valtrex

DIABETES

First consider:
Tylenol

If not effective, consider:
Tricyclic antidepresssant (Elavil)

NIGHT LEG CRAMPS

First consider:
Elevate legs

If not effective, consider:
Quinine sulfate

KIDNEY STONES

First consider:
NSAID *plus* Vicodin

If not effective, consider:
Percodan *plus* NSAID

RHEUMATOID ARTHRITIS

First consider:
NSAID (Relafen, Daypro, Naprosyn, etc.)

If not effective, consider:
NSAID in combination with Rheumatrex (methrotrexate) and Plaquenil (hydroxy-chloroquine). Many experts now recommend initial treatment with all three medications to prevent bone destruction and inflammation.

NSAIDs FOR OSTEOARTHRITIS AND OTHER PAINFUL DISEASES

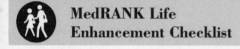 **MedRANK Life Enhancement Checklist**

Generic Name	Trade Name	Usual Dosage and Comments
Aspirin (plain, buffered, or enteric coated)	**Bayer** and many others	2.4–6.0 g daily, by mouth, in four divided doses
Salicylates		Aspirin can interact with many different medications
Diclofenac	**Voltaren, Cefaflan**	50 mg twice or three times daily; 75 mg twice daily
Diflunisal	**Dolobid**	500 mg twice daily
Etodolac	**Lodine**	600–1,200 mg in divided doses
Fenoprofen	**Nalfon**	300–600 mg four times daily
Flurbiprofen	**Ansaid**	200–300 mg in divided doses, twice, three, or four times daily
Ibuprofen	**Advil, Motrin, Nuprin, Rufen,** others	200–800 mg four times daily
Indomethacin	**Indocin**	25 mg three or four times daily; 75 mg twice daily (slow-release preparation)

Generic Name	Trade Name	Usual Dosage and Comments
Ketoprofen	Orudis, Oruvail	50 mg four times daily, or 75 mg three times daily
Meclofenamate	Meclomen	50–100 mg four times daily
Mefenamic acid	Ponstel	250 mg four times daily
Naproxen	Naprosyn, Anaprox, Aleve	250–500 mg twice daily
Nabumetone	Relafen	1,000–2,000 mg once or twice daily
Oxaprozin	Daypro	1,200 mg once a day, or 1,800 mg in divided doses
Piroxicam	Feldene	10 or 20 mg once daily
Sulindac	Clinoril	150–200 mg twice daily
Tolmetin	Tolectin	200–400 mg four times daily

CHAPTER 18

PAPA'S GOT A BRAND-NEW PILL

Medications for Prostate and Potency Problems

Symptoms caused by prostate enlargement affect more than 8 million American men. As men grow older, their prostate glands undergo changes that can compromise the normal flow of urine. These changes, which are not cancerous, are usually called benign prostatic hyperplasia (BPH), which is just another way of saying that there has been an overgrowth of certain elements in the prostate gland.

In fact, autopsy studies show that nearly all men develop BPH if they live long enough. This excessive growth of prostate tissue produces such symptoms as obstructed urinary flow, decreased size or force of the urinary stream, dribbling, hesitancy, and incomplete emptying of the bladder. You can use a questionnaire developed by the American Urological Association, called the BPF Symptom Index, to rank the severity of your symptoms and establish a baseline for your condition. You should ask your physician if you can complete this questionnaire if you suspect that you are having prostate problems.

Not all cases of BPH have the same underlying cause. In some men, the prostate is very enlarged, and there is excessive growth of so-called epithelial cells, while in other men, the prostate is much smaller, and an overgrowth of muscle cells lining the prostate is the cause of the problem. Both situations can produce the kind of urinary symptoms described above.

For many years, the only effective approach was surgery, which was expensive and invasive and, like any procedure, carried a risk of serious complications. Recently, the value of medications for relieving symptoms associated with BPH has been clarified. Although pills cannot *cure* BPH, they certainly can reduce the severity of such symptoms as decreased urinary stream, burning, and urgency to urinate. In addition, if these medications are effective, they can delay the need for surgery, sometimes for as long as three to five years. The question as to which drugs produce the best results is controversial.

Two drug classes are approved for BPH: the alpha reductase inhibitors, and the peripheral alpha-one blockers. Alpha reductase inhibitors, such as finasteride (Proscar), inhibit the enzyme that is responsible for the development of the prostate gland. Accordingly, these drugs are used to treat people who have urinary symptoms caused by BPH. But the effectiveness of Proscar in the treatment of patients with BPH is much debated. Although it appears to cause a rapid reduction in the size of the enlarged prostate in most patients, fewer than half of patients treated with this drug experience an increase in urinary flow or improvement in their symptoms. Six to twelve months of treatment may be required to determine whether you will respond to this medication.

The peripheral alpha-one blockers (Cardura, Hytrin) are more effective for increasing urinary flow in patients with symptoms of BPH.

Consequently, they are recommended as the *initial* drug of choice for most men with symptoms severe enough to treat. For a complete discussion of medications used for BPH, you should consult the MedRANK Checklist "Pills for Urinary Symptoms in Men with Prostate Enlargement."

Infections of the prostate can afflict both young and older men. This condition, called prostatitis, is treated with antibiotics. If you are younger than 35 and have been diagnosed with acute prostatitis, you will require treatment for gonorrhea, which—especially in younger men—is a frequent cause of this problem. Fortunately, there are many "one dose cure" treatments for gonorrhea, including Ciprofloxacin, Cefixime, Zithromax, and Floxin, all of which are recommended. At the same time, I recommend that you be treated for chlamydia infection, which is another possible cause of prostatitis in men under 35. The best "less is more" oral treatment for uncomplicated chlamydial infection is one dose (1 g) of Zithromax.

For men who are older than 35, the treatment of acute prostatitis is slightly different, because different bacteria are involved. The most effective regimens require a two-week course with either Cipro or Septra DS (trimethoprim sulfa). Septra is much less expensive, but may not be quite as effective.

Cipro is the best approach to treating chronic bacterial infections of the prostate, in both younger and older men.

Six weeks—and sometimes up to twelve weeks—of therapy are required to eradicate symptoms. Finally, a syndrome called prostatosis is the most common cause of symptoms associated with prostate inflammation. No bacteria can be identified, but experts suspect that infecting organisms are involved. A two-week course of doxycycline is the treatment of choice.

The Viagra revolution

Whether or not it is destined to become "Prozac for the penis," the introduction of Viagra into the physician's arsenal has brought a new therapeutic paradigm to the practice of medicine. This new equation threatens to undermine time-honored healing principles used by physicians to optimize quality of life for their patients. The fact is, although Viagra has become an essential medication for enhancing sexual function in men who suffer from impotence, many managed care organizations still view this $9 wonder pill as an "optional" form of drug therapy (a luxury), rather than "standard equipment" (a necessity) for treating patients who complain of less-than-adequate sexual performance.

In the age of managed care, or in the case of Viagra, what threatens to become an era of "managed castration," there already have been vigorous attempts to curb use of a drug that is known to improve quality of life. Why? The problem is, although there are clinical "measurement scales" that can quantify severity of "erectile dysfunction" (ED), up to 60 percent of men who will benefit from Viagra have so-called psychogenic impotence—in other words, theirs is a sexual dysfunction for which no organic disease (diabetes, prostatectomy, spinal cord injury, etc.) can be identified. Put simply, in the overwhelming majority of cases, erectile dysfunction is simply *not* quantifiable: it is not a hard and fast diagnosis that begins at one cyclic GMP level (the molecule that increases blood supply to sex organs) and ends abruptly at another. This means that identifying who can benefit from Viagra requires evaluating what are fundamentally *subjective* impressions offered by the patient.

And herein lies the rub. Your subjective impressions may not coincide with the subjective impressions of health care actuaries charged with rationing Viagra pills among health plan members in order to save dollars.

In the real, flesh-and-blood world, in which the goal is to make patients like you feel better, physicians have to rely on patients' perceptions and confidential sexual histories in order to determine whether a prescription for Viagra is justified. Analyzing the complex mind-body interplay that determines penile vigor and stamina is not like taking your temperature, measuring your blood pressure, or getting your blood cholesterol level. By definition, assessment of sexual function is in the mind—and body—of the *beholder*: you! If compassionate health care as we know it—and compassionate almost always means drug therapy that is *customized* for the patient—is to survive, your needs must take precedence over the perceptions of number crunchers who are trying to keep down pharmacy costs and, indirectly, run the risk of dampening your zest for life.

Of course, it is reasonable to ask: Should the quality of life improvements—the enhanced self-esteem, the positive impact on marital life, and reduced anxiety—that accompany adequate sexual function be viewed as a health care "right" or "privilege"? The history of medicine in this country suggests sexual wellness should be viewed as a physiological necessity on par with any other "target" organ—the heart, ovaries, brain, or lungs—that is not functioning at maximal efficiency.

Based on this logic, it can be argued that physicians and health plan administrators should not be discriminating against one target organ in favor of another. But with Viagra at the center of this debate, that day has already come. Hamstrung and pressured by their plans' cost-containment measures, physicians are apt to say to their patients: "I'm sorry, Mr. Jones, we have very strict criteria for approving Viagra in our health plan . . . from what I can tell, you're strong enough 'down there' to support the weight of a washcloth . . . there's no reason you need to be hard enough to bear the weight of a beach towel. I'm sorry, your Viagra request has been rejected by our S.P.S.C., that is, our Sexual Performance Standards Committee."

The fact is, orgasm quotas are not written into health insurance policies because if they were, there would be no buyers. But market-driven Viagra, due to its cost and potential for runaway demand, has put a wrench into time-honored precedents that place a priority on patient well-being. Managed care organizations, so slavishly attached to cost considerations, are trying to make sexual function an exception to well-accepted healing and prescribing principles that take patient input into account as part of the decision-making process for drug therapy.

One can only wonder whether health plans that are tightening the screws on Viagra use in *men* would be willing to take such a strong stand against reimbursement for Viagra prescriptions in *women*—if and when this drug is approved for enhancing sexual performance in this population. Would they be willing to take on the increasingly influential Women's Health Care movement and to restrict the use of this medication in females who, in most cases, would be required to present their physicians with nothing more than subjective impressions of less-often-or-less-intense-than-desired sexual function or sub-

optimal gratification. Probably not. The political consequences of titrating sexual activity or fulfillment in women would be too hot to handle. In this sense, the "ration Viagra" movement that is gaining momentum represents a curious form of sexual—and health—discrimination against *men*, and all should be aware of the implications.

Whether it is heart failure or, in the case of Viagra, hard failure, it is symptoms that drive medication use and make doctors put pens to their prescription pads. Up until now, health plans have not asked doctors to deny their patients antihistamines if they "feel like they need something for the burning and itching in their eyes." And they haven't restricted use of antidepressants in patients who tell their doctors that they "are sad to the point of not being able to work or participate in family life." As physicians, we oftentimes rely on *subjective* impressions to press medications into service on behalf of our patients' medical problems. This is as fundamental to the practice of medicine as the Hippocratic Oath itself.

And Viagra should be no exception. Physicians should have the freedom to do what is necessary to keep blood flowing to vital sexual organs that have the capacity to give our patients pleasure and fulfillment with their loved ones. Viagra-mediated improvements in sexual function have health- and psyche-enhancing benefits as important as those offered by other medications, many of them less effective and more toxic. After all, who is to say that optimal functioning of the heart is any more or less important to any individual patient—or sexually active couple, for that matter—than optimal functioning of the family jewels? As physicians, our role is to improve the health of any and all target organ our *patients* identify as a potential problem.

For the time being, however, managed care organizations and health insurers are willing to impose measures that limit Viagra to only those individuals who occupy the most severe end of the erectile dysfunction spectrum. In turn, they are setting the stage to play Big Brother in the bedrooms of sexually impaired or less-than-optimally satisfied Americans. The diagnosis of sexual dysfunction, in most cases, is a patient-centered diagnosis. There are many gray areas, and health plan managers should not be playing hardball with soft calls. One can only imagine physicians and pharmacists paying late night visits to the homes of our patients, tiptoeing up to their bedroom with clipboards and rulers in hand, commenting to the couple who has just ducked for cover under the sheets: "Sorry to interrupt you, we're just here to see whether or not you meet our strict indications for Viagra therapy."

Approaches that limit physicians' abilities to respond to the subjective symptoms and impressions of their patients will be a setback to a health care system that has prided itself on improving quality of life for a wide range of conditions, from headache to heartache. In a free-to-choose society, where health enhancement, especially in the area of "personal pharmacology," has been elevated to high art and science, sexual dysfunction should be medicated—with Viagra when necessary and appropriate—not legislated or bureaucratized as recent trends suggest may soon be the case.

GO WITH THE FLOW
Pills for Urinary Symptoms in Men with Prostate Enlargement

 MedRANK Life Enhancement Checklist

Pills of Wisdom: For many years, surgery was the primary approach for relieving bothersome symptoms caused by BPH. These procedures involved removal of part of the overgrowth of prostate tissue through direct incision, laser therapy, electrosurgical vaporization, ultrasonic coagulation, or other techniques. Although these approaches are still sometimes necessary, there has been a growing movement toward using *medications* as a means for delaying surgical intervention. These medication-based therapies have been shown to be very safe and effective.

Medications used to treat symptoms of BPH fall into two main categories: (1) alpha-one adrenergic antagonists, such as Cardura (doxaozosin) and Hytrin (terazosin), which relax the smooth muscle of the prostate gland; and (2) alpha reductase inhibitors, such as Proscar (finasteride), which actually shrink the prostate gland by blocking formation of the androgen dihydrotestosterone. There has been a rather intense debate as to which category of medication—the alpha-one blockers or the alpha reductase inhibitors—produces better relief of BPH symptoms. The issue is not entirely settled, but recent studies suggest the *alpha-one blockers are probably the pills of choice for going with the flow.*

A reasonable approach is as follows: If you have

urinary symptoms compatible with BPH, and your doctor tells you your prostate is not enlarged, Cardura (or Hytrin) is the best first choice. If you have symptoms and your prostate is enlarged (as it is in about 20 percent of men over 60), then treatment with Cardura (or Hytrin) *or* Proscar should be considered. There appears to be no advantage from using a combination of medications.

Remember, if you have *no* symptoms, you don't need a medication, no matter how big your prostate is. On the other hand, if you have *severe* symptoms, surgery may be the best approach. You and your physician should make these decisions together. Finally, remember that many of the symptoms that cause BPH can also be caused by cancer of the prostate. Be sure you have had a complete physical exam (including a digital exam of the prostate) and necessary laboratory studies (the PSA test) prior to starting pills for relief of BPH symptoms.

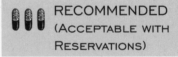

RECOMMENDED (ACCEPTABLE WITH RESERVATIONS)

Hytrin (terazosin)

Like Cardura, Hytrin is an alpha-one blocker that has been proven very effective for relieving symptoms caused by BPH. The first dose should be taken at bedtime because, on rare occasions, there is an exaggerated first-dose effect that causes low blood pressure. The main side effects are dizziness, headache, and fatigue.

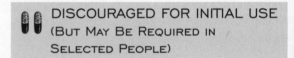

DISCOURAGED FOR INITIAL USE (BUT MAY BE REQUIRED IN SELECTED PEOPLE)

Proscar (finasteride)

Proscar has had its ups and, most recently, its downs, as an initial drug for treating symptoms of BPH. It reduces the concentration of dihydrotestosterone in the prostate gland, thereby shrinking its size. About 20 percent of men who have BPH symptoms also have an enlarged prostate gland. If you fall into this category, Proscar has a greater likelihood of relieving your symptoms than if your prostate gland is normal in size. In most cases, however, I would still recommend Cardura or Hytrin as the intial drug.

The only important side effects of Proscar are related to sexual function. When you take the placebo effect into account, about 4 percent of men on Proscar report a decrease in libido, and about 2.5 percent report impotence.

OPTIMAL (HIGHLY RECOMMENDED/ BEST OF CLASS)

Cardura (doxazosin)

Cardura should be considered first for treatment of BPH. This medication is indicated for two kinds of symptoms that are caused by BPH: (1) obstructive symptoms, including weak urine stream, dribbling, hesitancy, and incomplete emptying of the bladder; and (2) irritative symptoms, which include burning during urination, urinating at night, and frequent urination during the day.

This once-daily medication relaxes the smooth muscle in the prostate, which is why it improves urinary symptoms. Its dose needs to be adjusted upward gradually over a period of one to four weeks. The main side effects are dizziness, weakness, fatigue, and headache.

Minipress (prazosin)

Once routinely used for the treatment of high blood pressure, Minipress has fallen out of favor because of its side effects and requirement for multiple daily dosing. It can produce sudden drops in blood pressure with the first dose, and it is not approved for relief of symp-toms associated with BPH. Bypass this drug and use Cardura instread.

PLANT EXTRACTS

Saw palmetto
Bladderwrack
Beta-sistosterol

There is no scientific evidence confirming the effectiveness of these plant derivatives.

PILLS FOR IMPOTENCE

MedRANK Life Enhancement Checklist

Pills of Wisdom: Although Viagra is the best and most effective drug available for the treatment of male impotence, anyone considering use of this medication must be aware of both its upsides and downsides. Riding a wave of media coverage, Viagra exploded into the mainstream in the spring of 1998, shattering new product launch records, cornering the market on impotence treatments, and spawning dozens of questions and concerns.

Virtually every major newspaper, magazine, and television feature covering Viagra usually did so in glowing terms. Yet despite the extensive coverage, there are still many questions to be answered, and even though the manufacturer has warned physicians of the possible side effects and, especially, the danger of prescribing this drug in combination with nitroglycerin-like medications, many of these warnings have been drowned out by the sheer volume of media coverage.

At the time that this book went to press, six deaths in patients who had been taking Viagra were reported, but it was unclear whether or not these deaths were related to Viagra. What is clear is that, like any medications, Viagra has its downsides and certain precautions apply when considering this medication for treatment of impotence.

First, Viagra should *never* be taken in combination with any medications containing nitrates, nitrites, dinitrates, or nitroglycerin. Most of these medications are used to treat chest pain associated with angina, and include the following: Nitro-Bid, IMDUR, Nitroguard, amyl nitrite, nitroglycerin, Nitrocine, Nitrol ointment, Nitrostat, Nitrolingual spray, Sorbitrate, Deponit, Dilarate SR, Isordil, Monoket, Nitrolingual, Transderm Nitro, and many others. If you are on any of these medications—or any other nitrate-containing drugs—the combination of Viagra plus these medications can cause serious reductions in your blood pressure that have the potential to be life-threatening. Consequently, if you have ever been told you have heart disease, you *must* ask your physician if you have been prescribed a nitrate for your condition; and if you have, Viagra is simply not for you. No ifs, ands, or buts about it.

Second, although Viagra is commonly prescribed for middle-aged and older individuals—both with and without heart disease—it should be used cautiously in people, especially the elderly, with advanced heart disease. Because sexual intercourse requires physical exertion, and because this exertion can, in some patients, produce heart symptoms such as angina, Viagra should be used cautiously in people who are borderline compensated as far as their cardiac reserve is concerned. If you have heart disease, but have not had sexual activity for a long period of time, and are considering the use of Viagra, start low (i.e., use the lowest dosage, 25 mg) and go slow (don't overdo it) the first time around. On the other hand, elderly patients who are otherwise physically active, have good aerobic exercise tolerance, and are able to tolerate the physical exertion of sexual activity without problems are excellent candidates for this drug.

Third, although Viagra is safe and effective when used in the appropriate patient, there are side effects that need to be mentioned. The side effects are related to the dose of the drug—mildest and less frequent at the 25 mg dose and more frequent at the 100 mg dose—and include headaches (up to 16 percent of patients), flushing (10 percent), indigestion (7 percent), nasal congestion (4 percent), and visual disturbances/blue coloration (3 percent).

OPTIMAL (HIGHLY RECOMMENDED/ BEST OF CLASS)

Viagra (sildenafil)

More convenient and effective than other impotence medications such as Muse (a medication which requires insertion of a pill into the male urethra), Viagra has been shown in clinical trials to improve sexual performance in clinically diagnosed impotent men. In studies involving more than 3000 impotent men, 35 percent to 80 percent of those who took the drug reported improved sexual performance, while only 20 percent of those in the placebo (inactive pill) group cited improvement. Men who were diagnosed with impotence and who improved on this medication include those with a wide range of problems: psychogenic impotence, post-prostatectomy, diabetes, spinal cord injury, and other groups.

How does Viagra work? Unlike previous treatments for impotence, Viagra affects the response to sexual stimulation. The drug enhances the smooth muscle relaxant effects of nitric oxide, a substance that is normally released in response to sexual stimulation. This smooth muscle relaxation then allows blood to enter the penis and produce an erection.

Is Viagra safe? Yes, it is safe as long as used appropriately. This means it should never be used in combination with nitrates (see "Pills of Wisdom") and should be used cautiously in men known to have advanced heart disease, congestive heart failure, irregular heart rhythms, or anginal chest pain with exertion. As with any drug, some people do experience side effects. The most important are headache, flushing, stomachache, nasal congestion, and color perception changes. All of these side effects are reversible.

How do you take Viagra? Viagra is typically prescribed as one 50 mg tablet, once a day, and is taken about one hour prior to anticipated sexual activity. It may, however, be taken anywhere from 30 minutes to four hours before sexual activity. Some individuals may need higher doses (100 mg) to achieve the desired level of sexual function. Currently, the drug should not be taken more than once per day.

How much does Viagra cost? You should do

comparison shopping among pharmacies, but the price per pill will range from $9 to $12. Most insurance companies will not fully cover the cost of this medication.

Will Viagra enhance performance in men who have "adequate" sexual function? That is the $64,000 question. Although the manufacturer has not published studies reporting on the effects of Viagra in men who are not impotent but who want to improve their performance, anecdotal reports have surfaced suggesting that Viagra can enhance erectile properties in this group.

Does Viagra affect sexual function in women? Because Viagra increases blood flow to sexual organs in both women and men, there is good reason to think that it can improve sexual function in females. Although at present the drug is not approved for use in women, early small studies in women suggest the drug can be of benefit as far as increasing lubrication and other sexual responses. Currently, using the drug in women is an "off-label" indication.

CHAPTER 19

—

SMOOTH PASSAGE

Medications for the Postmenopausal Years

A wide range of natural and synthetic hormones are used to treat a broad spectrum of conditions that occur commonly in postmenopausal women: among them diabetes, thyroid disease, asthma, and arthritic disorders. Estrogens, a group of related sex hormones, are available as injections, tablets, and vaginal creams. Although both men and women have estrogens in their bloodstream, as medications they are used primarily to treat a number of symptoms and disease entities in women, including hot flashes associated with menopause; for estrogen replacement after failure of the ovaries due to menopause, disease, or surgical removal; and vaginal tissue breakdown. They are also used to relieve symptoms of cancer in some men and women, especially those with widespread disease. In men, estrogenlike hormones are used to treat

advanced androgen-dependent cancer of the prostate gland. Conjugated estrogens, such as Estradiol, are used to prevent loss of bone mass that accompanies menopause.

☼ *There are many unlabeled uses for estrogens, and therefore you should consult your physician if you are taking them for a condition for which they are not indicated.*

Although hormone replacement therapy (HRT) in postmenopausal women has been a topic of intense debate, the risks and benefits of HRT have recently been clarified. For complete pill-by-pill recommendations, you will want to consult the MedRANK Checklists "Estrogen: Pill for a Lifetime" and "Troubleshooting Estrogen Therapy" in this chapter.

☼ *At the outset, all postmenopausal women should be considered candidates for HRT. Of course, the final decision as to whether estrogen therapy is appropriate should be made by the patient and her physician after weighing all the relevant factors.*

For example, the only true, absolute contra-indication to estrogen use is a history of breast cancer or other estrogen-sensitive malignancy. Although a history of blood clots is a common, relative contraindication, it should not always exclude a woman from the benefits of long-term estrogen replacement. In women who have had a hysterectomy, for whatever reason, the benefits of HRT almost always outweigh the risks, because there is no risk of endometrial cancer and no annoying recurrence of menstrual bleeding.

☼ *In postmenopausal women who still have a uterus, progestins should generally be added to the estrogen regimen in order to minimize the risk of endometrial cancer.*

At present, there is no evidence that this combination decreases the beneficial lipid-lowering effects of estrogen. You should be warned that the standard cyclical estrogen/progestin regimen frequently results in withdrawal bleeding, which can adversely affect quality of life and compromise long-term compliance. The use of *continuous* low-dose progesterone along with daily estrogen can decrease the frequency of bleeding and thereby improve the tolerability of HRT. If you have continued heavy or irregular bleeding, it should be investigated by your physician. As a rule, doses of conjugated estrogen (or its equivalent) greater than 1.25 mg per day should be avoided.

☼ *As you may gather, the administration of estrogen during the postmenopausal years is still somewhat controversial. But evidence supporting its routine use has rapidly mounted in recent years.*

On the positive side, estrogen replacement therapy significantly reduces the rate of postmenopausal osteoporosis, and as a result decreases the number of hip fractures in elderly women. The reduction in hip fractures has been reported to be as great as 60 percent. In addition, a number of studies strongly suggest that HRT can reduce the risk of heart disease in postmenopausal women by as much as 50 percent. On the downside (although the results are conflicting), epidemiological data suggest that hormone replacement therapy may *slightly* increase the risk of breast cancer in postmenopausal women. Other studies, however, fail to confirm the link between estrogen replacement therapy and breast cancer. We have known for quite some time that there is a clear link between estrogen replacement therapy and the risk of endometrial cancer, although this increase can largely be *prevented* by the concomitant use of progestins.

☺ *Those physicians and public health experts who support estrogen replacement therapy argue that even if it increases the rates of endometrial and breast cancer, these detrimental effects are largely outweighed by its substantial beneficial effects on osteoporosis, heart attacks, and perhaps even stroke.*

Admittedly, if you have greater concerns about the more immediate potential increases in cancer than about the long-term protective effects on the heart and bones, you may be reluctant to start hormone replacement therapy. Consequently, the decision must be individualized for each patient. Perhaps the most compelling reason in favor of using estrogen is the dramatic reduction in heart attacks, both fatal and nonfatal, and in deaths from all causes related to vascular disease. The benefits of estrogen therapy are greatest if these medications are started immediately after menopause.

So what is the bottom line regarding estrogen replacement therapy? Based on currently available studies, virtually all postmenopausal women should be considered candidates for estrogen replacement. As emphasized, you should make the final decision in consultation with your physician, after weighing all of the relevant medical and nonmedical risks. If you have a previous history of breast cancer or another estrogen-sensitive malignancy, it would be reasonable to avoid chronic estrogen re-

placement. On the other hand, if you have had a hysterectomy, have risk factors for heart disease, and have no previous history of breast cancer, the benefits of estrogen replacement therapy will almost always outweigh the risks. In women without a hysterectomy, progestins should be added to the drug regimen to minimize the risk of endometrial cancer.

The standard recommended cyclical estrogen/progestin regimen (0.625 mg conjugated estrogen on days 1–25 each month, along with 10 mg medroxyprogesterone on days 13–25) may cause withdrawal bleeding. To overcome this problem, the use of continuous low-dose progesterone (2.5 mg per day medroxyprogesterone) along with estrogen can greatly reduce the frequency of bleeding and thereby improve toleration of the drug regimen.

☺ *A comprehensive, **life-prolonging** approach for women is based, to a great extent, on preventing the diseases that accompany the aging process.*

You will want to study the MedRANK Checklist "Pills for Maintaining Health and Feeling Great After Menopause" on page 305 for a complete listing of prevention-oriented pills that have been shown to improve well-being and prevent conditions such as osteoporosis, heart disease, Alzheimer's disease, and depression.

ESTROGEN
Pill for a Lifetime*

  MedRANK Life Prolongation and Enhancement Checklist

HORMONE REPLACEMENT THERAPY: PROS AND CONS

HEALING: HERE'S THE GREAT NEWS

The misery of menopause.

"Look, Ma! No pain." Four main types of symptoms are associated with the decrease in estrogen that accompanies menopause: (1) the core temperature problems that produce hot flashes and perspiration; (2) the gradual loss of glands and thinning of the vaginal wall, which leads to loss of lubrication and discomfort during sexual intercourse, which can lead to a reduction of sexual activity that perpetuates this vicious cycle; (3) the changes that occur in the bladder and urethra that lead to frequent episodes of burning with urination, the urge to urinate frequently, and bladder infections; and (4) the "psychological" symptoms that include insomnia, and a vague deterioration in mental well-being.

The bottom line is that estrogen relieves, to a significant and life-improving degree, all these symptoms. Take-home lesson: Take estrogen, you'll feel better.

Broken bones and broken backs.

As women age, their risk for breaking bones in the back and hips increases. Long-term estrogen therapy protects women against osteoporosis which is the principal cause of these problems. This is an important personal health priority, because fractures that result from weak, calcium-deficient bones not only produce discomfort, they frequently cause disability and cosmetic deformities, and can lead to depression and other complications that *shorten life expectancy.*

From the perspective of bone protection and building, you will get the greatest benefits from estrogen if you start taking it *immediately after the onset of menopause and continue for at least seven years after menopause.* It also appears that older women who start estrogen replacement later, and continue it for at least two years, begin to show some protective effect, but less than if estrogen is taken immediately after menopause. Put simply, really decreasing the risk of broken bones (fractures of the back and hip) requires long-term treatment. Discontinuing estrogen is followed by an accelerated rate of osteoporosis, equivalent to that seen in women who don't take estrogen at all. So once you start, it's best not to stop—as long as you don't develop a complication or another condition that would make estrogen use harmful.

---

* For specific recommendations, dosages, delivery systems, and pill rankings, please see the MedRANK Checklist "Pills for Maintaining Health and Feeling Great After Menopause" on page 305.

☺ *Heart saver.*

When women get old enough, they die of heart attacks just as men do. But estrogen has been shown to decrease women's risk of getting a heart attack by as much as 50 percent! That is very impressive. The *more* heart disease risk factors (a family history of heart attacks, smoking, obesity, diabetes, sedentary lifestyle, high blood pressure, elevated cholesterol) you have, *the more you need estrogen.* Take estrogen and save your heart—and your life. If you're an appropriate candidate, it's that simple.

☺ *Stroke of luck.*

Although the jury is still somewhat out on this issue, recent studies show a trend toward reducing the risk of stroke in women who have been on estrogen therapy. If this is confirmed, estrogen could be the ultimate heart-brain rescue drug.

☺ *Fat chance.*

Many of the heart- and life-promoting effects of estrogen are probably the result of *lowering* cholesterol levels. When estrogen is used alone (that is, unopposed by progestin hormones), it lowers the bad (LDL) cholesterol and raises the good (HDL) cholesterol. Estrogen delivered by skin patches may have *less* effect on cholesterol levels than estrogen taken by mouth.

For a while, we were not sure whether the addition of progestogen would counteract the benefits of estrogen on blood cholesterol. For now, it appears that estrogen-progestogen combined therapy also protects against heart disease. Although estrogen has a positive effect on cholesterol levels, it's not a cure—get your cholesterol levels checked. If they are high enough, you may need another medication—perhaps a statin such as Lipitor, Zocor, or Pravachol—to get your cholesterol levels down into the life-prolonging range.

☺ *Heads up.*

Although not yet confirmed in large studies, preliminary investigations have suggested that the onset of symptoms due to Alzheimer's disease may be *delayed* in women who have taken estrogen therapy. These studies need to be confirmed in larger clinical trials, but for now, since estrogen has so many other benefits, there's no harm in recommending it to women with a family history of Alzheimer's disease.

HARMING: HERE'S THE BAD NEWS (MAYBE)

☺ *Breast case, worst case.*

The issue of increased risk for breast cancer is not fully resolved. Some studies report a slight increase in the risk of breast cancer, while others firmly conclude that when estrogen is given at a dose of 0.625 mg or less per day, there is no increase in risk for breast cancer. Because of the potential association, however, most doctors feel that women who have had breast cancer should be disqualified from estrogen therapy.

It should be stressed, however, that others disagree and argue that a history of breast cancer—especially if the woman has survived a ten-year cancer-free period, has severe menopausal symptoms, and has two or more risk factors for heart disease—should not *automatically* disqualify a woman from taking lifelong estrogen. Certainly, if you fall into a higher risk group because of breast disease, one way to safeguard your health is to get regular mammograms and breast exams. These are some of the issues you will weigh when discussing the pros and cons of estrogen use with your physician.

☺ *Cancer (endometrial) of the uterus.*

There is no doubt that estrogen use increases the risk of cancer in the lining of the uterus (endometrial cancer). But this problem is easily correctable—that is, your doctor can eliminate the increased risk entirely—simply by adding minidose progestogen pills (Provera) for at least 12 days in every 25-day cycle of estrogen. This can be done as a "cyclical" dose (you get the progestogen only on the 12 days) or a "continuous" dose (you get a little bit of progestogen on each of the 25 days, along with your estrogen pill). When progestogen is added in "cyclical" fashion, about 90 percent of women get withdrawal bleeding (which many find disturbing enough to prompt discontinuation of

their estrogen program), whereas the continuous-dose approach is associated with less breakthrough bleeding and better compliance.

☺ *When to proceed with caution.*

The other factors that usually will disqualify you from taking estrogen include: (1) fibroids (noncancerous growths) in the uterus; (2) endometriosis (estrogen may produce a recurrence of pain); (3) migraine headaches (many women have migraines that are triggered by estrogen); (4) pregnancy; (5) a history of having blood clots while on birth control pills; (6) serious liver disease; and (7) any estrogen-sensitive tumor. You are not disqualified from estrogen if you have a history of cervical cancer, certain types of ovarian cancer, or cancer of the vagina.

HEALING VERSUS HARMING: THE FINAL SCORE

If you are a postmenopausal woman, you should take estrogen, unless you and/or your physician identify a compelling reason (see "Harming") not to take it.

TROUBLESHOOTING ESTROGEN THERAPY
Solutions to Common Pitfalls and Problems

MedRANK Life Problem and Side Effects Checklist

☼ **Pills of Wisdom:** Estrogen therapy does not always go smoothly. But some of its side effects can be eliminated—or at least reduced in severity—by making slight modifications in the treatment regimen.

Here is a list of the most common pitfalls and questions, and possible solutions to them.

NAUSEA

The nausea that sometimes accompanies the start of estrogen therapy *usually goes away* on its own after 2–3 months of treatment. If your nausea does not go away, it may be diminished by taking your estrogen (or estrogen-progestogen combination) with *food* or at bedtime. If this is not successful, you and your physician should try switching brands of estrogen—for example, from Premarin to Estrace or vice versa—or using a transdermal patch.

BREAST TENDERNESS

Estrogen sometimes stimulates breast glands enough to produce tenderness or mild pain. This problem is best addressed by *decreasing* your estrogen dose—for example, taking it only on Monday through Friday. Other approaches that can be considered include switching to a different progestogen, decreasing caffeine intake, or using a very low dose of a diuretic. This approach should only be considered if lowering the estrogen dose does not improve your symptoms.

MOOD SWINGS

Mood swings occur most commonly when progestogens are given according to a "cyclic-combined estrogen-progestogen" regimen. These ups and downs can be regulated by changing brands, reducing the progestogen dose, or converting to a "continuous-combined" regimen. (See the MedRANK Checklist "Pills for Maintaining Health and Feeling Great After Menopause" on page 305.) Not infrequently, mood swings may be due to depression, in which case a combination of counseling, social support, and antidepressant medications may be necessary.

BLOATING

Bloating is a symptom that is usually related to progestogen and that may respond to changing formulations or a low-dose diuretic.

WHAT IF I HAVE A UTERUS BUT CANNOT TOLERATE PROGESTOGEN?

Unopposed estrogen should *not* be given to women with an intact uterus. But the reality is that some women simply cannot tolerate progestogens. In this case, if estrogen is prescribed for you—and you may very well need it because of bone wasting, heart disease, or other compelling reasons—you probably should have a uterine biopsy every year, and anytime bleeding occurs.

WHAT IF I CAN'T TAKE ESTROGEN, BUT HAVE TERRIBLE HOT FLASHES?

Other drugs may work, including clonidine (Catapres), androgens, or medroxyprogesterone. Consult with your physician about these options.

DO I NEED A BIOPSY OF MY UTERUS BEFORE STARTING ESTROGEN THERAPY?

Some gynecologists take a biopsy (a tissue sample that can be examined for abnormal cells) before starting *anyone* on estrogen, but this is *not* routinely recommended. The majority of experts recommend a biopsy only in women who have abnormal bleeding while taking estrogen.

AT WHAT AGE SHOULD I START ESTROGEN, AND HOW LONG SHOULD I TAKE IT?

Estrogen therapy should be started as soon after menopause as possible and continued for your lifetime—assuming, of course, that you have no medical conditions that would make prolonged treatment unsafe.

How well do women comply with lifelong estrogen replacement?

Unfortunately, not very well. Recent studies from the Kaiser Foundation Health Plan show that about one-third of women stopped their estrogen after the first prescription, and that 75 percent stopped by the end of the third year. To a great degree, this reflects the failure of the medical profession and pharmaceutical industry to develop an estrogen-progesterone formulation that is associated with long-term continuation rates.

Given the undisputed preventive health benefits of estrogen, more work needs to be done. A good place to start is your physician's office, where you should take the time to address all your concerns, so that adjustments in your pill program can be made that encourage better compliance.

PILLS FOR MAINTAINING HEALTH AND FEELING GREAT AFTER MENOPAUSE

  MedRANK Life Prolongation and Enhancement Checklist

Pills of Wisdom: Designing a life-prolonging and mood-enhancing medication program for women in their postmenopausal years requires careful consideration of many factors. Discuss all your concerns with your doctor in detail. Generally speaking, you will want to consider a "cocktail" that includes estrogen (with or without progestogen, depending on whether you still have a uterus), calcium supplementation, and low-dose aspirin, especially if you are 50 or older and have strong risk factors for heart disease. This MedRANK Checklist also ranks pills that are frequently pressed into service for problems—insomnia, depression, and the like—that are associated with the postmenopausal period.

Overall, estrogen is a highly recommended, life-prolonging and -enhancing medication that should be strongly considered—and reviewed carefully for use—in all postmenopausal women. Prior to taking estrogen, you must be sure that you have no current or previous medical condition(s) that would make estrogen therapy potentially unsafe for you. In other words, your doctor must carefully consider your current and past medical conditions, your family history, and lifestyle issues that might disqualify you from being a candidate for hormone replacement. Please refer to the MedRANK Checklist "Estrogen" on page 301 for a complete discussion of these issues.

Once you and your physician have determined that estrogen replacement therapy is right for you, the next step is to decide what kind of estrogen pills or formulations are best for you and, most important, whether you need to take a progestogen hormone along with your estrogen. This depends primarily on whether you still have a uterus or have had it removed surgically (hysterectomy).

The critical pill-selection decision essentially boils down to this: If you have had your uterus surgically removed, you are an excellent candidate for unopposed estrogen replacement—which means taking estrogen alone, i.e., without progesterone (Provera). On the other hand, if you still *have* a uterus, certain modifications in your hormone replacement program will be required. Unopposed estrogen (Premarin, Estrace, etc.)—is not advised for most women with a uterus. This group should have progesterone added to the estrogen in order to decrease the risk of uterine cancer.

Finally, other medications, including aspirin, estrogen creams, calcium supplements, ointments, and antidepressants, are commonly used in women in this age group. They are discussed in the checklist as well.

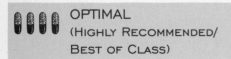

OPTIMAL
(Highly Recommended/ Best of Class)

Estrogen Replacement Therapy for Women Who Do Not Have a Uterus

Premarin 0.625 mg (conjugated estrogens) each day
OR
Estrace 1 mg (estradiol) each day

This is the preferred regimen for women who do not have a uterus. It's simple, it's once-a-day, and compliance is very good.

Continuous-Combined Estrogen-Progestin Replacement Therapy for Women Who Still Have Their Uterus

Prempro
OR
Premarin 0.625 mg each day *plus*
Provera (medroxyprogesterone) 2.5 mg each day
OR
Estrace 1 mg each day *plus* **Provera 2.5 mg each day**

Prempro is the simplest and most reliable approach for women with a uterus. My preferred regimen is "continuous-combined estrogen and progestin." I recommend this approach because compliance is good or improved when you take the same two pills at the same dose each day. The "cyclic-combined estrogen and progestin" regimen is also effective and is discussed in the "Recommended" category. Because Prempro combines estrogen and progesterone into a *single* pill, it is the *preferred* medication for estrogen replacement in women who still have their uterus.

Note: The use of progesterone along with estrogen is complicated by breakthrough bleeding, which many women find disturbing. The frequency of this side effect is *reduced* with the continuous-combined approach, and as many as 80 percent of women have no bleeding after one year of hormone replacement.

Calcium Supplements

Calcium nutritional supplements are advised for postmenopausal women, inasmuch as studies suggest that elderly women who take calcium and vitamin D have a lower risk of breaking a hip than those who do not. The beneficial effects of calcium supplements are enhanced in women who exercise regularly, because physical activity appears to retard osteoporosis. In addition, most of the other medications—estrogen, Fosmax, and the like—recommended to prevent bone wasting have been proven beneficial in women who were also taking calcium supplementation.

How much calcium do you need to take? A panel of experts from the National Institutes of Health recommends 1,000 mg per day for women 25 to 50 years old and for women 51–65 years of age who are taking estrogen. If you are older than 65, this panel recommended a daily intake of 1,500 mg of calcium, which is far in excess of what most women get in their daily diet. In fact, the average diet provides less than 800 mg per day, which means that to ensure adequate calcium intake, women over 50 should take one 500–600 mg tablet per day, and women over 65 should take two.

Calcium carbonate (Caltrate 600, Os-Cal 500, Tums 500)

The calcium carbonate regimens are optimal because they are the simplest and most convenient to take. These supplements are usually well tolerated, although gastrointestinal symptoms such as constipation and bloating are sometimes seen.

Calcium citrate (Citracal, Citracal + D)

Equally convenient. See "calcium carbonate" for details.

VITAMIN D SUPPLEMENTATION

Vitamin D

I recommend vitamin D (a daily dose of 400 International Units), along with calcium supplementation, to prevent and treat the bone wasting caused by osteoporosis.

ASPIRIN

Aspirin (many preparations available)

Many experts recommend low-dose aspirin (81 mg/day Bayer Aspirin, Low Strength) for all individuals who are 50 or older. Given the low risk of bleeding associated with low-dose aspirin, this is a reasonable strategy for reducing the risk of a first heart attack, especially in men.

The role of aspirin in prevention of first heart attacks in *women* is less clear, especially since women (a) are likely to be on hormone replacement therapy, which itself exerts a powerful protective effect against heart disease, and (b) have a higher risk of bleeding strokes, which can potentially be worsened by aspirin use.

Overall, however, many postmenopausal women should strongly consider taking long-term, low-dose aspirin. If you are a woman over 50 and (a) are unable or unwilling to take estrogen replacement, or (b) have one or more risk factors for heart disease (smoker, obesity, sedentary lifestyle, high blood pressure, diabetes, elevated cholesterol), you should ask your physician to consider your suitability for chronic, low-dose aspirin therapy to prevent heart disease.

ESTROGEN CREAMS

When used judiciously and not in excess, these creams can provide extraordinary relief for symptoms associated with vaginal wall thinning and urinary infections caused by urethral problems. (See "Estrogen: Pill for a Lifetime" in this chapter.) Always use the lowest dose required to achieve results, whether to improve vaginal lubrication or to relieve urinary discomfort.

Estrace
Premarin
Ortho Dienestrol
Ogen

These creams require 1–2 weeks of intensive daily therapy, followed by intermittent use for several weeks and a gradual tapering over three months. Vaginal bleeding is the most common side effect.

RECOMMENDED
(ACCEPTABLE WITH RESERVATIONS)

These regimens for estrogen replacement are called "cyclic-combined estrogen and progestin." They are just as effective and safe as the "continuous-combined" regimen discussed in the "Optimal" category, but they are *downgraded* to the "Recommended" category for convenience reasons only.

THE CYCLIC-COMBINED REGIMEN FOR ESTROGEN REPLACEMENT THERAPY IN WOMEN WHO STILL HAVE THEIR UTERUS

Premarin 0.625 mg each day is taken on days 1 through 25, *plus* on days 13 through 25, a low-dose progestogen is taken

The cyclic-combined estrogen-progestin approach to hormone replacement therapy is less convenient than the continuous approach described in the "Optimal" category. The use of progesterone along with estrogen is sometimes complicated by breakthrough bleeding, which many women find disturbing. The frequency of this side effect is reduced with the continuous-combined approach. Women who have breakthrough bleeding on the cyclic regimen can be *switched* to the "continuous" regimen in order to eliminate this troublesome symptom. As many as 80 percent of women have no bleeding after one year of hormone replacement. For additional information, please see discussion in "Optimal" category.

DISCOURAGED FOR INITIAL USE
(BUT MAY BE REQUIRED IN SELECTED PEOPLE)

"Estrogen patches" (transdermal estradiol patches combined with either oral progestogen or progestogen patches)

Many women simply cannot tolerate the inconvenience or cosmetic implications of three daily estrogen skin patches. Specifically, 15–20 percent of people who use this system complain of irritation or redness at the site where the patch is applied. This approach to estrogen replacement is *not* recommended because of convenience problems.

MEDICATIONS FOR TREATING MENOPAUSE-ASSOCIATED DEPRESSION

Fortunately, many of the uncomfortable symptoms of menopause—flashes, insomnia, perspiration, and the like— are effectively relieved with estrogen replacement. Whether or not there is a specific depression syndrome associated with menopause per se—like a postpartum depression—the fact is, menopause is frequently associated with a number of life events, physical changes, and medical problems that can lead, at least, to a situational depression. Overcoming it may require counseling, therapy, and—not uncommonly—treatment with antidepressant medications. If you have not had a serious episode of depression prior to menopause, but your physician feels you need to start an antidepressant, it is oftentimes reasonable to stay on it for about twelve months and consider gradual discontinuation after that time.

Some studies show a relationship between depression and bone mineral density (a measure of a bone's health and strength). Women who are depressed have weaker bones that are more susceptible to hip fractures. This may be due to decreased physical activity associated with depression.

In any event, depression during menopause should be treated aggressively, not only to improve psychological well-being but, perhaps, to improve bone density. The serotonin-selective reuptake inhibitors (SSRIs)—the most widely used and safest antidepressants for postmenopausal women—produce excellent results. Treatment should be individualized; some women will report better results with one pill than another.

SSRI Antidepressants

Zoloft (sertraline)
This drug is recommended as the initial choice because it appears to have a lower risk of producing drug interactions, tends to be slightly less stimulating than Prozac, and is slightly less sedating than Paxil. Because drug interactions seem to be less of a problem, Zoloft is preferred for people who take multiple medications.

Prozac (fluoxetine)
This effective SSRI may be especially appropriate for people who are overweight, since it has mild appetite-suppressant properties. Because it may be a bit more stimulating than Zoloft or Paxil, it may be slightly less advantageous in people who have insomnia as a prominent, disabling symptom of their depression. On the other hand, its stimulatory properties may be of great benefit to others.

Because drug interactions may be more of a problem with Prozac than with Zoloft, people on multiple medications may be able to reduce their risk of drug interactions by using Zoloft instead.

Paxil (paroxetene)
Paxil is as effective as the SSRIs Prozac and Zoloft. It may be slightly more sedating, however, and there is still a potential for drug interactions.

INSOMNIA OF MENOPAUSE

The insomnia or sleeplessness that accompanies menopause is usually improved with estrogen therapy. Many women, however, continue to have irregular and unsatisfying sleep patterns and require medication to produce a sound sleep. Although pills may eventually be required, the preferred approaches to most sleep problems are nonpharmacological: exercising, avoiding daytime naps, regularizing sleep patterns, and avoiding substances that interfere with sleep such as caffeine, alcohol, and other medications. This approach may be more helpful than drugs, which can be associated with dependence and side effects. When estrogen replacement is not possible, safe, or advisable, the following medication can be used for sleep.

Ambien (zolpidem)
This rapidly acting medication appears to preserve normal sleep "architecture," that is, Stages 3 and 4 (deep sleep) and REM sleep, producing more restorative sleep. It may be less likely to produce tolerance or physical dependence. But this medication has been associ-

ated with next-day drowsiness, dizziness, and a "drugged" feeling in some people. Mental functions and memory appear to be preserved the next day after use.

SKIN CHANGES

Renova (retinoin emollient cream)

Some of the skin changes that accompany menopause are improved with estrogen therapy. Although Renova has been FDA approved—and shown to be effective—for producing cosmetic improvements related to "fine wrinkling," skin "roughness," and skin pigment discoloration, its effectiveness is not established in people 50 and older, or in individuals with moderately or heavily pigmented skin.

Despite this, if you have skin changes unrelated to menopause that you would characterize as "fine wrinkling" or "coarse skin," it is not unreasonable to experiment with Renova and evaluate its possible benefits.

 AVOID IF POSSIBLE
(NOT RECOMMENDED)

All menopause-related therapies, unless indicated for your specific condition.

CHAPTER 20

—

SEX AND THE SINGLE PILL

Contraceptives and Related Medications

As you are well aware, sex hormones are used for contraception. Oral contraceptives based on hormone therapy are more effective than mechanical, chemical, or rhythm methods. Generally speaking, there are two kinds of birth control pills: the mini-pill, which contains progestin only, and the combination pill, which consists of estrogen-progestin combinations.

☺ *As a rule, because of the association between estrogen and the risk of blood clots, the estrogen dose in the combination pill should be as low as possible.*

You may wish to discuss this matter with your physician. On occasion, doctors may prescribe an oral contraceptive as a postcoital contraceptive (or morning-after) pill. Following suspected conception, you may be asked to take more than one pill at a time for a limited number of days. Compliance is absolutely essential for maintaining the effectiveness of oral contraceptives. If you have any questions about what to do if you miss a pill, consult the package information and/or call your physician or pharmacist.

In addition to daily contraceptive medications, new, long-term, reversible birth control systems are also available, using the hormone lovonorgestrel (the Norplant System). These *implants* can prevent pregnancy for up to five years and should be removed by the end of the fifth year. New implants may be inserted at that time if continuing contraceptive protection is required. This method of contraception is not uniformly accepted; some people complain of bruising and irritation over the implant site.

A number of vaginal douche products are available, usually for general cleansing of the vaginal genital areas, for deodorization purposes, and to relieve minor itching, burning, and swelling. Generally speaking, vaginal douches are not contraceptive agents. If irritation, odor, or discharge occurs or persists during vaginal douching, you should discontinue use and call your doctor.

☺ *Spermicides, on the other hand, are topical contraceptive agents that are generally reliable if properly used. Their contraceptive properties are enhanced when they are used in combination with a diaphragm, condom, or other barrier method.*

The active ingredient in most spermicides is nonoxynol-9 or octoxynol, which immobilizes sperm cells by rupturing or removing their outer membrane. The gel, foam, or jelly vehicle that carries the spermicide also serves as a barrier to the union of sperm and egg by covering the opening of the cervix.

Overall, spermicides are less effective than oral contraceptives, but they have the advantage of not producing systemic side effects. The vaginal contraceptive sponge, which contains nonoxynol-9, absorbs semen and releases spermicide even during multiple acts of intercourse. As a rule, the sponge is effective for about twenty-four hours and should be kept in place for six hours following intercourse.

The Centers for Disease Control (CDC) recommends the use of condoms to prevent sexually transmitted diseases (STDs). If properly used, condoms can help prevent infection caused by *Chlamydia trachomatis*, *Ureaplasma urealyticum*, *Candida albicans*, and *Herpes simplex* I and II. Protection against other STDs, such as human papillomavirus and AIDS, is also afforded by condom use. To maximize either the spermicidal, contraceptive, or anti-infective properties of vaginal preparations, consult the package instructions included with each product.

A number of fertility agents have been shown to be effective in stimulating ovulation and the development of eggs in the ovaries. The most popular of these, clomiphene citrate (Clomid), produces a "false signal" that estrogen levels are low. In response, the body increases the secretion of hormones that stimulate the ovaries, which increases production of eggs. This medication is used to treat female infertility when pregnancy is desired. Unwanted effects include multiple pregnancy and minor side effects.

BIRTH CONTROL FOR YOUR SPECIFIC NEEDS*

 **MedRANK Life
Prevention Checklist**

Pills of Wisdom: The great advance in birth control pills (BCPs) has occurred in the area of estrogen dose reduction. In high doses, estrogen increases the risk of blood clots, especially in smokers. We now have pills that are just as effective as the old higher-estrogen BCPs but that are much less likely to cause blood clots and other problems. Equally important, we have identified which women are good candidates for BCPs and which ones are not.

With respect to side effects and safety, the use of BCPs is associated with an increased risk of blood clots, stroke, heart attack, gallbladder disease, and liver cancer. But the risk of serious problems is very small in generally healthy women who do not have underlying lifestyle or disease risk factors that would predispose them to such problems. In this regard, cigarette smoking clearly increases the risk of heart disease—including heart attacks—in women taking BCPs, and the risk of life-threatening complications increases with age (over the age of 35) and with heavy smoking (more than fifteen cigarettes per day). Stated simply, women who smoke should not be on BCPs. Other conditions that increase the likelihood of serious complications with BCPs include high blood pressure, high cholesterol levels, obesity, and diabetes.

As far as safety is concerned, the bottom line is that BCPs are best suited for young, healthy, non-smoking women. Women over 35 are at higher risk of complications. But because of the risks of pregnancy and possible complications—infection, bleeding, and blood clots—associated with pregnancy termination in older women, the benefits of BCPs may outweigh the risks in this population—but only in healthy, older, nonsmoking women. The mini-pill may be an excellent option for this group.

What should you do if you miss a dose of a combined estrogen-progestin BCP? Although there is little likelihood that you will become pregnant if only one pill is missed, there are no guarantees. The likelihood of ovulation (producing an egg that can be fertilized) increases with each successive day that pills are missed. Anytime you miss one day or more of active tablets, you should use another form of contraception for the balance of the cycle. If you have any questions, you should discuss them with your physician.

The mini-pill (progestin only) has a higher failure rate than combined estrogen-progestin BCPs but may be well suited for women over 40, for breast-feeding women, and for those who can't take estrogen. If you miss one mini-pill, take it as soon as you remember, and then take the next tablet at the regular time. If you miss two consecutive tablets, do not take both missed tablets at once; discard them and take the next tablet at the regular time (for Micronor and Nor-Q.D.). If you miss three consecutive tablets, discontinue BCPs immediately and use another form of contraception.

BCPs are also highly effective as a postcoital contraceptive (or morning-after) pill. Following an

---

* Oral contraceptives should not be taken by women who have a previous history of stroke, blood clots, heart attack, and conditions predisposing them to these problems. They should not be used in smokers older than 35, in those with known or suspected breast cancer, in women suspected or known to be pregnant, in women with liver disease, and in women with undiagnosed vaginal bleeding.

episode of unprotected intercourse, you will need to take more than one pill at a time for a limited number of days. If you have any questions about what to do in the event you have missed a pill, you should consult your physician.

In addition to daily contraceptive medications, long-term, reversible birth-control systems are also available. Implants with the hormone levonorgestrel (Norplant System) can prevent pregnancy for up to five years but should be removed by the end of the fifth year. New implants may be inserted at that time if continuing contraceptive protection is required. This method of contraception is not uniformly accepted—some people complain of bruising and irritation over the implant site. Finally, the hormone medroxyprogesterone (Depo-Provera) is a long-term injectable contraceptive that is administered at three-month intervals.

BCPs do not protect against HIV infection or STDs, but they do decrease the risk of developing fibrocystic disease and fibroadenomas of the breast, acute pelvic infections, cancer of the uterus, and ovarian cancer. In nonmonogamous relationships—and in monogamous relationships where there is a risk—barrier methods (condoms) should be used in combination with oral contraceptives to enhance prevention of sexually transmitted diseases, including HIV infection.

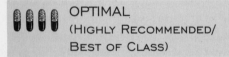

OPTIMAL
(HIGHLY RECOMMENDED/ BEST OF CLASS)

COMBINATION PILLS CONTAINING LESS THAN 30 MCG ESTROGEN

Loestrin 1/20 21, 28
Loestrin 1.5 /30 21, 28
Lo/Ovral
Desogen
Ortho-Cept 21

Their low estrogen content makes these the preferred medications among combination pills. The failure rate is 3 percent with typical use, 0.1% with perfect use. They protect against ovarian and endometrial cancer, ovarian cysts, pelvic inflammatory disease (PID), fibrocystic breast disease, iron-deficiency anemia, and dysmenorrhea. Blood clots and stroke are extremely rare with low-estrogen formulations.

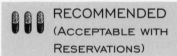

RECOMMENDED
(ACCEPTABLE WITH RESERVATIONS)

COMBINATION PILLS CONTAINING 35 MCG ESTROGEN

Triphasil-21
Ortho Tri-Cyclen
Ovcon 35 21, 28
Genora 0.5/35 21, 28
Modicon 21
Nelova 10/11 21
Ortho-Novum 7/7/7 21

The estrogen content of these pills is also low, although not as low as that of the pills in the "Optimal" category. They provide the same benefits at, perhaps, a somewhat greater risk.

MINI-PILLS (PROGESTIN ONLY)

Orvette
Nor-QD

The mini-pill must be taken daily at the same time of day. Failure rates are higher in younger women than in older women. The mini-pill causes irregular, unpredictable bleeding in some women. It is an excellent choice for breast-feeding women, for women over 40, and for women with serious medical conditions, such as diabetes with vascular problems and heart disease.

DISCOURAGED FOR INITIAL USE
(BUT MAY BE REQUIRED IN SELECTED PEOPLE)

COMBINATION PILLS CONTAINING 30 MCG ESTROGEN BUT HIGHER DOSES OF PROGESTIN

Levelen 21
Nordette 21

The higher doses of progestin (.15 mg of levonorgestrel) are less desirable. You should

consider upgrading to pills in the Optimal category, which contain lower doses of progestin.

AVOID IF POSSIBLE
(NOT RECOMMENDED)

COMBINATION PILLS CONTAINING 50 MCG ESTROGEN

Ovral
Ovcon 50
Demulen 1/50 21

Women on these pills should be switched to oral contraceptives with lower estrogen doses, as listed in "Optimal" category.

NON-ORAL CONTRACEPTIVE SYSTEMS*

MedRANK Life Prevention Checklist

Pills of Wisdom: Among the other hormone-based methods for contraception, the best known is the levonorgestrel implant (the Norplant System). During the first seven days of menstruation a total of six capsules are implanted in the midportion of the upper arm. The implant system is a long-term (up to five years) reversible contraceptive system. The main side effect are bleeding iregularities, including prolonged bleeding, many bleeding days, and spotting. The capsules can be removed at any time. About 30 percent of women discontinue their implants each year over the five-year period.

The Progestasert System is a T-shaped intrauterine device (IUD) containing progesterone. Implanted in the uterus, it enhances contraception by continuously releasing progesterone into the uterine cavity. There is an increased risk of pelvic infection with this device, and therefore it is recommended in women who are in a stable, mutually monogamous relationship and have no previous history of pelvic infections. Contraception effectiveness is maintained for one year, after which time the system must be replaced for continued contraception. You should notify a physician if you miss a period, develop abnormal or excessive bleeding, detect an abnormal vaginal discharge, or develop a fever.

* Barrier methods (condoms) should be used in combination with contraceptives to enhance prevention of sexually transmitted diseases, including HIV infection.

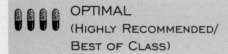

OPTIMAL
(Highly Recommended/ Best of Class)

None

(See "Optimal" category in the MedRANK Checklist "Birth Control for Your Specific Needs" on page 313.)

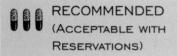

RECOMMENDED
(Acceptable with Reservations)

PROGESTIN IMPLANTS

The Norplant System

This skin implant is effective for five years. There may be removal problems, and menstrual irregularities are common. Skin problems and potential scarring may occur at the implant site. Another side effect is weight gain.

Its effects are reversible upon removal. It is useful for noncompliant adolescents, in whom pregnancy protection may be difficult to achieve with other methods.

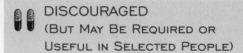

DISCOURAGED
(But May Be Required or Useful in Selected People)

INJECTIONS

Depo-Provera (medroxyprogesterone acetate)

The hormone medroxyprogesterone (Depo-Provera) is a long-term injectable contraceptive that is administered in women at three-month intervals. It can cause menstrual irregularities.

INTRAUTERINE DEVICES (IUDs)

Progestasert (progesterone T)

This device is effective, although there is an increased risk of ectopic pregnancy if the woman becomes pregnant. The IUD must be replaced every year. It is not to be used by women who have no children or who have a history of cervical or pelvic infections. Less menstrual blood is produced than with the copper T 380A.

Paragard (copper T 380A)

This IUD provides excellent contraception and is effective for up to ten years. It can cause menstrual irregularities. Intrauterine devices are not to be used in women who have never given birth or who have a history of cervical or pelvic infections.

MORNING-AFTER CONTRACEPTION
Preventing Pregnancy After Unprotected Intercourse

 MedRANK Life Prevention Checklist

 Pills of Wisdom: You may want to consider these approaches if you have had intercourse and a barrier method failed (broken condom, dislodged cervical cap or diaphragm), or you did not use your primary form of contraception and had unprotected intercourse.

OPTIMAL
(HIGHLY RECOMMENDED/ BEST OF CLASS)

Mifepristone (RU-486)

This is a well-tolerated approach to "morning after" pregnancy termination. The pregnancy rate is zero if it is used according to the instructions. The abortion controversy has delayed marketing of this drug in the United States. This debate aside, RU-486 is a low-risk, highly effective, user-friendly approach to preventing unwanted pregnancies and inducing therapeutic abortions.

 RECOMMENDED
(ACCEPTABLE WITH RESERVATIONS)

Ovral, 4 tablets (2 tablets given 12 hours apart)

This method is associated with side effects of nausea, vomiting, and headache.

Lo/Ovral, Nordette, or Levlen, 8 tablets (4 tablets given 12 hours apart)

Same as above.

 DISCOURAGED AND TO BE AVOIDED
(BUT MAY BE REQUIRED IN SELECTED PEOPLE)

OTHER ESTROGEN PREPARATIONS

PILLS FOR PREGNANCY TERMINATION
Alternatives to Surgically Induced Abortion

 MedRANK Life Prevention Checklist

 Pills of Wisdom: Abortion is a highly controversial issue. The debate has been characterized by widely varying emotional, moral, medical, religious, and political positions. Women who wish to consider abortion for health or other reasons should be aware that there are safe, effective alternatives to surgically induced abortion. These medication-based methods must all be used under a doctor's supervision.

OPTIMAL (HIGHLY RECOMMENDED/ BEST OF CLASS)

Mifepristone (RU-486)

RU-486 is well tolerated and, when used as prescribed, virtually eliminates all pregnancies. The abortion controversy has delayed the marketing of this drug in the United States. This debate aside, RU-486 is a low-risk, highly effective, user-friendly approach to preventing unwanted pregnancies and inducing therapeutic abortions.

 RECOMMENDED (ACCEPTABLE WITH RESERVATIONS)

Folex (methotrexate)
Cytotec (misoprostol)

These medications are not approved by the FDA or indicated for termination of unwanted pregnancies. However, they have been used successfully by women who have not had their period for 40 to 65 days. First, the methotrexate is given as an intramuscular injection once, followed 5 to 7 days later by 800 mcg of Cytotec (misoprostol), given as an intravaginal suppository. About 85 percent of women will abort completely within twenty-four hours. Those who don't receive a second dose of misoprostol.

This method is very effective. Overall, only about 5 percent of women will fail in this noninvasive medication approach to therapeutic abortion. Side effects include cramping, heavy bleeding, and on occasion, nausea, headache, and diarrhea.

 DISCOURAGED (BUT MAY BE REQUIRED IN SELECTED PEOPLE)

OTHER MEDICATIONS

CHAPTER 21

—

FOREVER YOURS

Pills and Lifestyle Changes for Life Prolongation

"At my age I don't even buy green bananas," chuckled the 84-year-old gentleman in the examining room. "Why in the world would I want to take pills to prolong my life? On the other hand, if you've got something that'll cure this nasty toenail infection, count me in." When it comes to medications, people pay much more attention to cures than to prevention. In all fairness, this is understandable.

Cures, after all, are the stuff of high drama. They are about disease and redemption, instant fixes, surviving against all odds. At their best, cures can signal transformations of mythic proportions. Call it *The Book of Cures*? We all know someone who, after a vanity-smashing, life-draining bout with chemotherapy, has come out the other side of the tunnel, "cured" of their cancer. We have seen our children, after feverish and fussy battles with bacterial ear infections, suddenly normalize their temperature, stop their vomiting, and become one of the joyful living again. We have heard about men with crushing chest

pain who, sweaty and limp, go into the hospital and miraculously recover after a clot-busting drug has been injected into their veins. And we have shared meals or had conversations with people on antidepressants who have journeyed from the depths of quiet desperation into a brighter and better world. Cures speak. Even on a smaller scale, there are few things as gratifying as seeing a skin infection clear up, getting rid of your child's head lice, or finding a dandruff shampoo that actually works.

We live in a "Me Zoloft, you Xanax" world of mood elevators, one-dose-cure "gorillacillin" antibiotics, and miracle arthritis cures. But although pills that work "magic" usually steal the show, something else is even more important and enduring: *preventing disease* and *promoting wellness*. Medicate and *modify*—this is the simple two-step plan to life prolongation. And when it comes to life prolongation and disease prevention, there are so many pills that work. I am talking about the "quiet" pills that, year after year, do little things that are big enough, in the grand cradle-to-grave scheme of things, to keep the Grim Reaper at bay and add pain-free years to your life.

In chapter after chapter of this book, you have read about pills that prevent medical catastrophes: the daily dose of aspirin that prevents heart attack and stroke and reduces the risk of colon cancer; the estrogen pill that reduces the risk of breaking a hip, having a heart attack, or fracturing your back; the beta-blocker that prevents heart attack and abnormal, life-threatening heart rhythms; the statin drug that lowers cholesterol; the ACE inhibitor that keeps you from having congestive heart failure; the cocktail of antiretroviral medications that prolongs life in HIV-infected individuals; the blood thinner that prevents clots from wedging in the brain; and many other medications that, if carefully chosen, can keep you off the slippery slope to that blackened, never-never land that waits on the other side.

☼ *But medications alone are* **not enough** *—you must also modify lifestyle habits and patterns that are injurious to your health and that are known to decrease your lifespan.*

You know what they are. To make pills work for you, you have to work for yourself. It is your doctor's responsibility to medicate—and your responsibility to modify. Specifically, this means achieving an ideal body weight, stopping smoking, increasing your daily exercise, avoiding excessive consumption of alcohol, having protected sex when appropriate, and reducing your intake of fat and cholesterol if you are at risk of heart disease. It also means eliminating cigarette smoke from your child's environment. Approaches to lifestyle modification are beyond the scope of this book, but suffice it to say that these changes are essential for maximizing the benefits you will get from your personal pharmacology.

☼ *Kicking the Habit: Smoking Cessation. Among the medications used to aid in smoking cessation, the majority contain nicotine, among them Nicotrol, ProStep, and Nicorette chewing gum, usually available over-the-counter.*

Nicotine treatment should be used as part of a comprehensive behavioral smoking-cessation program that includes a smoking-cessation support group, physician consultation, and other lifestyle modifications. Nicotine-based smoking deterrents are based on their ability to help prevent physical signs of nicotine withdrawal after the sudden discontinuation of cigarettes. The instructions for using these products should be studied carefully. In the case of Nicorette chewing gum, most people will require ten to twelve pieces per day during the first month of treatment. Nicotine gum should *not* be used until you have stopped smoking completely. Nicoderm, Nicotrol, and Habitrol are patches that are applied once daily to nonhairy, clean, dry skin on the upper body or upper outer arm. Dosages may vary according to the individual patient. Generally speaking, therapy should continue for no more than five months. Individuals should not smoke while taking smoking-cessation products.

☺ *Home Testing Kits. Clearly part of disease prevention, home testing kits are available for a wide number of clinical conditions.*

Some of them, such as those used to monitor blood or urine glucose, are used by diabetics to monitor their need for drug therapy and to detect deterioration in their health status. A new saliva test for detecting the HIV virus is available in many parts of the world and will soon be available in the United States. Health fairs frequently screen for blood cholesterol levels and high blood pressure. Occult blood tests, used to measure the presence of hemoglobin in the gastrointestinal tract, are used as screening methods in patients who are at high risk for developing cancer of the colon, and for those who may have peptic ulcer disease.

☺ *If you wish to avoid pregnancy, or monitor windows of opportunity for fertilization and conception, you can use ovulation tests.*

Pregnancy tests now provide reliable home screening, as do testing kits that indicate the presence of urinary tract infection. Although home testing kits are generally quite accurate, confirmation and follow-up by your physician are usually advised. Generally speaking, diagnostic or therapeutic decisions should not be based on any single test result determined at home. If you have any questions regarding your test results, you should always contact your doctor.

☺ *Blood sugar tests are helpful for monitoring blood glucose levels in diabetics, indicating possible need for modifications in their medication regimen, diet, or exercise program.*

These tests can also prevent complications and problems during pregnancy, which may be associated with poor diabetic control. All blood glucose test strips require a finger prick. For most tests, a single blood drop is placed on a test strip. When the test pad is covered completely, timing begins. At the end of the timed reaction, the blood drop is wiped from the test strip. It should be stressed that timing is critical, and that the wiping or blotting technique and the recommended tissue paper or cotton for blotting will vary according to the manufacturer. The results are then read from the meter display, and the test is read against a color key.

☺ *Self-monitoring of blood sugar is considered a mainstay of management for patients with diabetes, particularly those with insulin-dependent diabetes.*

Commonly, however, readings obtained from home testing kits vary significantly from those obtained in the office or clinic setting. In this case, your physician must determine whether the difference represents erroneous self-monitoring or transient increases in blood sugar levels that do not accurately reflect the degree of glucose control.

☺ *Although home glucose monitoring can be an extremely valuable tool for the management of diabetes mellitus, it is not appropriate or beneficial for all individuals.*

For example, it makes little sense for a family member to partake of an inconvenient, somewhat painful, and costly procedure if the information they obtain from it is neither reliable nor valuable for changing treatment regimens. Unfortunately, a significant proportion of individuals monitoring at home are using improper techniques that yield inaccurate measurements. This becomes a problem of "bad data is worse than no data at all," particularly if the information is used to adjust your medication program.

☺ *If you have diabetes and decide to start home glucose monitoring, be sure you are provided with thorough, detailed instructions and that you undergo periodic assessments of how well you are performing these monitoring techniques at home.*

Another major cause of erroneous measurements is the cognitive or visual defects that are common among diabetics. It may be necessary to enlist the help of family members or visiting nurses to perform the monitoring tests. Finally, it should be emphasized that even if your monitoring technique is good, there is still the potential for disparity between home and office glucose readings. The explanation for this phenomenon, called "white coat hyperglycemia," remains unclear.

☺ *Blood glucose monitoring is especially useful if your blood sugar is consistently out of control, or when you feel symptoms of blood sugar that is either too high or too low.*

In addition to tracking their blood sugar levels, diabetic patients will benefit from education programs that help them understand diabetes and all aspects of its treatment, including exercise, diet, and signs of clinical deterioration. These education materials can be obtained through your local chapter of the American Diabetes Association.

Colon cancer is one of the leading causes of death in American men and women over the age of 55. Studies have shown that the detection of so-called occult or hidden blood in the stool (feces) is an important screening method for detecting colon cancers at an early, treatable stage. Testing for occult blood is accomplished with a number of different products, including Hematest, Early Detector, and Hemoccult. You should be aware that presence of occult blood does not necessarily indicate that you have a malignancy. Occult blood can also be an indication of minor illnesses such as hemorrhoids and gastrointestinal infections, as well as diverticulitis, fissures, and gastric ulcers.

☺ *Nevertheless, hemoccult screening is recommended for persons over 40 years of age and for those who have a strong family history of lower-intestinal disorders, including familial polyps, as well as colorectal cancer.*

These tests do not replace regular physical and rectal examinations by your physician, but they may indicate the need for more invasive investigation. To enhance early detection of colorectal cancer, the American Cancer Society currently recommends a digital rectal examination every year for patients over 40 and annual fecal occult blood testing and sigmoidoscopy every three to five years for patients older than 50.

Unfortunately, there is no general consensus about these recommendations. In fact, some experts argue that fecal blood testing alone is an effective way to screen for colorectal cancer and that it has the advantage of eliminating a sigmoidoscopic examination—a test that is often uncomfortable and costly and has poor patient acceptance. Although it has been difficult to identify the exact benefits and limitations of hemoccult screening, patients at high risk for colon cancer should be instructed in its use.

Ovulation tests, available for purchase in most pharmacies, are used to predict the time of ovulation and fertility. They can aid in planning pregnancy and in determining fertile periods during the menstrual cycle. Many home pregnancy tests are available, all of which detect the presence of human chorionic gonadotropin (HCG) in the urine. HCG usually appears at measurable levels in the urine one to three days after the first menstrual period is missed.

Although these tests are relatively accurate, false positive results can occur—that is, the test result is positive, but no pregnancy actually exists. False negative results are those in which pregnancy is present but the test indicates there is none. False positive and false negative results can occur for a variety of conditions. For home pregnancy tests, in the event you get a negative result, it is advisable to repeat the test in three to seven days. It is possible that insufficient HCG has accumulated to cause a positive result. In the event that you do get a positive result, you should contact your doctor to confirm the result and determine a plan of action (such as prenatal care).

Finally, urinary tract infections—infections in the kidney or bladder—can be detected using test strips that detect white blood cells and nitrites in the urine. As a rule, nitrites are detected in the first-morning urine specimen in up to 90 percent of all people with urinary tract infection. Accompanying symptoms include lower back pain, frequent urination, painful or burning urination, and a feeling of urinary urgency. If you get a negative result with a test kit, it does not rule out the possibility that you have a urinary tract infection. If you have the aforementioned symptoms but your home test indicates a negative result, you should consult your physician.

WEIGHT-LOSS PILLS AND APPETITE SUPPRESSANTS FOR OBESE INDIVIDUALS*

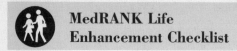

MedRANK Life Enhancement Checklist

Pills of Wisdom: One out of every three American adults is now considered to be overweight, and obesity-related conditions are responsible for an estimated 300,000 deaths annually. Obesity now ranks second only to smoking as a preventable cause of death. The yearly economic costs of obesity in the United States are equally staggering: $68 billion from excess medical expenses and lost income, in addition to the $30 billion spent on diet foods, products, and programs.

Given the powerful incentives to manage obesity, it is not surprising that weight-loss medications have been the subject of intense interest on the part of both physicians and patients. Between 1973 and 1996 no new medications for obesity treatment were approved by the FDA, but between 1992 and 1998 the number of prescriptions written for Pondium (fenfluramine) increased from about 60,000 to more than 1 million. Eventually, in 1997, Redux was removed from the market, because of concerns about heart valve abnormalities.

Until more is known, all weight-loss pills should be avoided for weight-reduction.

If and when safe, effective drugs become available, they *cannot* be recommended for *routine* use in obese individuals, although they may be helpful in *selected* patients. Only certain people should be considered for drug treatment of their obesity. For example, the North American Association for Study of Obesity recommends that drug therapy be considered only in people who have a body mass index (which is the person's weight in kilograms divided by the square of their height in meters) of 27 kg/m^2 or greater. The American Society of Bariatric [Obesity] Medicine believes it should be considered for women who have more than 30 percent of their weight as body fat, and for men whose body fat exceeds 25 percent. The Committee on Nutrition of the Massachusetts Medical Society considers medically significant obesity to include adults who have gained more than 30 pounds since they were 18 years of age. These are all minimal eligibility criteria. Generally speaking, drug treatment should be entertained only if other dietary and lifestyle modifications have failed to produce satisfactory results.

How well have weight loss drugs worked? Not all that well, if one pools all the studies together. After one year of treatment, overall long-term weight loss that can be attributed to weight-loss medications alone is only 4 to 22 pounds. Weight loss tends to plateau by six months, and many studies show partial weight gain despite continued treatment. Stated simply, these have never been magic pills. In fact, most of the differences between active drugs and placebo pills are modest.

* There are no "Optimal" or "Recommended" medications for the treatment of obesity, since few studies are available that have evaluated the safety or efficacy of these medications for more than one year. In general, the National Task Force on the Prevention and Treatment of Obesity does not recommend routine use of any of these agents in obese individuals, although it does acknowledge the value of these medications in *selected* individuals with significant obesity. (Hence, they appear in the "Discouraged" category.) All of these medication programs must be accompanied by a behavioral program (diet and exercise) directed at weight loss.

As far as safety is concerned, there are considerable differences among approved medications. As a rule of thumb, anorexiant drugs (drugs that decrease appetite) fall into two classes: (1) those that affect the catecholamine system, which includes the amphetamines, benzphetamine, phendimetrazine, phentermine, mazindol, diethypropion, and phenylpropanolamine, and (2) those that affect the serotonergic system, which include fenfluramine, dexfenfluramine, fluoxetine, sertraline, and other antidepressants.

Amphetamines and related drugs are *not* recommended for treatment of obesity because of their high potential for abuse. The serotonergic medications such as dexfenfluramine (Redux) and fenfluramine (Pondimin) have been removed from the market.

In summary, long-term drug treatment, in combination with appropriate behavioral approaches, will help some obese patients to lose weight and maintain weight loss for one year. The main limitation of these pills is not their ability to produce initial weight loss but their ability to *maintain* weight loss over the long term. How well they do this simply is not known. What is clear is that short-term treatment with obesity pills generally is not advisable and that once a person is committed to therapy, medications will likely have to be continued for years. Until the safety and long-term efficacy of these pills are clarified, drug therapy for obese individuals should not be used.

OPTIMAL
(HIGHLY RECOMMENDED/ BEST OF CLASS)

None

Because the effectiveness and toxicity of these medications over the long term are still in question, no medications satisfy the criteria for "Optimal."

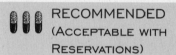

RECOMMENDED
(ACCEPTABLE WITH RESERVATIONS)

None

Because the effectiveness and toxicity of these medications over the long term are still in question, no medications satisfy the criteria for "Recommended."

AVOID IF POSSIBLE
(NOT RECOMMENDED)
ALL WEIGHT LOSS PILLS

Biphetamine (amphetamine/ dexamphetamine)

This drug has potential for abuse and for drug withdrawal syndrome.

Desoxyn (methamphetamine)

This drug also has abuse potential.

Didrex (benzphetamine)

This drug has potential for abuse and for drug withdrawal syndrome.

Bontril (phendimetrazine)
Piegene
Prelu-2
X-Trozine
Adipex-P (phentermine)

These drugs may cause insomnia, nervousness, and constipation.

Fastin
Oby-trim
Tenuate (diethylpropion hydrochloride)
Tenuate Dospan
Sanorex (mazindol)
Mazanor

Dexatrim (phenylpropanolamine)
This drug may cause an increase in blood pressure, and other side effects.

Acutrim
This drug has questionable efficacy over the long term.

SMOKING CESSATION*

  MedRANK Life Prolongation and Enhancement Checklist

Pills of Wisdom: Smoking cessation is most effective when counseling, behavior modification, and nicotine-containing medications are combined into a comprehensive treatment program. Because smoking produces nicotine addiction, medications containing nicotine are used to "ease" people through a withdrawal period that accompanies smoking cessation. Some nicotine formulations are more convenient than others.

OPTIMAL
(HIGHLY RECOMMENDED/ BEST OF CLASS)

NICOTINE PATCHES
Patches are better tolerated than gum and therefore are considered Optimal for this lifestyle modification.

ProStep
Smallest patch size. Recommended.

Habitrol
Nicoderm
Nicotrol
All patches will be used for 6 to 12 weeks. They can cause mild skin irritation.

 RECOMMENDED
(ACCEPTABLE WITH RESERVATIONS)

ANTIDEPRESSANTS

Zyban
Wellbutrin (bupropion)
This drug is helpful in selected smokers who do not respond to nicotine patches. Its long-term effectiveness is unclear.

NICOTINE GUM

Nicorette DS (4 mg)
Nine to twelve pieces must be chewed each day for effectiveness. The maximum number of pieces per day is twenty. Side effects include gas, nausea, indigestion, hiccups, and unpleasant taste. Mild withdrawal symptoms

* None of these medications produces perfect results, but the medical complications associated with cigarette smoking are so devastating that smokers should be encouraged to try pharmacological aids, including nicotine patches and gum, when indicated. The effectiveness of these medications is enhanced by counseling, although even without counseling, about twice as many people using nicotine patches are able to stop smoking as those who do not use this method.

may occur after discontinuation. Six months of use is recommended.

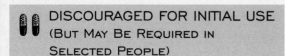

DISCOURAGED FOR INITIAL USE
(BUT MAY BE REQUIRED IN SELECTED PEOPLE)

NICOTINE GUM

Nicorette (2 mg)

The 2 mg dose appears to be much less effective than the 4 mg dose.

ANTIANXIETY DRUGS

BuSpar (buspirone)

This drug may be helpful in selected smokers who do not respond to nicotine patches. Its long-term effectiveness is unclear.

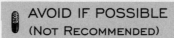

AVOID IF POSSIBLE
(NOT RECOMMENDED)

ANTIHYPERTENSIVE DRUGS

Catapres (clonidine)

Its effectiveness is questionable. Side effects (drowsiness, sedation) are common.

PART III

THE 12-WEEK ACTION PLAN: GETTING THE BEST AND SAFEST PRESCRIPTION DRUGS

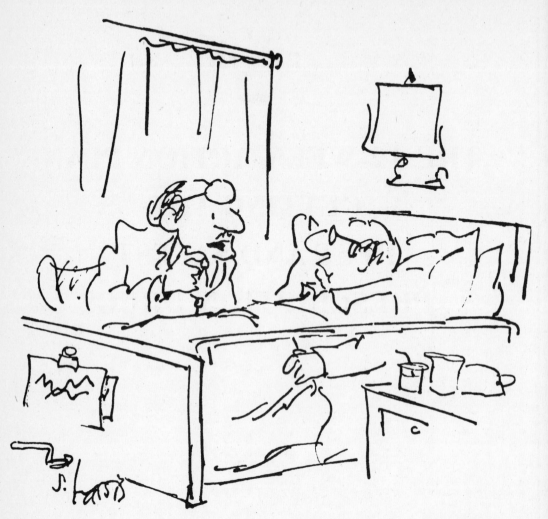

"FEWER THAN ONE IN TEN THOUSAND — SOMETHING LIKE ONE IN FOURTEEN THOUSAND — GETS THESE SIDE EFFECTS. HARDLY ANYBODY GETS THESE SIDE EFFECTS. THEY'RE EXTREMELY RARE. YOU SHOULD BE VERY PROUD."

CHAPTER 22

GOALS AND GUIDELINES OF THE 12-WEEK ACTION PLAN

☼ *The 12-Week Action Plan detailed in this and the next two chapters provides proven strategies for eliminating, consolidating, or replacing unnecessary, inappropriate, and unsafe prescription drugs.*

The goal is to produce maximal results with the best drugs currently available, while *minimizing* the number of prescription medications required to get the job done. The Action Plan helps you identify medications that you feel may not be working, that are too expensive for long-term use, or that are causing side effects that interfere with your sexual function, sleep, or emotional state. Finally, it highlights the importance of risk factors such as generic medications, drug interactions, too many physicians, age, cost, dose levels, health plan policies, and duration limits in shaping your drug therapy program.

Naturally, this drug-reduction and -substitution Action Plan is not something patients should undertake alone. Although there may be times when you feel you know more than your doctor about the specific options available for your particular needs, it is important to collaborate closely with him or her. By referring to the MedRANK Checklists in Part II, you will be able to work *with* your physician to select the *least toxic, most effective medication at the lowest possible dose required to treat your condition*. In addition, you will be able to identify medications that are customized for your age, condition, and family history. Because improving your medication program is a *collaborative* process, maintaining communication with your physician about side effects, costs, and how you are feeling is of paramount importance.

☼ *The purpose of this program is not to bulldoze your physician into a "medication clear-cutting" operation in which he or she simply axes all the drugs you are taking.*

Be firm—but you'll get the best results if you

tell your physician that the only drugs you want changed are those deemed, on the basis of a careful review, to be unnecessary, less than optimal, redundant, outdated, unnecessarily given for excessively long periods, or prescribed at an inappropriately high dose. Moreover, inform your doctor that you'll be much more comfortable with this medication-reduction plan if your health status, symptoms, and other relevant parameters (such as blood pressure, cholesterol levels, and sleeping patterns) are carefully monitored during the twelve weeks it takes to carry it out. You are the patient, the client, the customer, and the consumer. It's your body, so you should control the speed at which you would like these medication changes to be made.

☺ *Almost without exception, encourage your physician to go slow. Gradual is better.*

Inform him or her that your preference is to eliminate, modify, or replace no more than one or two drugs per Action Plan cycle. Once you feel comfortable with the alterations made during the first twelve-week cycle, you and your physician can target other medications for possible modification and substitution during a second cycle.

MISSION STATEMENT

What should you expect to accomplish with the 12-Week Action Plan? The primary short-term goals of this program include the following:

- Eliminating prescription drugs that you may no longer need or that may have been started with inadequate indications
- Decreasing the total number of pills that you are taking each day, in order to improve compliance with your medication program
- Decreasing the dose of one or more of the drugs you are currently taking, in order to decrease the cost and minimize side effects
- Combining two or more medications into a single more versatile drug, in order to simplify your drug regimen
- Replacing suboptimal medications with safer and more effective medications.

☺ *In broad terms, one of the most important objectives of the 12-Week Action Plan is to minimize any real-world barriers (including cost, side effects, efficacy problems, and compliance pitfalls) that stand between your medications and an optimal outcome.*

The Action Plan can steer your practitioner toward the construction of a safe, lean, and user-friendly medication regimen that will permit you to complete the journey from prescription pad to clinical cure and health maintenance.

☺ *The long-term goals of this medication-reduction plan include improving your sense of well-being, implementing lifestyle modifications that will reduce your dependence on prescription medications, and minimizing the possibility of drug interactions.*

Finally, one of the most important objectives

of this plan is to ensure that you are taking advantage of medications that are known to *prevent* serious illnesses, such as heart disease, stroke, cancer, and osteoporosis.

....

ARE YOU A CANDIDATE FOR THE ACTION PLAN?

Everyone's health needs are different. Some people require pills to treat sinus infections and asthma, whereas others require them to manage anxiety and obesity. Regardless of which problem concerns you the most, it is certainly reasonable for you to ask: "What can the 12-Week Action Plan do for me and my family? And who will benefit most from this approach? Me? My aging parents? My children? My spouse?" The answer is, *all* of these people will benefit. In fact, any individual who is currently taking a drug for a chronic or recurrent problem, or who has risk factors for certain diseases, can improve their health status using the 12-Week Action Plan. Review the following checklist, and identify which categories apply to you.

ACTION PLAN CHECKLIST OF COMMON CONDITIONS TREATED WITH MEDICATIONS

Are you or a family member taking pills to treat any of the following problems or health states?

....

_____ Infections
_____ Allergies
_____ Asthma
_____ Skin rashes
_____ Sinus problems
_____ High blood pressure
_____ Heart disease
_____ Diabetes
_____ Arthritis
_____ Pregnancy prevention
_____ Menopause
_____ Depression
_____ Anxiety
_____ Insomnia
_____ Cholesterol problems
_____ HIV infection
_____ Herpes
_____ Heart attack
_____ Alzheimer's disease
_____ Obesity
_____ Blood clots
_____ Irregular heart rhythm
_____ Stroke
_____ Schizophrenia

If you have checked *any* of these categories, the Action Plan offers something for *you*. Some people will benefit much more than others; among the best candidates are people on multiple medications, the elderly, and those with more than one disease requiring drug therapy. Certain drug-intake patterns can also place people at high risk for medication-related problems. But even if you are taking only *one* prescription (or nonprescription) medication, or if you have a child who requires drug therapy for common conditions such as ear infections, asthma, or allergies, or if you are over 60, the chances are good that this program will improve your health. Moreover, if you are young and healthy, but have a family history of cancer, arthritis, depression, heart disease, or diabetes, you can still benefit by considering medications that may be suitable for *preventive* therapy.

If you meet any of the criteria in the checklist below, consider beginning a collaborative medication-evaluation and -reduction plan with your physician immediately.

PRIME CANDIDATES FOR THE ACTION PLAN

Place a check mark on the appropriate line if any of the following apply:

____ You are taking two or more prescription drugs

____ You are 65 or older

____ You are receiving medications from more than one prescriber

____ You have a history of unexplained fatigue, decreased interest in sex, cough, mood disturbance, insomnia, or gastrointestinal problems

____ You have made six or more physician visits within the past year

____ You have a history of previous drug reactions or interactions

____ You feel your medications are too costly

____ Your current regimen contains one or more medications that have to be given more than once daily

____ You have a tendency not to take your medications exactly as prescribed (i.e., skipped doses, doubling up on doses)

____ Your physician has had to increase the dose of your medication on more than one occasion

____ You are taking one or more medications at the highest recommended dose level

____ You are taking more than eight pills per day

____ You are taking primarily generic medications for heart problems or neurological conditions

____ You are a postmenopausal woman and are not taking estrogen replacement therapy

____ You are over 60 and are not taking low-dose aspirin for prevention of heart disease

____ You have a history of depression, panic attacks, anxiety, or other mood disorders

____ Your blood pressure has been well controlled for three or more years using only a single medication, and you have never been considered for a step-down program

____ You feel your sense of well-being or quality of life has deteriorated in some way since having a medication started or having the dose of any of your medications changed

____ You have been on a medication for more than three years and are not sure if it is still needed

____ Your physician has switched your medications more than three times over the past year

Not surprisingly, given the widespread use of prescription drugs in modern society, most people turn out to be prime candidates for the 12-Week Action Plan.

THE THREE PHASES

The 12-Week Action Plan is divided into *three* distinct, four-week "phases." Although they do overlap, these phases can basically be described as assessment, implementation, and evaluation. Once you tell your physician you are interested in working on the 12-Week Action Plan, you will need to make contact with your physician again (either in an office visit or by telephone) at the end of weeks four, eight, and twelve.

☺ *PHASE ONE: ASSESSMENT.*
During the first phase, you and your physician should explore a number of features about your current drug regimen.

First you should express your interest in collaborating with your physician on a program of medication refinement. Explain to him or her that in approximately four weeks you will be bringing in a number of Action Plan Checklists that will set the stage for a program of medication elimination and replacement.

Sometime during this first four-week period, you should carefully complete the following Action Plan Checklists in this book:

* Drug Chronicle
* Medication Compliance
* Medication Evaluation
* Side Effects
* Quality of Life

The first three of these checklists appear later in this chapter; the last two can be found at the end of Chapter 24. You should also examine the drug-for-disease MedRANK Checklists (see Part II) that apply directly to you.

If you complete these checklists honestly and accurately, you will have done yourself and your physician a great service. You will have provided your practitioner with valuable information about your current drug regimen. Based on this information and the MedRANK Checklists, your physician will be able to design a customized, highly effective, patient-friendly, and safe drug regimen tailored to your specific medical problems and health goals. The modifications will be made in phase two of the 12-Week Action Plan cycle.

☺ *PHASE TWO: IMPLEMENTATION.*
During this second four-week phase, you will consider with your doctor each of the drugs you are taking and pose to him or her as many of the fundamental questions as possible, as detailed in Chapter 23.

The Medication Precaution Checklist that concludes that chapter will help summarize major areas of concern.

During this period you will also want to fill out the following Action Plan Checklists in Chapter 24:

* Simplifying Your Drug Regimen
* Drug Elimination
* Dose Reduction
* Inappropriate Medications for the Elderly
* "Mental Manglers"
* Medication Time Bombs

- Drugs with Possible Duration Limits
- Selected Medications with Significant Risks of Drug-Drug Interactions
- Generic Medications
- "Versatile Drugs"

These checklists will help you and your physician focus on specific problem areas that need attention, whether they be excessive use of generic drugs, high-dosage medications, unnecessary medications, inappropriate medications, or failure to use versatile or top-of-the-line medications. Your physician may not agree with all of the potential problems or issues raised in these checklists, but the chances are excellent he or she will find at least a few very important problems and suboptimal prescribing patterns that have fallen through the cracks. These checklists will set the stage for specific Action Plan objectives.

Your physician has several options during the implementation phase of the Action Plan. He or she may decide to lower a dose of one of your drugs, taper a medication gradually, consolidate two into a single more versatile drug, or add a medication for the purpose of disease prevention. Regardless of the kind of intervention, you and your physician will have to keep close tabs on your progress during the evaluation phase.

☼ *PHASE THREE: EVALUATION. The purpose of this final four-week phase is to evaluate your medical, psychological, and symptomatic response to the modifications made during the implementation phase.*

Between weeks ten and twelve you should complete (once again) the three checklists in this chapter (the Drug Chronicle Checklist, the Medication Compliance Checklist, and the Medication Evaluation Checklist), as well as the two checklists at the end of Chapter 24 (the Action Plan Side Effect Checklist and the Four-Point Quality of Life Survey).

Once you have filled out these checklists, you and your physician can sit down and compare impressions of your well-being, your quality of life, and your medication program *before* and *after* the changes were made to your drug regimen. These checklists will also help determine whether your attitudes about drug therapy have improved or deteriorated since the first physician visit. If the medication changes meet with your approval, it is appropriate to evaluate new opportunities and begin a second 12-Week Action Plan cycle.

••

BEFORE YOU START

The Drug Chronicle can provide you and your doctor with a baseline of your current drug intake. It will be important for your physician to compare this Drug Chronicle against his or her records in order to identify possible discrepancies between drugs you are supposed to be taking and those you actually are taking. Before you fill out this checklist, you should make a photocopy of it, because you will want to fill it out again at the end of each of your Action Plan cycles, to keep current with your medication regimen as changes are made.

After completing the Drug Chronicle and the two other checklists in this chapter, you will be armed with some of the most important information for optimizing your personal pharmacology program.

DRUG CHRONICLE CHECKLIST

1. Please list the prescription medications you are currently taking, the time of day you take them, and their purpose. (You may use your medication bottles or any other sources to find this information.)

Medication   1 _____
Time of Day Taken   _____
Purpose of Medication _____

Medication   2 _____
Time of Day Taken   _____
Purpose of Medication _____

Medication 3_____
Time of Day Taken   _____
Purpose of Medication _____

Medication   4 _____
Time of Day Taken   _____
Purpose of Medication _____

Medication   5 _____
Time of Day Taken   _____
Purpose of Medication _____

Medication   6 _____
Time of Day Taken   _____
Purpose of Medication _____

Medication   7 _____
Time of Day Taken   _____
Purpose of Medication _____

2. Please list the over-the-counter (OTC) medications you are currently taking, the time of day you take them, and their purpose. (You may use your medication bottles or any other sources to find this information.)

OTC Medication   1_____
Time of Day Taken   _____
Purpose of Medication _____

OTC Medication   2_____
Time of Day Taken   _____
Purpose of Medication _____

OTC Medication   3_____
Time of Day Taken   _____
Purpose of Medication _____

OTC Medication   4_____
Time of Day Taken   _____
Purpose of Medication _____

One of the most important concerns about drug regimens is compliance. If you are complying with yours, you should make this clear to your physician. If you are not taking the medications as prescribed, you need to state this unambiguously. To help identify the specific objective and subjective features that may be preventing you from taking your drugs as requested, you should complete the Medication Compliance Checklist on page 338. If there are specific reasons for your noncompliance, jot them down for future reference. This checklist will also give you the opportunity to express your preference for trying other medications that might produce the same results with fewer side effects and lower cost.

MEDICATION COMPLIANCE CHECKLIST

1. For the most part, do you take your medications exactly as prescribed? _____
   (If your answer to this question is "no," "maybe," "some of the time," or something similar, you should complete Question 2.)
2. In your view, what are the factors that best explain your failure to take your medications?

(Please check all those that apply.)

_____ They are too expensive.
_____ I have to take them too often.
_____ I don't like the way they make me feel.
_____ They don't seem to be working.
_____ They make me feel worse than I did before starting them.
_____ I don't think I need as much medication as I once did.
_____ They don't seem to work as well as they once did.
_____ I am a forgetful person.
_____ It's too complicated to take them the way they are prescribed.
_____ I have never been told exactly how my medications should be taken.
_____ I haven't been given written instructions on how to take them.
_____ In general, I just don't like taking pills.
_____ I believe there may be better medications available to treat my condition.
_____ I have heard that one or more of my medications produce undesirable side effects.

3. Would you be interested in having your medications adjusted so you could take fewer pills less frequently? _____
4. Would you be interested in trying other medications that produce fewer side effects? _____

Although the Action Plan identifies which drugs in your regimen need to be considered for possible modification, it is just as important to get your own gut feeling about which drugs might be causing problems. This Medication Evaluation Checklist can help you clarify what your feelings are. Knowing your current level of satisfaction will also help steer your physician toward some drug options and away from others. As important, by filling out this checklist, you will convey to your practitioner just how serious you are in participating in this collaboration.

MEDICATION EVALUATION CHECKLIST

1. Are there any medications in your drug regimen that you would prefer not to take? If so, which one(s)? _____
   Why? _____
2. Are you happy with your current drug regimen? _____ If not, please explain why. _____
3. Are there any medications in your regimen you think are too expensive? _____ If yes, which one(s)? _____
4. Would you be interested in trying other medications that are just as effective for your medical problem(s) but much less likely to cause side effects? _____

5. Would you be interested in medications that are less expensive than the ones you are currently taking? _____

6. Would you be willing to make regular visits to your physician over the next several weeks to eliminate or replace medications in your drug regimen? ____

7. Is there any single medication you feel you absolutely must stay on because it has produced dramatic improvements in your health? _____

8. Is there any single medication you feel you should absolutely stop taking because it has produced such a dramatic worsening in your condition or in your quality of life? _____

☺ *Once you have filled out these checklists, you are ready for your first physician visit. Present them, along with the Action Plan Side Effect Checklist and the Four-Point Quality of Life Survey on pages 375 and 376, to your physician about four to five weeks after your first contact.*

Using the information in these checklists, you and your physician are now ready to make specific drug eliminations, additions, replacements, or dosage adjustments.

....

PILLS AND PITFALLS: THE IMPORTANCE OF PSYCHOLOGICAL PREPARATION

As motivated as you may be to begin this Action Plan for getting off pills, the process does require some psychological preparation.

The fact is, streamlining your medication regimen is much easier said than done. But one thing is certain: Your cooperation is of the utmost importance. No matter how logical, practical, or justified a change in your regimen may seem, you must be willing and confident enough to put the plan into action.

Many people are reluctant to make changes in their drug regimens, for a variety of reasons. First, although many drugs do more harm than good, individuals often may depend heavily on them for reasons that may not seem logical or scientific. For example, if you are middle-aged or older and have been taking multiple medications for quite some time, you may cling to your regimen as if it were a pharmacological security blanket. The elderly, in particular, are creatures of habit when it comes to medications. If you are in this age group, you may feel reluctant to have medications removed from your drug list—or even have dosages reduced—despite the clinical wisdom of such modifications.

Through no fault of your own, you may feel more secure taking your current medications, and you may perceive that more drugs, rather than fewer, can better control symptoms that otherwise might be incomprehensible, painful, or frightening. If this is the case, you may strongly resist attempts to wean yourself off unnecessary or inappropriate medications. This is a very natural and common response, and it does not mean that the Action Plan will not work for you. In fact, just the opposite is true.

☺ *One of the main objectives of the Action Plan is to introduce you to medications that can service all of your health needs but with smaller doses, less frequent administration, and better tolerability.*

This "less is more" orientation is now the driving force in pharmaceutical development, so the quicker you become comfortable with it, the better prepared you will be for future developments in drug therapy. On a more immediate level, the sooner you accept the notion that you can minimize drug therapy to maximize your health benefits, the more productive your Action Plan will be.

☺ *Although the Action Plan is designed to produce more streamlined, better-tolerated medication programs, like any medical intervention it has potential risks.*

For example, there is always the risk that your physician will discontinue a medication that you need. Usually this can be avoided if your doctor is careful to avoid eliminating necessary drugs, by closely reviewing your medical records and thoroughly investigating why you were started on the medication in the first place.

Once a medication is discontinued, you should be closely observed. If you have heart disease, lung problems, or a psychiatric condition, for example, discontinuation of medications such as digoxin, antidepressants, or corticosteroids requires careful clinical monitoring. If you inappropriately discontinue an antidepressant such as Prozac, Zoloft, or Paxil,

you may notice a recurrence of your depressive symptoms. But a recurrence is less likely if you were originally started on the antidepressant to treat an episode of situational depression (caused by a stressful event in your life, such as a death in the family, a divorce, or loss of a job) and if you have had no more than one episode of serious depression over the past five years. Your health status can deteriorate not only from abrupt cessation of a medication but from a reduction in drug dosage.

Drug elimination and replacement also have the potential to produce unexpected side effects and drug interactions. But these complications are rare, since the Action Plan itself identifies medications with fewer side effects and drug interactions. Whenever drug changes are made, it is always possible that the new regimen will not be as effective as the original. If this is the case, you and your physician should not give up on the basic goals of the Action Plan. For example, let's say you are taking a diuretic and a beta-blocker for your high blood pressure, and your physician decides to substitute an ACE inhibitor for these two medications. If the ACE inhibitor doesn't provide adequate control of your blood pressure, it may be worthwhile to try another antihypertensive drug such as a calcium channel blocker before you go back on your old two-drug regimen. Reduced effectiveness is a potential liability of any reconstructed regimen. Therefore, careful clinical monitoring is mandatory whenever Action Plan modifications are made.

A WORD OF CAUTION ON COSTS

When it comes to money, the Action Plan brings good news and bad news. The good news is that streamlining your drug program can save you considerable money through drug elimination and dose reduction. If your physician is able to delete a drug like theophylline, digoxin, Cytotec, Cognex, a sedative, an anti-ulcer medication, or Persantine, you will be spared years of unnecessary expenditures. These drugs can cost up to $400 per year merely for maintenance therapy. Consequently, over many years, the amount of money you will save from eliminations recommended by the Action Plan is considerable.

But the replacement of existing drugs with better ones is another story, since better drugs usually carry a higher price tag and may actually cost you more. In such cases, the savings derived from the Action Plan may not seem obvious at first. But take heart: The long-term balance sheet is on your side. Even if costlier drugs are required, you should remember that the benefits they can bring— such as quality-of-life improvements, simplified dosing, better compliance, and reduced risk of drug interactions—usually are well worth the price. In addition, your improved overall health status will mean that the total amount of money you will have to spend on medical problems in the future will be reduced substantially. In other words, an ounce of pharmacological prevention is worth several pounds of pharmacological cure.

 Many studies confirm the cost-effectiveness of superior drugs like those advocated by the Action Plan.

As reported in the March 21, 1996, *Wall Street Journal*, the Health Management Outcomes Institute in Salt Lake City found that when HMOs permitted their physicians to prescribe medications without any restrictions, the overall cost of providing health care for their subscribers was reduced. In other words, practitioners who were free to prescribe superior medications produced better health outcomes for their patients and, in turn, saved their plans lots of money.

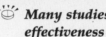 ***Moreover, the majority of patients in health plans and HMOs are insulated from most of the additional expense of better medications.***

Even the elderly on fixed incomes who have been absorbed into Medicare-sponsored managed care plans can obtain medications with only minimal copayments, ranging from $5 to $10 per prescription. Consequently, if your physician substitutes a more expensive drug for a cheaper one, your copayment may stay the same or increase by only a few dollars per prescription.

Your health is your most important asset. As a health care consumer, be persistent in your insistence that prescribing the best and safest medications should be your practitioner's primary goal. The MedRANK Checklists in Part II can steer you and your physician toward optimal, best-of-class medications.

CHAPTER 23

ASKING THE RIGHT QUESTIONS

Taking Control of
Your Personal Pharmacology

There is no better way to protect yourself against unsafe, inappropriate, and ineffective drug therapy than to ask your doctor the right questions about your drugs. Preferably, you should ask the questions in this chapter before you embark on any medication program, but you should certainly ask them during the Action Plan, both about drugs you are already taking and about any new substitution drugs that your doctor prescribes for you. The "describe before you prescribe" approach is based on sound principles. Know what you are getting into, then decide for yourself whether you want to embark on the new medication program. Ask first, take your pills later.

☼ *What class does this drug belong to?*
One of the first things you will want to ask your doctor is what class the drug you have been prescribed belongs to. Some classes of medications produce excellent results with reasonable convenience and minimal toxicity, like the ACE inhibitors for high blood pressure,

HMG-CoA reductase inhibitors for cholesterol-lowering, and proton pump–blocking drugs for ulcer disease. Classes of drugs that are held in somewhat lower esteem include thiazide diuretics, tricyclic antidepressants, and antacids.

It is also useful to know the lay terms that are used for the drug. For example, because diuretics reduce the water content of the blood and increase urine volume, they are often called "water pills." Sympathomimetic medications, such as bronchodilators, may be described as "drugs that make breathing easier by widening certain breathing passages of the lung."

Detailed information about biochemical mechanisms of action, pharmacology, and pharmacokinetics is beyond the scope of this book. For the most part, however, this kind of information is not especially useful in making practical decisions about your medication intake. For the sake of information and education, however, you may want to learn how a medication works and what its mechanism of

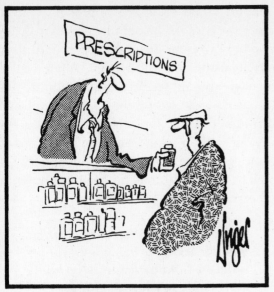

"Read the instructions very, very, very, very carefully."

action is. This kind of information is available in any standard home drug reference.

☼ For what illness or illnesses is this medication indicated? Are there unlabeled or off-label uses for this drug that are currently considered appropriate?

One of the most fundamental questions you must ask about any medication is whether it is indicated for the condition for which it has been prescribed. Sales representatives from pharmaceutical companies sometimes recommend medications for off-label purposes, prompting physicians to use a drug without supporting clinical trials. If, however, your physician or pharmacist tells you that the drug you have been given is not indicated for your problem, there is no need to panic.

Having FDA approval for a specific indication means a drug has been shown to be ef-

fective for that condition. Generally speaking, when a drug carries an FDA-approved indication, researchers have conducted placebo-controlled, double-blind studies that confirm its usefulness for that particular medical condition.

In practice, however, medications that have been in use for a number of years and with which physicians gain considerable experience over time may eventually be shown to be effective for conditions for which official approval has not been granted. Unlabeled uses are usually the result of years of such practical, trial-and-error experience. Good results over time can lead to a general consensus of medical opinion that a drug is, in fact, useful for a condition, even without an official indication. Be sure your drug has undergone a level of scrutiny that is sufficient to support its use for an off-label purpose.

☼ The reality is that prescribing drugs for unlabeled indications is one of the most important and potentially controversial areas in modern-day drug therapy.

From a practical perspective, the fact that a drug is prescribed for an unlabeled indication doesn't mean that it isn't effective for that condition; it simply means that the drug doesn't carry official FDA approval for that condition. Even though formal trials have not been conducted to prove its effectiveness, experience is frequently so broad and so deep that its use for an unlabeled indication is well justified. If you are taking a drug for an unlabeled use, however, it is reasonable to inquire about any evidence that the medication produces more harm than benefit for its unlabeled indication.

Unlabeled uses apply to medications from a wide variety of therapeutic classes. For example, although they are not officially indicated for postpartum depression or premenstrual syndrome, the SSRI antidepressants (Prozac, Zoloft, and Paxil) appear to produce significant relief among people with these syndromes. In another example, doctors may occasionally prescribe the drug nitroglycerine to help reduce the workload on the heart in patients who have had heart attacks or congestive heart failure. Doctors may also prescribe nitroglycerine ointment (along with other medications) for the treatment of Raynaud's disease.

Cimetidine (Tagamet) has been used to treat a wide variety of medical conditions for which it is not indicated, including chronic hives, allergic skin reactions, and abnormal hair growth in women. Unlabeled uses for anticonvulsants such as Dilantin include control of irregular heart-beat and management of the pain associated with trigeminal neuralgia (tic douloureux). Unlabeled uses are especially common with drugs used to treat nervous system disorders such as depression, obsessive compulsive disorder, panic attacks, bulimia, and obesity. Once again, although these unlabeled uses are generally safe and appropriate, consulting your pharmacist or physician is prudent in most cases.

 As for labeled uses, be aware that specific medications within a drug class frequently have indications that differ from one another.

For example, in the benzodiazepine class of anti-anxiety medications (which includes Valium), some drugs are approved to treat panic disorder and anxiety associated with depression, whereas others are approved to treat anxiety associated with alcohol withdrawal or management of seizures. Thus, alprazolam (Xanax) is indicated for the treatment of panic disorder but not for seizures, whereas diazepam (Valium) is indicated for symptoms of acute agitation, tremor, or delirium tremens, as well as for convulsions (in combination with other medications).

 If you determine that a medication you are taking is being used for an unlabeled indication, it is certainly reasonable to consult with your doctor and ask about the evidence supporting its use for your condition.

The following list identifies commonly used therapeutic classes containing drugs with variable indications. If you are taking a drug that belongs to any of these classes, you will want to ask your physician whether it is indicated for your particular medical problem.

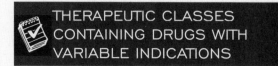

THERAPEUTIC CLASSES CONTAINING DRUGS WITH VARIABLE INDICATIONS

- Beta-blockers
- Calcium blockers
- SSRI antidepressants
- Cholesterol-lowering drugs (HMG-CoA reductase inhibitors)
- Sedatives
- Anti-anxiety medications
- Macrolide antibiotics

- Cephalosporin antibiotics
- Penicillinlike antibiotics

It is also helpful to ask your physician whether the medication prescribed for you is useful as a primary drug for your particular illness or as an alternative medication. If you have been prescribed a drug that is indicated as an alternative treatment, it certainly is reasonable to ask your physician if another medication is preferred and, if there is, why the alternative drug was selected in your particular case.

☺ *Finally, note that in some cases the uses of a medication will differ depending upon whether you are using a prescription or over-the-counter product.*

For example, in the case of histamine H2-antagonists (used to treat ulcer disease), the prescription drugs cimetidine, famotidine, and ranitidine are indicated for the treatment of gastric and duodenal ulcers as well as for the management of gastroesophageal reflux. In contrast, the OTC formulations of cimetidine and famotidine (which are weaker) are approved for the prevention of heartburn, acid indigestion, and sour stomach. Because the dosage strength of OTC drugs is generally less than that of prescription medications, you usually cannot substitute therapy of one with another.

☺ *What dosing and timing considerations should I be aware of?*

Although many drugs are prescribed for consumption on a scheduled basis—that is, you must take the pills on a more-or-less precise schedule—many others are taken on an as-needed basis for relief of acute problems or to prevent worsening of a chronic disease. As-needed pill intake commonly is used for managing specific pain syndromes in people with migraine headaches, arthritis, or cancer, and for individuals with asthma, allergies, and heart conditions. If you take a pill on an as-needed basis, it is important that you know when to take it in relation to the onset of symptoms, how many doses you can take, and what the maximum permissible dose is for any single attack or situation. In some cases alternate-day therapy can lower the risk of side effects while retaining the beneficial effects of the drug. To take advantage of this dosing schedule, consult your physician.

In addition, some drugs are available in both tablet form and in injections. For example, sumatriptan (Imitrex), used for the immediate treatment of migraine headaches, is available both in tablet form and as an injection. The tablets can be taken without regard to food, as a single dose with fluids, as soon as the patient notices migraine symptoms. If this dose is unsuccessful and symptoms return, a second dose may be taken, but no sooner than two hours following the first dose. Patients should not take more than 300 mg in any twenty-four-hour period. But the use of the injectable preparation is different. The injection is given as soon as symptoms of migraine appear, but it may be administered at any time during an attack. Moreover, a second injection may be given if symptoms come back, with no more than two injections in any twenty-four-hour period.

☺ What are the major side effects I should watch for?

Every drug is capable of producing side effects, although many patients may never experience them even with chronic therapy. The frequency and severity of side effects depend on many factors, including the dose of the medication, how long you take the drug, and your own individual susceptibility.

Side effects may affect the digestive tract, nervous system, circulatory system, respiratory system, skin, urinary tract, eyes, and other organs. Side effects that relate to the digestive tract may include upset stomach, vomiting, constipation, indigestion, and similar discomforts. Those involving the nervous system may vary widely, including sleeplessness, headache, drowsiness, dizziness, mood changes, unstable emotions, and other impairments.

Side effects that pertain to the circulatory system are potentially serious problems, among them changes in blood pressure (elevations or decreases), palpitations (abnormal pounding in the chest), fast heartbeat, flushing, and unexpected chest pain. Side effects involving the kidney or urinary tract can include an increased risk for urinary tract infections, painful urination, inadequate urinary stream, and a propensity to cause kidney stones.

☺ On rare occasions, a drug may have to be withdrawn from the market because of side effects that are very serious or even, if rarely, life-threatening.

Because of their propensity to cause very serious side effects, some medications are indicated only for life-threatening medical conditions or as last-resort drugs, in cases where their benefits may outweigh their risks. Examples of medications that should be restricted to patients who have life-threatening problems include anti-arrhythmic agents such as flecainide, mexiletine, and moricizine. In some medications, the side effects may be so serious that hospitalization is required when starting them.

☺ It should be emphasized that many medication-induced side effects are worsened by alcohol intake, excessive coffee ingestion, and over-the-counter medications.

For example, if your doctor has you on a prescription nonsteroidal anti-inflammatory drug (NSAID), the gastrointestinal irritation and heartburn that are sometimes experienced with these drugs can be worsened by alcohol intake or simultaneous intake of an over-the-counter NSAID, such as Motrin or Advil. Even commonly used nonprescription medications, such as Benadryl, cimetidine, aspirin, and over-the-counter flu remedies, have the potential to increase the severity of troublesome side effects of prescription medications. You may find that you are better able to tolerate your prescription drugs simply by reducing your intake of alcohol, certain foods, or over-the-counter drugs.

Unfortunately, it may be very difficult to distinguish between the side effects of a medication and the symptoms of a disease. Nevertheless, if you notice the onset of troublesome side effects or new symptoms shortly after beginning a medication and you suspect your medication may be the cause, you should trust your intuition and consult your physician or pharmacist in order to determine whether there is a possible association.

☺ Can the drug cause physical dependence?

Addiction is associated with a number of undesirable social, emotional, and psychological behaviors. It is critical that you know when a drug you are taking has the capacity to produce chemical dependence: that is, a craving for the medication that goes beyond mere psychological need, accompanied by the development of tolerance, such that the longer you use the medication, the more intense and consistent the craving becomes.

☺ *Drug dependence is possible with a number of medications, including narcotics and anxiety-reducing medications. Be sure that your physician warns you about the potential for abuse or dependence with any medications prescribed for longer than one week.*

For example, virtually all central nervous system stimulants—including amphetamines and Ritalin—can cause extreme dependence and even severe social disability with chronic abuse. People have a tendency to increase their intake of these amphetaminelike drugs gradually to many times the recommended dose. Abruptly stopping them can cause a severe withdrawal syndrome, which can manifest as extreme fatigue, mental depression, and changes in sleep habits. These drugs should always be taken under a doctor's supervision.

If your condition requires a medication with a potential for producing addiction, you should be observant for signs and symptoms associated with drug withdrawal. Your physician should provide you with a description of the withdrawal phenomenon, including the timing and severity of symptoms, and characteristics of the recovery period associated with drug dependence.

For example, narcotic pain relievers are commonly used analgesics that have abuse potential. The withdrawal syndrome associated with them is usually related to the abruptness of the withdrawal and the specific drug that is being used. Generally speaking, withdrawal symptoms develop around the time the next dose is ordinarily given. Thus, patients who are withdrawing from morphine have symptoms that gradually increase in intensity, reach a maximum in thirty-six to seventy-two hours, and then subside over the next five to ten days. In contrast, methadone withdrawal is much slower in onset, and the patient may not fully recover for six to seven weeks. Meperidine withdrawal often runs its course within four to five days, whereas hydrocodone (Vicodin) withdrawal peaks at forty-eight to seventy-two hours.

☺ *Early symptoms of withdrawal from narcotics include yawning, tearing, runny nose, restlessness, and sweating. More severe symptoms include flushing, increased heart rate, appetite loss, irritability, and dilated pupils.*

The late and most severe symptoms include fever, nausea, and diarrhea, among others. If you develop any of these symptoms while taking a medication that can produce physical dependence, it is essential that you consult your prescribing practitioner as soon as possible.

☺ Should I be wary of transient side effects or a "first-dose" effect?

When it comes to starting a new medication, patience can be a virtue. To be sure, some medications produce such disagreeable and intolerable side effects from the outset that you will have no choice but to bail out and ask your physician to consider a new medication. Many drugs, however, produce initial side effects that are transient. That is, they may be quite prominent during the first few days of therapy but eventually diminish over time. There is something to be said for plowing through this rough period and withholding final judgment until you give the drug a few days to "work the kinks out."

Transient side effects often result from taking blood pressure–lowering medications or antidepressants. For example:

- Patients who are being treated for high blood pressure often feel tired and run down for a few days or weeks after beginning drug therapy. It may take time for the body to adjust to lower blood pressure. Generally speaking, you should continue taking your blood pressure medication, even though you may not feel entirely normal.
- Similar changes in energy level can be seen when starting antidepressants. Zoloft, a commonly used antidepressant, can produce diarrhea and other gastrointestinal symptoms during the first few weeks, but these side effects almost always disappear shortly thereafter.

More often than not, the first few days of most medications will require a period of adaptation. You should always check, however, with your doctor or pharmacist during this initial period for any new symptoms that arise. You will want to be sure that these side effects are an expected consequence of the new drug.

Some medications can produce a so-called "first-dose" effect, which means that the initial symptoms or side effects are serious enough to cause harm. Always ask your doctor if a medication prescribed for you has a tendency to produce first-dose effects, and if so, what strategies are available for dealing with them. For example, the alpha-one adrenergic blocking agents (Hytrin) used to treat high blood pressure and enlargement of the prostate can produce a first-dose effect that consists of dizziness, fainting, and falling. This is probably due to the sudden decreases in blood pressure seen after the first dose. These symptoms are more likely to occur when the patient rises quickly from a seated or lying position, if the dose is increased suddenly, or if therapy is stopped and then started again. To lessen the chances of these problems, the first dose should be given at bedtime; in addition, you will be encouraged to sit or lie down if you feel light-headed.

First-dose effects can occur with a number of other medications, including anti-allergic medications, drugs used to treat asthma, psychoactive drugs, and other blood pressure–lowering medications. Although first-dose effects do not always produce serious complications, they can produce symptoms that are disturbing enough to deter you from wanting to continue with drug therapy. Be assured that such symptoms are frequently transient in nature and will disappear once you get accustomed to taking your medication on a regular basis.

☺ Does the prescribed drug come with any special precautions?

An ounce of prevention is worth a pound of cure. Special precautions are readily available to your physician in the package insert for the medication. This information—which includes indications, contraindications, and warnings—is also published in modified, extracted, or complete form in the *Physicians' Desk Reference (PDR)*, *Drug Facts & Comparisons*, and similar resources, many of which are available at your public library. As emphasized in an earlier chapter, however, it is simply impossible for your doctor to know as much about your family history, coexisting medical conditions, over-the-counter medications, and other prescription medications in your regimen as you do. In practical terms, you are your own best, last line of defense.

☺ Some drugs should not be used under any circumstances in some individuals. In other cases, use of a drug may be permissible but only with caution.

For example, the antibiotic erythromycin should not be used when the patient is allergic to erythromycin or to any component of the medication, or if either of the antihistamines astemizole (Hismanal) or terfenadine (Seldane) are also being taken. In fact, no drug should be used if the patient has a known allergy to it or to any of its components.

☺ For some drugs, warnings about their use will apply if the patient has had a certain previous or existing medical condition or is taking a drug for which there is a potentially significant drug interaction.

Issues about which you will want to ask include warnings related to breast-feeding and pregnancy; possible cautions for young children or the elderly; and underlying medical conditions that may be worsened by the medication. In other cases, cautionary warnings may pertain to a drug's use in combination with certain kinds of foods.

What should you do if you suspect that special precautions are associated with a drug you've been prescribed? Contact your doctor or pharmacist for clarification immediately. If a special precaution does pertain to your situation, do not panic. It may very well be that the drug has been prescribed for you because its benefits far outweigh any potential harm.

☺ Does my drug regimen require laboratory monitoring?

Many medications require not only careful monitoring of levels of the drug in the blood but also surveillance of other blood parameters, including the blood count and liver function tests, among others. These lab tests are performed to ensure that the medication is not at toxic levels. Even if it is at an appropriate level, however, other lab tests may be required during treatment, to ensure that it is not causing toxicity to other susceptible organs. Some drugs—including anticonvulsant medications, diuretics, lithium, theophylline, antiviral medications used for HIV infection, chemotherapy drugs, blood thinners, and lipid-lowering medications—may require complete blood counts, liver and kidney function tests, and blood levels of the medication to monitor drug therapy.

CHECKLIST FOR MEDICATIONS REQUIRING LABORATORY MONITORING

____ Digoxin
____ Theophylline
____ Coumadin
____ Warfarin
____ Lithium
____ Antiviral drugs (HIV infection)
____ Tacrine
____ NSAIDs
____ Chemotherapy drugs
____ Ketoconazole
____ Anti-arrhythmic drugs
____ Antidepressants
____ Cholesterol-lowering agents
____ Diuretics
____ Ticlopidine
____ Anticonvulsants

You should ask whether your medication is known to be associated with drug dependence, or, if you are using other medications, if you risk a potentially life-threatening drug interaction. You should ask whether you can change from one dosage form of the medication to another. Ask if your medication can produce sensitivity to sunlight, or if it has a propensity to cause staining of tooth surfaces, tooth restorations, or the tongue. Finally, some drugs contain sulfite preservatives, which can cause allergic reactions in certain individuals.

How should I discontinue the medication? Prescribed drugs should not be discontinued without your doctor's approval.

To minimize the risk of withdrawal symptoms, unexpected reactions, rebound symptoms, and serious complications, always ask if discontinuing your medication may cause serious consequences. The fact is, suddenly stopping a medication may carry a great risk of harm. It has the potential to cause a number of serious complications, including rebound elevations in blood pressure, uncontrolled diabetes, and hormonal imbalances that, in turn, can cause serious—sometimes even life-threatening—problems. For example:

- People taking long-term oral corticosteroids (so-called steroid medications, such as prednisone, which is widely used for treatment of arthritis, asthma, allergies, emphysema, and many other conditions) may lose the ability to produce their own natural corticosteroid hormones. This can cause a serious withdrawal illness characterized by low blood pressure, acidosis in the blood, and life-threatening elevations of potassium. If you have been taking a corticosteroid at high doses or for several weeks or longer, your physician will advise you to taper off the medication gradually.

- Sudden discontinuation of beta-blockers may worsen chest pain associated with angina or produce sudden elevations in blood pressure.
- Abrupt withdrawal of calcium channel blockers may also cause a withdrawal syndrome characterized by chest pain and rapid heart rate.

Similar warnings apply to the sudden discontinuation of antidepressants (including Zoloft, Paxil, Effexor, and Elavil), blood pressure medications, drugs used to treat angina, sedatives (Xanax and Valium), pain medications (narcotics), oral sulfonylureas, insulin, and many other drugs. In general, these problems can be minimized if drugs are slowly tapered off, under medical supervision.

In some cases it may be necessary to stop one medication and start another. In fact, replacing inferior medications with better pills is an important part of the Action Plan. A transition or tapering period may or may not be necessary. An overlap period may also be required, during which you taper off one medication as you start taking its replacement. For example, to prevent withdrawal side effects, beta-blockers should be tapered slowly and overlapped for eight to ten days when starting a calcium channel blocker such as amlodipine, nicardipine, or nifedipine. Your doctor should provide clear—and preferably written—instructions that will help you make the transition from one to another.

☺ Is this the safest drug in its class for my condition?

Even among similar medications, significant safety differences exist. Although decisions regarding the safety of your medication rest primarily with your doctor and pharmacist, this book can point you toward medications within the same drug class that are associated with a lower risk of side effects or complications. These safety differences can be quite pronounced, especially in the case of NSAIDs, birth control pills, antidepressants, anticonvulsants, antibiotics, antihistamines, calcium channel blockers, and drugs used to treat abnormal heart rhythms.

Oral contraceptives are a good example. Three kinds of combination contraceptive pills exist. The so-called monophasic pill has the same dose of estrogen and progestin in each pill. In contrast, the biphasic and triphasic pills have varying amounts of these hormones. The mini-pill contains only progestin. Because estrogen use is associated with the risk of blood clots—especially in patients who are smokers or have other vascular disease risk factors—you should request a combination pill with an estrogen dose that is as low as possible. You can ask your doctor to ensure that your contraceptive contains the lowest estrogen dose that is effective for your contraceptive needs.

☺ Is it safe to substitute or interchange brands?

As I mentioned in Chapter 2, some group care practices may encourage their doctors to change medications from one brand to another within the same class. Generally speaking, these substitutions are profit- rather than patient-motivated, directing physicians toward medications that presumably have the same benefits but lower costs. Many states permit such substitutions, especially if a patented drug is replaced by a generic formulation, or if the patient's doctor signs off on the substitution. Experience shows, however, that different brands of related medications can have very different effects in an individual.

Safeguards that prevent inappropriate substitutions are not always followed. Even if a pharmacist notifies the prescriber about an inappropriate substitution, the prescriber may be pressured to give quick approval rather than take time to perform a detailed evaluation of the proposed substitution.

☺ Ask your physician about the safety of making brand interchanges with the drugs you are taking.

Brand interchanges are not always safe, and in many cases they should be discouraged. Many organizations, including the American Academy of Family Practice, discourage brand interchange for many medications used to treat heart disease, seizures, and other neurologic disorders. Most experts discourage patients who are taking cardiac glycosides (digoxin) from changing from one brand of digoxin to another without first consulting a pharmacist or physician.

Generally speaking, brand interchanges are discouraged for anticonvulsants (Dilantin), antidepressants (Prozac, Zoloft, Paxil), drugs used to treat abnormal heart rhythms (quinidine formulations), and antipsychotic medications such as Navane, Stelazine, and Haldol. Because products manufactured by different companies may not be equally effective, it is preferable to stay on the medication you have been taking over the long term and to permit brand interchanges only when recommended by your prescribing practitioner.

☺ How important is the drug's "delivery system" to its effectiveness?

Medications are frequently available in a number of different formulations, including liquid suspensions, tablets, capsules, and powders. In addition, crushing, chewing, or breaking can affect their rate of absorption and cause serious adverse or toxic side effects. In some cases, altering a medication can decrease its effectiveness. Be sure to ask your doctor or pharmacist if the dosage form you have been prescribed can or cannot be crushed or chewed.

A delivery system is the route by which an active prescription ingredient can be introduced into the body. Nasal sprays, pills, ointments and creams, implants, and inhalation are all delivery systems. One of the most important advances in drug therapy today involves the introduction of new delivery systems. Specific precautions and timing issues are critical to the success of products with particular delivery systems. For example, the Norplant contraceptive requires certain precautions to ensure its safety and efficacy.

Some medications can be administered through a variety of delivery systems. For example, anti-anginals (medications for chest pain of angina), such as nitrates, are available as inhalants, sublingual tablets, translingual sprays, transmucosal tablets, topical ointments, transdermal nitroglycerine patches, and sustained-release oral nitroglycerine. To maximize the benefits of each preparation, and to ensure its safe use, be sure you are given specific instructions on how to use your drug dosage forms.

For example, nitroglycerine inhalants should be used only when lying down. In contrast, sublingual tablets should be dissolved under the tongue—but not crushed, chewed, or swallowed. Transmucosal tablets should be placed between the upper lip and the gum above the front teeth, or between the cheek and the gum. Topical nitroglycerine ointments must be applied in a uniform layer over a certain skin area of the chest or back, whereas transdermal nitroglycerine patches require rotation in order to avoid undue skin irritation.

Medications that should not be crushed, chewed, or divided include Glucotrol XL, a drug used to lower blood sugar in noninsulin-requiring diabetics. It should be swallowed whole. You should not be alarmed if the tablet shell appears in the stool, since this delivery system is designed to release the medicine slowly and then expel the empty shell from the body.

Information pertaining to drug delivery should be discussed thoroughly, and you should follow instructions step-by-step in order to maximize the potential benefits of the medication under discussion.

What are the precise chemical ingredients of the medication?

Knowing the precise chemical ingredients is an essential prerequisite for evaluating your drug regimen. Although most medications consist of a single chemical ingredient, a sig-

nificant percentage of formulations—both prescription and nonprescription—currently available are so-called combination drugs, comprising two or more active ingredients. Because each ingredient in a combination drug is capable of producing its own side effects, drug interactions, and so forth—as well as benefits—it is essential that your physician provide you with information that breaks down any combination medication you are taking into its respective primary ingredients. If you are experiencing side effects while taking a combination drug, it may be that these problems are caused by only one of the ingredients contained in the formulation, but not the other. If this is the case, your doctor will have the option of trying you on some other medication that excludes the problematic ingredient.

Combination products are frequently used to treat conditions such as asthma, bronchitis, infections, high blood pressure, and chronic pain. For example, antihypertensive drug combinations include the following "link-ups":

- Thiazide diuretics and beta-blockers
- Thiazide diuretics and ACE inhibitors
- Calcium channel blockers and ACE inhibitors
- Thiazide diuretics and clonidine

These "fixed-dose" combination products (with so much of one drug and so much of another) may present several problems.

You simply may not need all the components

in the product. Perhaps only one of them is actually providing the benefits. Or you may need all the components, but in different strengths or at different dosing intervals. The risk of drug-drug and drug-disease incompatibilities is also increased because of multiple ingredients.

Combination products are frequently used to treat minor viral respiratory conditions in children. An asthma drug may contain a stimulating xanthine derivative as well as a sympathomimetic drug that widens the bronchial airways to permit easier breathing. In contrast, a combination used to treat upper respiratory symptoms may include a decongestant, an antihistamine, an analgesic, or an anticholinergic drug. A cough preparation may include an antitussive (cough suppressant) or expectorant as well as ingredients to relieve other symptoms. Any or all of the ingredients in these combinations have the potential to produce side effects.

Because of the potential problems, I generally advise *against* using combination medications unless absolutely necessary.

☺ *Are lifestyle and dietary considerations crucial factors in determining the effectiveness of the medication?*

Consumption of alcoholic beverages, sun exposure, and nonprescription drug use may all affect the efficiency of many medications. You can maximize the safety and effectiveness of your medications by adhering to lifestyle habits that are appropriate for them. These lifestyle activities will vary from one medication to another. For example:

- It is preferable to avoid aspirin and alcoholic beverages if you are taking a nonsteroidal anti-inflammatory drug (NSAID). Moreover, NSAIDs should be taken with food, milk, or antacids to reduce gastric irritation. NSAIDs can cause sensitivity to sunlight, and therefore prolonged exposure should be avoided. You should use sunscreens and wear protective clothing until you determine your level of tolerance.

- A strategy for preventing hypoglycemia can improve the effectiveness of antidiabetic agents (insulin preparations and oral sulfonylureas such as Glucotrol and DiaBeta). Diabetic patients should be encouraged to understand the symptoms of low blood sugar levels, to eat a healthful diet and not miss meals, and to monitor their blood sugar levels to see whether dosing adjustments might be required.

- Mood-elevating medications of the monoamine oxidase inhibitor (MAOI) class should not be taken with tyramine-containing foods. Foods with high tyramine content have the capacity to produce significant increases in blood pressure in patients who are taking MAOIs. You should also avoid consuming alcoholic beverages and excessive amounts of caffeine, using narcotics such as meperidine (Demerol), and self-medicating with cold, hay fever, or weight-reducing medications.

FIRST, DO NO HARM

In summary, a number of issues must be clarified before you start taking a drug. The two most important potential considerations are: Will the drug cause harm if used in combination with other medications you are taking? And will the drug cause harm in the presence of underlying illnesses from which you may suffer? The following list summarizes the conditions, concerns, and criteria for drug safety that you should bring up with your physician before starting a medication.

MEDICATION PRECAUTIONS CHECKLIST

____ What class of drug is it?

____ Is the drug indicated for my condition?

____ What is its success rate in my condition?

____ Is it being used for off-label purposes? If so, why?

____ Are there medical conditions for which this drug should not be used?

____ Is this a primary drug used to treat my problem, or is it an alternative medication?

____ Are special dosing and timing considerations involved with this drug?

____ What are the most common side effects I should watch out for?

____ Will I develop a tolerance or build up a resistance to the effects of this medication?

____ Can it cause physical dependence or addiction?

____ Does it have any transient or first-dose effects that I should be aware of?

____ Are there any special contra-indications or warnings about this drug?

____ Does it have any interactions with prescription or OTC medications that may be harmful?

____ Do we need to schedule lab tests to monitor any of the effects it may be having on my body?

____ How should I discontinue the drug, if necessary?

____ Are there significant withdrawal symptoms if I discontinue it suddenly?

____ Is this the safest drug in its class for my condition?

____ Are brand interchanges permitted?

____ Is the prescription itself written accurately and legibly?

____ Is this the safest, most effective, and convenient form and delivery system for this medication?

____ Does the drug contain multiple chemical ingredients? If so, what are they?

____ Are there any dietary incompatibilities with this medication?

____ Can it be taken during pregnancy? Up to what trimester?

____ Can it be taken while breast-feeding?

CHAPTER 24

GETTING THE BEST PRESCRIPTION DRUGS FOR YOU AND YOUR FAMILY

Implementing and Evaluating the 12-Week Action Plan

In this chapter you will learn about specific approaches to streamlining your regimen. Armed with the Action Plan Checklists you completed in Chapter 23, and by referring to the MedRANK Checklists in Part II, you will be ready to guide your physician toward a medication program that will prevent disease, improve the quality of your life, and reduce your overall health care costs.

To achieve these goals step-by-step, you will need to know all the options that are available for refining and customizing a drug regimen. These options include:

- Simplifying your regimen by introducing medications with more convenient dosing and that require a shorter duration of therapy
- Eliminating unnecessary, inappropriate, suboptimal, and relatively unsafe prescription and over-the-counter drugs

- Reducing the dose of your current medications, if possible and appropriate
- Replacing inferior drugs with superior ones
- Consolidating your regimen with versatile "smart" drugs that permit you to take fewer pills and yet accomplish the same objectives

....

A TEAM APPROACH

Although collaboration and communication with your doctor are keys to success, two cautionary notes are worth mentioning. First, it is important that you reassure your physician that your intention is *not* to prescribe medications for yourself, nor to be the architect of your drug regimen. You are not interested in practicing medicine on yourself! Rather, you should make it clear that your goal is to pro-

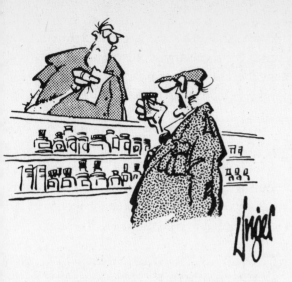

"Are there any side effects to these pills apart from bankruptcy?"

vide useful information that, you hope, will *help* your physician make medication choices more tailored to your needs. You also need to make it clear that you are willing to *cooperate* in a *collaborative* plan to meet this goal. The terms of cooperation include an agreement between you and your physician that when an attempt is made to eliminate, delete, or replace a medication, you will follow the Action Plan as directed and immediately report any concerns, unpleasant side effects, or deterioration in your health.

The second cautionary note is that if you have more than one physician, all of them should be informed about any changes in your medication regimen resulting from this Action Plan. Usually your primary care physician will be the person who facilitates your drug elimination and replacement program, and it is perfectly natural for him or her to call your other physicians to consult about

possible changes. On occasion, it may not be possible for your primary practitioner to coordinate all of your prescriptions. If this is the case, any other doctors participating in your care should write prescriptions only in their area of specialty; each practitioner should also notify the others when medications are added, changed, replaced, or deleted. In addition, all medications should be filled at one pharmacy. This will reduce the likelihood that multiple or duplicate medications will be prescribed for the same medical problem.

GETTING STARTED

The tools for embarking on the 12-Week Action Plan are now in your possession. The basic strategies, specific drug information, and preparation techniques have been outlined in previous chapters. You should complete the Action Plan Checklists and present them to your physician in order to target possible modifications, additions, and substitutions to your drug regimen.

But since every patient is different, your Action Plan must be tailored to your specific health needs. You will want to consult—and even study—the drug rankings in Part II of this book for detailed information about various medical conditions, specific drug options, prevention strategies, and lifestyle changes that are of special importance. The MedRANK Checklists identify versatile drugs, user-friendly medications, and drug-interaction problems that apply to various disease groups, as well as specific recommendations for almost anything that ails you. The information and recommendations are presented in a format that is easily incorporated into the Action Plan.

☺ *How rapidly can these medication changes be made?*

A twelve-week period is generally required to implement, monitor, and fully evaluate the impact of any single drug withdrawal, replacement, or addition. Twelve weeks is a prudent and conservative period. It is unusual that anyone would need more than twelve weeks to assess the full impact of a medication change. In some cases, however, your physician may feel comfortable moving along more quickly and, let's say, making a major medication modification within a ten-week or six-week or even two-week time span. If he or she explains clearly why this accelerated pace is justified and you are happy with the explanation, you should go along with the recommendation.

One final introductory comment: Never hesitate to ask for reassurance if you have any reluctance about changing your regimen. There are a number of things you should know that will prepare you for this program. First, just because you are feeling fine on your medications now doesn't mean that your regimen is safe or appropriate for your needs. Problems may surface quietly and gradually —or suddenly and without warning. As discussed in previous chapters, about 25 percent of people 65 or older are currently taking medications inappropriate for their age and health status. Many of these individuals may not even notice any problems until something unexpected and dramatic happens—they fall and break their hip because a drug caused excessive sedation; or they have gastrointestinal bleeding from an NSAID; or they develop congestive heart failure due to a calcium channel blocker. Constant reevaluation of your drug regimen is the only way to ensure that you are deriving maximal benefits, at the lowest possible risk, from it.

KEEP IT SIMPLE

Keep it simple. As straightforward as this may sound, the sad fact is that many practitioners neglect the real-world convenience—or as the case may be, inconvenience—factors that determine whether patients will take their drugs as prescribed. As we have seen, noncompliance increases the risk that your physician will add drugs to your program; conversely, good compliance is an important way to minimize your total medication burden. To this end, streamlining a drug regimen is the most effective way to enhance compliance with it.

Simplification takes many forms, from instituting once-daily dosing and reducing daily pill consumption, to implementing the Universal Compliance Precautions on page 359, to emphasizing one-dose or short-duration therapies. Issues that you should discuss with your physician to simplify your drug regimen are listed here.

ACTION PLAN CHECKLIST FOR SIMPLIFYING YOUR DRUG REGIMEN

- Reduce the total number of pills you have to take on a daily basis.
- Reduce the total number of prescription ingredients in your regimen.
- Construct your regimen using once-daily medications that can be taken together at the same time of day.
- Decrease the number of times per day that drugs have to be taken.
- Avoid medications with complex dosing schedules.
- Avoid medications that require special precautions (like food intake).
- Avoid medications known to produce drug interactions.

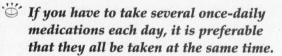 *If you have to take several once-daily medications each day, it is preferable that they all be taken at the same time.*

In addition, medications that require special precautions related to food intake or other factors should be avoided. One of the most important simplification techniques is to consider the Universal Compliance Precautions. These are steps that your physician should take to improve your compliance. Such precautions are necessary because it is very difficult to predict which patients will and which patients will not take their medications as prescribed. Consequently, the most prudent approach is to assume that all patients, including you, are poorly compliant.

UNIVERSAL COMPLIANCE PRECAUTIONS

- Use one-daily medications.
- Use short-duration therapy whenever possible.
- Use one-dose therapy if available.
- Educate the consumer regarding the medication and its side effects.
- Prescribe drugs with tolerable side effects.
- Arrange for follow-up visits to ensure the drug is working.

ELIMINATE PILLS THAT DON'T WORK

First and foremost, it's important not to eliminate medications that you need. Make it clear to your physician during your first visit that you would like him or her to eliminate only those medications that can be discontinued without adversely affecting your health. For the Action Plan, start with those drugs that have a very low probability of producing clinical deterioration if they are deleted from the regimen.

If you bring your Action Plan Checklists to your physician and present possible options for modifying your drug regimen, and your physician either disapproves or approves of specific changes, be sure you are offered credible reasons why.

Ask your doctor to prioritize which medications he or she thinks are most suitable for elimination or replacement. For some drugs, the original indications may have changed. Drugs that are no longer useful can be discontinued without adverse effects. Your practitioner should rank your drug list according to: (a) medications that can potentially be harmful; (b) drugs that, although they pose no harm, may not have worked as well as expected; and (c) drugs that, according to current standards, are obsolete (such as many generic medications) and ought to be replaced with better and more user-friendly medications.

Sometimes a drug can be eliminated because new clinical studies have shown that it really isn't as useful as originally suspected. For example, dipyrimadole (Persantine) is still widely used to prevent stroke and heart attacks, even though studies show that it isn't even as good as aspirin for these purposes. This rather costly medication can be discontinued in virtually all patients who are taking it. (A minor exception is that the drug may have some benefit for those with mechanical heart valves.)

A number of additional categories of medications (antiseizure drugs, heart pills, asthma drugs, the benzodiazepines, and the selective serotonin-reuptake inhibitors) deserve special attention when we are considering which medications to eliminate.

 When to stop: Antiseizure medications. The long-term use of antiseizure medications also is fiercely debated, especially since many of these drugs can produce very unpleasant side effects. Clearly, the majority of patients derive important benefits from them. Yet it is estimated that four million people in this country today who are taking the antiseizure drug Dilantin are excellent candidates for discontinuation. It should be stressed that blood levels of antiseizure medications should be carefully monitored by the physician and that any attempts to stop these drugs or reduce their dose should be made only under close medical supervision.

The most important group of seizure patients in whom drug discontinuation may be feasible are individuals who have had a long-standing diagnosis of an idiopathic (no specific cause can be identified) *seizure disorder, but who have been* free of any actual seizure episodes for more than three to five years *while taking Dilantin or any other anti-epilepsy drug.*

Remember, this is a select group of patients with mild epilepsy of unknown cause, who have been seizure free for a long time. Studies show that among patients in this select group, those who have their Dilantin discontinued are no more likely to experience a recurrence of their epilepsy than those who remain on it. Since the recurrence rate in this select group appears to be the same whether patients are on or off the drug, elimination of the medication appears to be well justified.

In children the relapse rate after medication withdrawal is about 20 to 35 percent, and it is 30 to 65 percent in adults. What this means is that 65 to 80 percent of eligible children who have their seizure medications eliminated, and 35 to 70 percent of adults, remain seizure free after permanent discontinuation of their antiseizure medications. (For additional options that can be applied to a wide range of neurological conditions, see Chapter 11.)

☼ *Heart stoppers: the cardiovascular drugs. Drugs used to treat irregular heart rhythms are some of the most dramatic examples of medications that potentially can be eliminated.*

Excellent studies show their lack of benefit in many patients and, in some cases, their increased risk for causing life-threatening complications. If you or a family member is taking a drug used to treat an irregular heart rhythm —these conditions are known as arrhythmias and the drugs are called anti-arrhythmics— you should consult with your physician to see whether it is absolutely needed.

Before the potential dangers of these anti-arrhythmic medications were fully appreciated, many older patients with irregular heartbeats known as premature ventricular contractions (PVCs) were started on these drugs, sometimes almost with impunity. Eventually cardiologists learned that these irregular beats were a normal part of the aging process and didn't pose any real health danger to patients. But the drugs *did.* Some of them even doubled the risk of sudden death in patients for whom they were prescribed. Consequently, if you or a family member have had an anti-arrhythmic drug started for a nonlife-threatening rhythm disturbance, the chances are excellent that the drug can be discontinued. Anti-arrhythmic drugs that require reevaluation for possible elimination include encainide, flecainide, quinidine, Norpace, Cordarone, Quinaglute, Mexitil, Tambocor, and many others.

☼ *Studies also show that up to 40 percent of people with a regular heart rhythm who have been on digoxin (Lanoxin) for many years, and have never had a documented bout of congestive heart failure, can be discontinued without adverse consequences.*

It is estimated that 6 million Americans may fall into this category, and you or your family member may be one of them. If you are on digoxin, consult with your physician to see whether you are a good candidate for a noninvasive test called an echocardiogram, which will confirm or dispel your need for this medication.

As mentioned earlier, there are numerous opportunities for streamlining and simplifying drug regimens for heart problems. If this is one of your Action Plan goals, evaluate the opportunities discussed in Chapter 5.

☼ *Waiting to exhale: the asthma medications. In many cases, certain medications can be eliminated because less harmful, less toxic, and less quality-of-life-impairing ones are available that produce equivalent results.*

For example, many asthmatics still take a medication called theophylline in order to reduce wheezing and improve their shortness of breath. This is unfortunate because theophylline and a similar medication, terbutaline, are known to produce a wide range of side effects, including nausea, shakiness, and stomach discomfort. When taken in high doses, these drugs can even produce life-threatening complications such as seizures and cardiac arrest. Although theophylline may be useful for very ill patients in the emergency room, for routine therapy, inhalers containing beta-agonists or corticosteroids are much *less toxic* and *more effective*. If you have asthma and have been put on theophylline without trying an inhaler first, you should talk to your physician and see whether it might be appropriate to replace the theophylline with a metered-dose inhaler.

☺ *Unfortunately, even inhalers are over-used, which means it may be possible to eliminate or reduce their use in selected patients as well.*

For example, an asthmatic may be prescribed an inhaler containing one ingredient, such as a beta-agonist, to open his or her airways. If the patient fails to improve with this first inhaler, the practitioner may prescribe another inhaler containing a different active ingredient—usually a steroid medication. Although on the surface it appears as if the second inhaler is needed, the prescription for the second inhaler is frequently unnecessary. Studies show that about one-third of patients don't get the full benefit of their inhalers simply because they haven't been instructed in how to *use* them properly. In fact, some people use these little handheld devices as if they were breath fresheners or room deodorizers and never get the full dose into their airways.

Consequently, if you are using more than one inhaler for your lung condition, especially asthma or bronchitis, it is possible that one of them can be eliminated. An inhaler that delivers steroid medications is your best bet for eliminating the need for other asthma medica-

tions. This should be your main protection against recurrent episodes of asthma. But to take the best advantage of inhaled steroids, you probably should consult your doctor to be sure you are using it correctly.

☺ *Calming down with the benzodi-azepines. Drugs used to treat anxiety, insomnia, and panic disorders require special caution.*

Sedative medications and so-called mild tranquilizers or hypnotics belonging to the benzodiazepine class initially should be prescribed for short durations only. These "Valley of the Dolls" medications, including Xanax, Ativan, Halcion, Restoril, and Valium, have the potential to become physically addicting. Consequently, if you are taking one of them, you should consult with your physician and, as part of the Action Plan, review the original reason for starting the medication. Unless there are compelling reasons to continue taking it, gradual discontinuation should strongly be considered, using strategies outlined below.

The benzodiazepines are very popular drugs. It is estimated that currently about 18 million Americans are taking Xanax or similar medications to treat anxiety and panic-related conditions. It should be stressed that some people, especially those with disabling panic attacks, require treatment with drugs such as Xanax, which has been proven to be effective for this disorder. Although the optimal length of treatment for panic disorder has not been established, it is reasonable to consider discontinuing this drug under a doctor's supervision after six to eighteen months of effective therapy (that is, no panic attacks). After someone has been free of disabling symptoms for at least six months, there are many reasons to consider stopping the drug, including the possibility of physical addiction and the fact that treatment may no longer be necessary. Although you might question discontinuing treatment with a drug that has been shown to be effective, the potential side effects, expense, risk of dependence, and long-term inconvenience justify attempts at discontinuation.

 ### *Anxiety-reducing drugs such as the benzodiazepines have a long and troubled history.*

Because so many people cling to them as antidotes to the edginess of modern life, the decision to discontinue their use can be difficult. After all, people frequently take these sedative-hypnotics for many years and come to depend on them for psychological and emotional stability. They often start them in response to short-term situational crises, but then the drugs become permanent fixtures in their lives. Oftentimes, a patient is unaware that physical or psychological addiction has occurred and may pressure the physician into long-term therapy. These cases are difficult to manage because the patient believes that the medication is still required for symptomatic relief even though it isn't. In addition, the doctor may be reluctant to discontinue a drug that has the potential for producing withdrawal symptoms.

 Without exception, the decision to discontinue any of the benzodiazepines should be a mutual one between you and your doctor. In many cases, discontinuing benzodiazepines can be accomplished without adverse consequences, but it is critical that you taper the medication slowly and gradually to minimize withdrawal symptoms.

Studies show that if these drugs are discontinued abruptly, almost 50 percent of patients experience recurrent anxiety, whereas less than 10 percent experience uncomfortable symptoms if the drugs are tapered gradually over a three- to six-month period. People are better able to tolerate discontinuation of benzodiazepines such as alprazolam, Valium, and Halcion if they know what to expect. If you do experience anxiety or panic symptoms during the discontinuation phase, be assured that they are not life-threatening and will usually go away within a few days.

 Ups and downs: the selective serotonin-reuptake inhibitors (SSRIs). Few drug classes have received as much attention or been as widely used across so many segments of society as the antidepressants belonging to the class of selective serotonin-reuptake inhibitors.

Prozac. Zoloft. Paxil. The names of these drugs have become household words. An estimated 26 million Americans now take antidepressants on a daily basis. Virtually every family has an immediate member or a friend who has had experience with one of these drugs.

With these user-friendly SSRIs, however, patterns of antidepressant use have changed dramatically. More and more, drugs such as Prozac and Zoloft are being used to treat panic disorders, the dysphoria associated with premenstrual syndrome, obsessive-compulsive disorders, and chronic anxiety, as well as other distressing syndromes associated with the trials of modern life. With so many people taking these drugs, it has become increasingly difficult to determine which individuals have a bona-fide depressive illness that requires long-term maintenance treatment and which can be discontinued once their situational crisis is resolved.

Even though the criteria for discontinuing these medications are controversial, some windows of opportunity and vulnerability can be identified. Generally speaking, depressive episodes—which are characterized by symptoms such as fatigue, low energy, crying spells, impaired concentration, withdrawal from social groups, low self-esteem, and inability to sleep—extend over a lifetime. For the majority of people, the risk of having future episodes of depression increases as the number of past episodes increases. Moreover, the length of the stay-well interval between episodes becomes progressively shorter. People who are older at the onset of their depression have a higher probability of future relapse if they are not maintained on drug therapy. As the number of episodes of depression grows and the person becomes older, their severity will often intensify and the benefits of medication may diminish or disappear. Fortunately, this destructive lifetime pattern can be modified in many, if not most, people who suffer from depression since antidepressants are effective in preventing most future episodes and preserving quality of life.

So what does this mean for you or for others you may know who have been taking these popular medications? Naturally, the decision to discontinue an antidepressant should take place in collaboration with your doctor as part of the Action Plan. And while most people on these drugs should probably not shift toward discontinuation, there are patients who clearly will do just as well without them.

Given the lifetime patterns associated with depressive illness, the most prudent philosophy is to consider discontinuation only in patients who were put on these medications for treatment of situational stress, mild panic attacks, or short-term anxiety-related problems. In contrast, lifetime maintenance is generally indicated for people who are 50 or older when they experience their first episode of depression; for those who are 40 or older who have had two or more prior episodes of depression; and for those with three or more episodes of depression in their lifetime, regardless of age. If discontinuation is attempted, the safest and most successful approach is to reduce the dosage by about 25 percent every three months.

☺ *Discontinuation of unnecessary medications is a cornerstone of the Action Plan.*

Your process of drug elimination should begin with a careful review of your current medication list. There are many indications for cessation of medications, all of which deserve careful consideration. Please fill out the following Action Plan Checklist, and review the opportunities that are available to you.

ACTION PLAN CHECKLIST FOR DRUG ELIMINATION

(Place a check mark if any of these situations apply to you or you are taking any of these drugs.)

....

- You were originally put on the medication for inadequate or marginal reasons. Examples include:

  ____ Digoxin
  ____ Valium
  ____ Cytotec
  ____ Tagamet
  ____ Blood pressure medications
  ____ Zantac
  ____ Sedatives
  ____ Theophylline

- You may be taking a drug that is no longer required. Examples include:

  ____ Tagamet
  ____ Zantac
  ____ Pepcid
  ____ NSAIDs
  ____ Antibiotics
  ____ Sleeping medications
  ____ Muscle relaxants
  ____ Seldane
  ____ Claritin
  ____ Hismanal

- New studies may show that a medication is not useful for the condition for which it was once thought effective. Examples include:

  ____ Persantine (dipyridamole)

  ____ Theophylline
  ____ Isoxuprine
  ____ Hydergine

- Less toxic and safer agents with fewer side effects may produce equivalent results. Examples for which better drugs may be available include:

  ____ Theophylline
  ____ Indomethacin
  ____ Benadryl
  ____ Amitriptyline
  ____ Valium
  ____ Verapamil
  ____ Erythromycin
  ____ Augmentin
  ____ Propranolol
  ____ Chlorpropamide
  ____ Ketoconazole
  ____ Diltiazem

- Your medical condition has been stable for a long time, and continued drug therapy may no longer be necessary. Examples include:

  ____ Dilantin
  ____ Steroids
  ____ NSAIDs
  ____ Tagamet
  ____ Zantac
  ____ Pepcid
  ____ Blood pressure medications
  ____ Theophylline
  ____ Anticonvulsants

- Less expensive, equally effective medications may be available. Examples include:

  ____   Ticlopidine
  ____   Persantine

- You are not taking a medication as prescribed, and therefore it is not producing good clinical results. Examples include:

  ____   Cholestyramine
  ____   Pentoxifylline
  ____   NSAIDs
  ____   Propranolol

As this checklist suggests, you may be able to discontinue some medications simply because the indications for starting them were questionable or insufficient in the first place.

••

HOW LOW CAN YOU GO: REDUCE YOUR DOSAGES

As part of your 12-Week Action Plan, you should also fill out the following Action Plan Checklist. It lists commonly used medications that have been shown to produce excellent therapeutic results at lower doses than originally recommended. If you are taking any of the drugs in this checklist, be sure to check with your physician that you are taking the drug at the lowest and safest effective dose.

ACTION PLAN CHECKLIST FOR DOSE REDUCTION

(Place a check mark if you are taking any of these drugs.)

••

  ____   Aspirin
  ____   Warfarin
  ____   Hydrochlorothiazide
  ____   ACE inhibitors
  ____   Antidepressants
  ____   AZT
  ____   Steroids
  ____   Coumadin
  ____   Heparin
  ____   Beta-agonist inhalers
  ____   Misoprostol
  ____   Synthroids
  ____   Prozac
  ____   Halcion
  ____   Diuretics
  ____   Cimetidine
  ____   NSAIDs
  ____   Digoxin
  ____   Zoloft

Medications amenable to dose reduction include those used to treat a number of common illnesses.

At one time physicians believed that, in patients with irregular heart rhythms (atrial fibrillation), stroke, and blockage in the deep veins of the leg, prevention of blood clots required the blood-thinning medication Coumadin (warfarin). The intent was to double the normal bleeding time. Since then we have learned that excellent results are achievable if the bleeding time is increased by only 30 to 50 percent. Reducing the dose of Coumadin maintains its therapeutic efficacy but dramatically reduces its potentially devastating hemorrhagic complications.

Because consumption of vitamin K–rich vegetables can affect this drug's action, patients who are taking it require regular monitoring of their blood-clotting time in order to ensure that their dose is in the appropriate range. Interestingly, the Coumadin dose-reduction saga is still in progress. More studies are under way to see whether even lower doses can be used without compromising its therapeutic effects. Accordingly, if you or a family member is taking Coumadin, you should check with your physician that you are taking the low dose currently in vogue.

Given the widespread use of antidepressants across many demographic groups and patient populations, determining their appropriate dosage is a particularly vexing problem. Prior to their release, these drugs and their dosage levels were never widely tested in people who, from a psychological perspective, resemble the millions of normal, nonclinically depressed Americans who now eat a breakfast that includes coffee, a croissant, and a Prozac. Quite the contrary: Initial trials evaluating dosage requirements for Zoloft, Prozac, and Paxil were conducted in individuals who were diagnosed as having a major affective disorder. In other words, dosage levels were determined based on mood improvements in patients who had suffered a major episode of clinical depression. These drugs are now widely used in patients who would never have qualified for entry into these original studies.

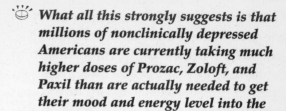 **What all this strongly suggests is that millions of nonclinically depressed Americans are currently taking much higher doses of Prozac, Zoloft, and Paxil than are actually needed to get their mood and energy level into the comfort zone.**

Both the medical literature and the lay press— the best-selling book *Listening to Prozac* drives home the point—have documented the pervasive use of antidepressants in young and middle-aged individuals who complain of chronic anxiety, lack of energy, and mild sleep disturbances. Although the majority of these individuals would not satisfy the criteria for a major affective disorder (like clinical depression), they nevertheless are being treated with SSRI antidepressants—and at doses, most experts believe, that are too high.

Another factor explaining the excessively high doses of these drugs is the fact that it takes at least six weeks— and sometimes much longer—for these medications to produce the desired effects.

Many practitioners fail to wait this long before adjusting the dose of the drug; instead they prescribe higher doses before the impact of the lower dose can be adequately assessed. You should be aware that although the antidepressants in the SSRI class are generally well tolerated, they are not entirely free of troublesome side effects, including edginess, tremors, shakiness, diarrhea, sedation, insomnia, and sexual dysfunction.

The implications are clear: Prozac-like drugs are being prescribed in many patients at inappropriately high doses. And you may be one of the victims. If you do not meet the strict criteria for a major affective disorder such as depression yet your physician has prescribed Prozac, Zoloft, or Paxil for you in order to treat a mood disturbance or medical condition, you should consult with your doctor as part of the Action Plan. In particular, you should investigate whether your antidepressant dose could be reduced by as much as 50 percent while still maintaining its mood-enhancing benefits. (For other opportunities to eliminate drugs or reduce dosages for medications used to treat mood disorders, anxiety, panic attacks, and depression, refer to Chapter 7.)

TWO AGAINST ONE

One of the most difficult issues in designing a drug regimen is whether it's better to stick with *one* drug at a *high* dose or to use *two* drugs at a much *lower* dose to get the job done. There are many factors to be considered. First of all, generally speaking, troublesome side effects are a function of increasing drug dose. Consequently, if your medications are being used at the maximal dosage permitted by the manufacturer, any unusual symptoms or complaints you may be having could be drug-related side effects. And because side effects tend to be dose-related, it is frequently difficult to decide which is better: to stay on the high dose of a single medication or to take two drugs at the lowest recommended dose.

The two-drug approach has the benefit of producing good results at *low* doses. On the other hand, a two-drug regimen may incur the additional *cost* of two prescriptions instead of one. In the end, the decision will depend on a number of factors, including side effects, cost, and compliance patterns. Whatever decision is made, you should be part of the process.

ALERT FOR THE ELDERLY

As helpful as physicians can be in refining drug treatment, the elderly, not infrequently, are their own worst enemies when it comes to medication use. Two years ago, while touring a skilled care facility for the aged, I encountered two elderly men playing poker. They were using their pills as gambling chips. One of the men pushed a medication capsule into the center of the table and said, "I'll see your two Valium, and raise you three Zoloft!" I have given you fair warning: Elderly Americans—and their physicians—occasionally gamble with their prescription medications.

If you or a family member is 65 or older, you can screen your drug regimen for possible problems by filling out the following two Action Plan Checklists. The first offers a comprehensive list of prescription drugs that are considered inappropriate or less-than-optimal for older individuals because better, safer medications are available that will accomplish the same goal.

ACTION PLAN CHECKLIST
FOR INAPPROPRIATE MEDICATIONS FOR THE ELDERLY

(Place a check mark if you are taking any of these drugs.)

____ Valium	____ NSAIDs	____ Ketoprofen
____ Dalmane	____ Meprobamate	____ Chlorpropamide
____ Librium	____ Pentobarbital	____ Propoxyphene
____ Muscle relaxants	____ Amitriptyline	____ Pentazocine
____ Benadryl	____ Doxepin	____ Cyclandelate
____ Aldomet	____ Propranolol	____ Isoxuprine
____ Reserpine	____ Indomethacin	____ Persantine
____ Verapamil	____ Ibuprofen	____ Theophylline
____ Terbutaline	____ Cimetidine	____ Seldane
____ Hismanal	____ Cyclobenzaprine	____ Orphenadrine
____ Methocarbamol	____ Carisoprodol	____ Trimethobenzamide

The following checklist identifies specific drugs that may have to be used in the elderly but are known to cause behavioral changes, mental slowing, or sedation—hence the term "mental manglers"—in individuals residing in chronic, skilled care nursing facilities.

ACTION PLAN CHECKLIST
FOR "MENTAL MANGLERS"

____ Halcion	____ Cimetidine	____ Reserpine
____ Restoril	____ Propranolol	____ Lithium
____ Ativan	____ Catapres	____ Tegretol
____ Valium	____ Narcotics (opioids)	____ Hypoglycemic drugs
____ Librium	____ Aspirin	____ Barbiturates
____ Dalmane	____ Anti-Parkinson's	____ Chloral hydrate
____ Navane	drugs	____ Meprobamate
____ Mellaril	____ Antispasmodics	____ Glutethimide
____ Thorazine	____ Elavil (amitriptyline)	____ Scopolamine
____ Haldol	____ Doxepin	
____ Benadryl	____ Beta-blockers	

....

REPLACE QUESTIONABLE DRUGS WITH BETTER ONES

Life never stands still. Your body is constantly changing over time, being affected by aging, alterations in your environment, emotional maturation, and so forth. Therefore, a drug that works predictably and reliably today may or may not promote the same bodily effects next month or next year. Some drugs may initially be well tolerated and produce no complications, but after several weeks or months, they may produce significant problems or toxicity. These medication "time bombs" can be hard to detect, as can drugs whose effectiveness gradually diminishes over time.

The following checklist shows a few drugs that may cause complications after long-term therapy. Place a check by any of them that you may be taking, and consult your physician or pharmacist.

ACTION PLAN CHECKLIST FOR MEDICATION TIME BOMBS

Medication (Primary Uses)	Possible Complications
____ NSAID (arthritis pain, muscle or joint strains)	Bleeding, kidney problems
____ Aspirin (heart attack and stroke prevention)	Bleeding
____ Redux (weight loss)	Lung disease
____ Coumadin (blood thinner, clot prevention)	Bleeding
____ Anti-arrhythmics (irregular heart rates)	Irregular heart rhythms, low blood pressure
____ Accutane (serious acne)	Visual disturbances, sight loss
____ Cognex (Alzheimer's disease)	Liver problems
____ Methotrexate (arthritis, psoriasis)	Liver problems
____ Ketoconazole (fungus infections)	Liver problems
____ Steroids (inflammatory conditions)	Bone wasting, obesity, infections, acne
____ Effexor (depression)	Elevated blood pressure
____ Nardil (depression)	Food and drug interactions
____ Depakene (seizures)	Liver problems
____ Clozaril (psychotic disorders)	Blood problems (serious)
____ Lithium (manic disorders)	Cardiac, neurological problems, drug interactions
____ Thorazine, Haldol (behavior problems)	Movement disorders

Medication (Primary Uses)	Possible Complications
____ AZT (HIV infection)	Blood disorders (low counts)
____ Stavudine (HIV infection)	Peripheral nerve problems
____ ddI (HIV infection)	Pancreatitis
____ Zalcitibane, ddC (HIV infection)	Neuropathy, pancreatitis, liver disease
____ Rifabutin (anti-infective)	Visual disturbances
____ Seldane (allergies)	Drug interactions, heart disturbances
____ Astemizole (allergies)	Drug interactions, heart disturbances
____ Thiazide diuretics (blood pressure)	Elevated cholesterol levels
____ Estrogen	Endometrial cancer

The following checklist shows medications your physician may be able to discontinue because they are no longer useful or indicated.

ACTION PLAN CHECKLIST FOR DRUGS WITH POSSIBLE DURATION LIMITS

(Place a check mark if you are taking any of these drugs.)

____ Cimetidine	____ Ranitidine	____ Famotidine
____ Nizatidine	____ Restoril	____ Halcion
____ Xanax	____ Valium	____ Librium
____ Prilosec	____ Dilantin	____ Diuretics
____ Antidepressants	____ Steroids	____ Cognex
____ NSAIDs	____ Antibiotics	____ Coumadin

BAD COMPANY: DRUG INTERACTION ALERT

When it comes to drug interactions, the bad news is that they do occur, and on rare occasions, they may even be fatal. The good news is almost all drug interactions can be *prevented*. Prevention first and foremost requires that you and your doctor communicate with each other. Virtually all drug interactions have been recognized and are well documented in drug information resources.

Protecting yourself against drug interactions requires you to tell your doctor or pharmacist if you are currently taking, or if you are planning to take, any over-the-counter or prescription medications in combination with a drug that is being prescribed for you. As previously emphasized, only rarely will a drug interaction be potentially fatal, but on many occasions the doses of one or both drugs may have to be modified, or a different drug may have to be prescribed, in order to prevent potential complications. Interactions can also occur between prescribed medications and alcohol and certain foods. It is crucial to disclose any and all prescription and nonprescription ingredients that you are likely to take in combination with a new drug that is being added to your regimen.

Although all medications have some potential for interactions, certain classes are associated with an increased risk for producing them. These classes of medications include: NSAIDs, digoxin, calcium channel blockers, MAO inhibitors, beta-blockers, antidepressants, anticholinergic medications, sedatives, hypnotics, macrolide antibiotics, antifungal agents, and histamine-2 antagonists such as cimetidine. If you have been taking medications that belong to any of these classes, and a new drug has recently been introduced into your regimen, it would be prudent to consult with your pharmacist or physician to determine whether these drugs pose any risk for interactions.

The following checklist targets medications that have a significant risk of undesirable drug interactions. If you are taking any of them, as part of the Action Plan you should have your physician screen your medications to ensure you are not using any combinations that may interact in harmful ways.

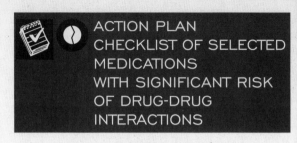

ACTION PLAN
CHECKLIST OF SELECTED
MEDICATIONS
WITH SIGNIFICANT RISK
OF DRUG-DRUG
INTERACTIONS

_____ Tagamet (cimetidine)
_____ Hismanal (astemizole)
_____ Seldane (terfenadine)
_____ Anti-arrhythmics
_____ Erythromycin
_____ Biaxin (clarithromycin)
_____ Antifungal drugs
_____ Lanoxin (digoxin)
_____ Coumadin (warfarin)
_____ NSAIDs
_____ Phenothiazines
_____ Metoprolol/acebutolol/propranolol/ beta-blockers
_____ Verapamil/diltiazem/calcium channel blockers
_____ Benadryl (diphenhydramine)
_____ Atenolol
_____ Quinidine
_____ Elavil/tricyclic antidepressants
_____ Thiazide diuretics
_____ ACE inhibitors
_____ Cipro (quinolone antibiotics)
_____ Nizoral (ketoconazole)
_____ Anticonvulsants
_____ MAO inhibitors
_____ Prozac
_____ Tranquilizers
_____ Corticosteroids
_____ Aspirin
_____ Muscle relaxants
_____ Benzodiazepines

AVOID GENERIC DRUGS

Complete the following checklist in order to identify any generic medications in your regimen that, in most cases, ought to be replaced with better, brand-name drugs. If you are taking more than one of these drugs, you should identify them for your physician during the first (assessment) phase of the Action Plan.

ACTION PLAN CHECKLIST FOR GENERIC MEDICATIONS

____ Verapamil
____ Diltiazem
____ Nifedipine
____ Hydrochlorothiazide
____ Propranolol
____ Clonidine
____ Doxepin
____ Glipizide
____ Reserpine
____ Prazosin
____ Cimetidine
____ Tetracycline
____ Erythromycin
____ Penicillin
____ Trazodone
____ Sulfamethoxazole
____ Methyldopa
____ Hydralazine
____ Amoxicillin
____ Doxycycline
____ Cephalexin
____ Amitriptyline
____ Nortriptyline

CONSOLIDATE YOUR REGIME

Minimizing medications to maximize results is the cornerstone of the Action Plan. To achieve this objective, versatile drugs that are able to treat multiple conditions, symptoms, or diseases are highly useful. Unfortunately, most doctors have not been trained to think in this manner. Consequently, you will likely have to educate your physician about the advantages of versatile drugs and suggest opportunities for using them in your therapeutic program.

Versatile drugs make it possible to reduce the number of prescription drugs you need. They are the smart bombs of the pharmacy, capable of doing more with less and at lower overall cost. Like smart bombs, versatile drugs also travel precisely to their targets and therefore obviate the need for a scattershot approach. And although smart bombs carry a princely price tag, launching a single expensive weapon can be more cost-effective than having to repeatedly use cheaper ones.

Like smart bombs, versatile drugs also have the capacity to target very specific diseases and symptoms. And like smart bombs with multiple warheads, they can hit many targets simultaneously. That is why you want your physician to identify these high-productivity medications: They possess the uncanny ability to treat a number of problems with only one active ingredient.

Versatile drugs can be used to treat a wide range of common conditions, including infections, heart disease, depressive disorders, and prostate problems, among many others. The final result of consolidating your regimen with these drugs is a reduction in your overall pharmacological burden. By using a few versatile drugs, you will decrease your risk of drug interactions, reduce your spending on drug therapy, and improve your compliance.

There are numerous examples of versatile drugs that you will want to bring to the attention of your physician. Stated simply, versatile drugs are the best drugs, and if you have the appropriate indications for their use, you will want to take advantage of them. Many of them are listed in the following Action Plan Checklist. Review this checklist very carefully: If you see drugs that match up with your medical problems, you should call your physician's attention to the possibilities of replacing dumb drugs with smarter agents.

ACTION PLAN CHECKLIST FOR VERSATILE DRUGS

Versatile Drug	Conditions Treated
Azithromycin (antibiotic)	Covers the most likely bacteria that are responsible for bronchitis, pneumonia, sinusitis, ear infections in children, and skin infections.
Amlodipine	Treats high blood pressure and chest pain caused by heart disease (angina).
Atenolol	Useful for treating high blood pressure and preventing recurrent heart attacks.

Versatile Drug	Conditions Treated
ACE inhibitors	Useful for people who have diabetes with kidney problems, high blood pressure, and congestive heart failure.
Doxazosin	Will treat high blood pressure and provide symptomatic relief for enlarged prostate glands (benign prostatic hypertrophy), before surgery is indicated. Particularly useful for elderly men who have these problems in combination.
Digoxin	Useful for treating congestive heart failure and the irregular heart rhythm called atrial fibrillation.
Aspirin	In small doses (as little as 80 mg/day), will prevent recurrent heart attacks and stroke.
Estrogen replacement	Prevents heart disease, stroke, osteoporosis, and troublesome post-menopausal symptoms; may even delay the onset of Alzheimer's symptoms in women.
Antidepressants (SSRIs: Zoloft, Prozac, Paxil)	Useful, in carefully selected patients, for treating depression, sleep problems, panic attacks, obsessive-compulsive disorders, and premenstrual dysphoria (sadness and agitation).

Although consolidating your regimen is an essential part of the Action Plan, it should be stressed that streamlining the regimen is not always going to be successful. The fact is, some people simply require two or three or more drugs to manage their complicated medical problems. But they are the exception to the rule. Streamlining will almost always work to some extent. In the majority of cases, consolidation strategies that replace inferior medications with versatile drugs are successful. The best results will be obtained if you work closely with your physician, and if you follow the step-by-step guidelines of the Action Plan.

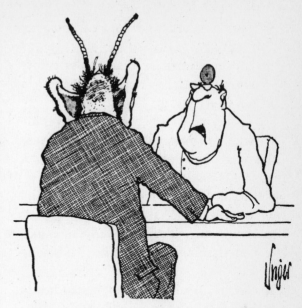

"If you remember, I did mention possible side-effects."

EVALUATING THE ACTION PLAN

The incremental approach to remodeling your drug regimen requires careful monitoring and follow-up. Many parameters, including your blood pressure, symptoms, sleep patterns, energy level, and sexual function, should be followed to assess the impact of the changes. Your physician should monitor objective measurements (as supplied by laboratory tests, electrocardiograms, urinalysis, and the like) related to your condition. You should also follow subjective, quality-of-life parameters that can give a more complete picture of your reconstructed regimen.

To help make these critical evaluations, complete the following checklist for side effects, as well as the four-point Quality of Life survey, both at the beginning and at the end of each twelve-week cycle.

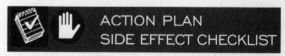

ACTION PLAN
SIDE EFFECT CHECKLIST

(Answer the following questions.)

1. Since being on your current medication program, have you noticed any significant changes in your energy level, zest for life, or desire for social engagement?

   _____

2. Are you sleeping the entire night? ____
3. Has your desire for sex decreased significantly? _____
4. Have you noticed any of the following symptoms: dry mouth, visual disturbances, difficulty voiding, constipation, excessive daytime sleepiness, or light-headedness? _____ If yes, which ones? _____

5. Have you noticed an unexplained cough? _____

6. Have you experienced shakiness, palpitations, anxiety, or rapid heart rate? If yes, which is most troublesome? ____

7. Have you experienced excessive fatigue, lethargy, or lack of energy? If yes, which symptom are you concerned about most? _____

8. Do you still have the desire to engage in hobbies and social activities? _____

9. Have you experienced any unusual, undesirable, or unexplained taste sensations? _____

10. Have you had any unexplained headaches? _____

11. Have you had difficulty concentrating?

12. Have you noticed any of the following gastrointestinal symptoms: burning in your stomach, nausea, constipation, diarrhea, abdominal discomfort, or dark stool? _____ If yes, which troubles you the most? _____

13. Have you noticed any unusual swelling in your legs? _____

14. Have you noticed the appearance of any new skin rashes? _____

15. Are there any medications in your regimen that you feel might be responsible for the symptoms or side effects you have identified in questions 1–14? _____ If yes, which medication(s) do you think might be responsible? _____

16. Are there any medications you are taking that do not agree with you? _____ If yes, which one(s)? _____

17. Has your appetite either increased or decreased significantly? _____

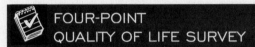

FOUR-POINT QUALITY OF LIFE SURVEY

1. In general, do you feel better or worse than you did before starting your current medication regimen?

2. Do you think you would feel better or worse if you were taken off all your medications?

3. Do you think your quality of life would improve if you were taking smaller doses of your medications?

4. In general, which makes you feel worse: your medical condition or your medications?

Because the step-by-step, pill-by-pill approach to drug regimen reform is gradual, be patient. It may take several weeks or even months to fine-tune your program. But this is a small amount of time considering that you may have to live with your regimen for years to come. In the process, not only will the 12-Week Action Plan produce more durable drug regimens, but you and your doctor will better be able to assess your attitudes and responses to the changes.

—

CLOSING THE INFORMATION GAP

Organizations Providing Information About Medication Use

Administration on Aging
200 Independence Ave., S.W.
Room 309 F
Washington, DC 20201
(202) 401-4543
Fax (202) 401-7741

AIDS Treatment Data Network
611 Broadway, Suite 613
New York, NY 10012-2809
(202) 434-3704
Fax (202) 434-3714

Alexandria Task Force on Elderly and Medications
6034 Richmond Highway, #206
Alexandria, VA 22303
(703) 329-0388

Alzheimer's Association
919 North Michigan Ave.
Suite 1000
Chicago, IL 60611
(312) 335-5786
Fax (312) 335-1110

American Association of Retired Persons (AARP)
601 E St., N.W.
Suite A6-300
Washington, DC 20049
(202) 434-3704
Fax (202) 434-3714

American Cancer Society
1180 Avenue of the Americas
New York, NY 10036
(212) 382-2169
Fax (212) 718-0193

American Dietetic Association
216 West Jackson Blvd.
Suite 300
Chicago, IL 50608-5995
(800) 745-0775
(312) 899-0040, Ext. 4759
Fax (312) 899-1739

American Health Care Association
1201 L Street, N.W.
Washington, DC 20005
(202) 842-4444
Fax (202) 842-3880

American Heart Association
7272 Greenville Ave.
Dallas, TX 75231-4596
(214) 373-6300
Fax (214) 706-1551

American Liver Foundation
1425 Pompton Ave.
Cedar Grove, NJ 07009
(201) 256-2550, ext. 228
Fax (201) 256-3214

American Lung Association
1740 Broadway
New York, NY 10019-4374
(800) LUNG USA
(212) 586-4872

American Pharmaceutical Association
2215 Constitution Ave., N.W.
Washington, DC 20003
(202) 429-7556
Fax (202) 428-0035

Arthritis Foundation
1330 W. Peachtree St.
Atlanta, GA 30309
(800) 283-7800, ext. 6222
Fax (404) 872-8694

Asthma & Allergy
1125 15th St., N.W.
Suite 502
Washington, DC 20017
(202) 486-7643, ext. 229
(202) 466-8940

The Better Sleep Council
1501 L St., N.W.
Suite 300
Washington, DC 20036
(202) 452-9428
Fax (202) 833-2471

Center for Medical Consumers
237 Thompson St.
New York, NY 20036
(212) 674-7105
Fax (212) 674-7100

Citizen Advocacy Center
1424 16th St., N.W.
Suite 203
Washington, DC 20006
(202) 462-1174
Fax (202) 265-6564

Citizens for Public Action on Blood Pressure & Cholesterol
P.O. Box 30374
Bethesda, MD 20824
(301) 770-1711
Fax (301) 770-1713

Epilepsy Foundation of America
4351 Garden City Dr.
Landover, MD 20785
(301) 459-3700
Fax (301) 577-2684

Gay Men's Health Crisis
129 West 20th St.
New York, NY 10011
(718) 351-1717
Fax (718) 667-8893

Lupus Foundation of America
1330 Piccard Dr.
Suite 200
Rockville, MD 20850-4303
(301) 670-9292, ext. 17
(800) 558-0121
Fax (301) 670-9486

Muscular Dystrophy Association
3300 East Sunrise Dr.
Tucson, AZ 87518-3208
(602) 529-2000
Fax (520) 529-5356

National Alliance for the Mentally Ill
200 North Glebe Rd.
Suite 1015
Arlington, VA 22203
(703) 516-7961
Fax (703) 524-9094

National Association of People with AIDS
413 K St., N.W.
7th Floor
Washington, DC 20005
(202) 898-0414
Fax (202) 898-0435

National Black Women's Health Project
1211 Connecticut Ave., N.W.
Suite 310
Washington, DC 20036
(202) 835-0117
Fax (202) 833-8790

National Cholesterol Education Month
P.O. Box 30105
Bethesda, MD 20824-0105
(301) 251-1222
Fax (301) 251-1223

National Condom Week
P.O. Box 30584
Oakland, CA 94504
(510) 891-0455

National Consumers League
1701 K St., N.W.
Suite 1200
Washington, DC 20006
(202) 835-3323
Fax (202) 835-0747

National Council of Advocacy
666 11th St., N.W.
Suite 810
Washington, DC 20001-4542
(202) 347-6711
Fax (202) 638-0773

National Council of Patient Information & Education
666 11th St., N.W.
Suite 810
Washington, DC 20001-4542
(202) 347-6711
Fax (202) 638-0773

National Headache Foundation
428 West St. James Place
Chicago, IL 60614
(800) 543-2256
Fax (312) 525-7357

National Heart, Lung & Blood Institute
P.O. Box 30105
Bethesda, MD 20324
(301) 251-1222
Fax (301) 251-1223

**National Mental Illness
Screening Project**
One Washington St.
Suite 304
Wellesley Hills, MA 02181-1706
(617) 239-0071
Fax (617) 431-7447

**National Women's Health
Network**
514 10th St., N.W.
Suite 400
Washington, DC 20004
(202) 272-3429
Fax (202) 504-2064

**Planned Parenthood Federation
of America**
810 Seventh Ave.
New York, NY 10019
(212) 541-7800
Fax (212) 247-6265

Poison Prevention Week Council
P.O. Box 1543
Washington, DC 20013
(301) 504-0580, ext. 1184
Fax (301) 504-0399

**President's Council on Physical
Fitness & Sports**
701 Pennsylvania Ave., N.W.
Suite 250
Washington, DC 20004
(202) 272-3425
Fax (202) 504-2064

**Public Citizen Health Research
Group**
1600 20th St., N.W.
Washington, DC 20009
(202) 588-1000

**RX Council of Western
Pennsylvania**
1701 Boulevard of the Allies
Suite 301
Pittsburgh, PA 15219

**Sickle Cell Disease Association
of America**
200 Corporate Pointe
Suite 495
Culver City, CA 90230
(310) 216-6363

U.S. Office of Consumer Affairs
50 17th St., N.W.
Suite 650
Washington, DC 20036
(202) 395-7900
Fax (202) 395-7901

APPENDIX B

FIGHTING PHARMA-CITY HALL

If you have questions or concerns about your medications or the availability of specific drugs, or if you would like drug information materials, you may want to contact health plan pharmacists, administrators, or physicians in your state, as listed below.

ALABAMA

Blue Cross/Blue Shield
936 S. 19th St.
Birmingham, AL 35205-3797
(205) 985-5590

Blue Shield/Blue Cross Alabama
450 Riverchase Pkwy. E.
Birmingham, AL 35244-2858
(205) 988-2100

Health Advantage
140 Riverchase Pkwy. E.
Birmingham, AL 35244-1887
(205) 786-0211

Health Choice
P.O. Box 830605
Birmingham, AL 35283-0605
(205) 916-2199

Health Partners of Alabama
600 Beacon Pkwy. W., Ste. 500
Birmingham, AL 35209-3115
(205) 942-5787

Premier Health Plans of Alabama
P.O. Box 18788
Huntsville, AL 35804-8788
(205) 539-7789

Prime Health
1400 University Blvd. S.
Mobile, AL 36609-2999
(334) 342-0022

United Healthcare
3700 Colonnade Pkwy.
Birmingham, AL 35243-2361
(800) 345-1520

ARIZONA

Regional Health Plan-AHCCS
1955 N. Casa Grande Ave., Ste. 116
Casa Grande, AZ 85222-1617
(520) 836-6000

Arizona Physicians IPA
3141 N. Third Ave.
Phoenix, AZ 85013-4345
(602) 274-6102

Blue Cross/Blue Shield Arizona
P.O. Box 13466
Phoenix, AZ 85002-3466
(602) 864-4100

FHP Health Care
P.O. Box 52078
Phoenix, AZ 85072-2078
(602) 244-8200

Health Partners
3141 N. Third Ave.
Phoenix, AZ 85013-4345
(602) 664-2600

Human Health Care Plans
2710 E. Camelback Rd.
Phoenix, AZ 85016-4317
(602) 381-4300

Intergroup HealthCare Corp.
1010 N. Finance Cr. Dr., #100
Tucson, AZ 85710-1361
(520) 721-1122

Phoenix Health Plan
2700 N. Third St., Ste. 3000
Phoenix, AZ 85004-1129
(602) 252-7997

USA Healthnet Inc.
7301 N. 16th St., Ste. 201
Phoenix, AZ 85020-5273
(602) 341-3880

Arizona Physicians IPA, Inc.
4539 E. Fort Lowell, Ste. 131
Tucson, AZ 85712-1108
(520) 881-6386

Cigna HealthCare
535 N. Wilmot Rd.
Tucson, AZ 85711-2604
(520) 571-8040

Intergroup Healthcare Corp.
2800 N. 44th St., Ste. 900
Phoenix, AZ 85008-1564
(602) 224-5528

University Physician, Inc.
575 E. River Rd.
Tucson, AZ 85704-5822
(520) 795-3500

ARKANSAS

Coordinated Arkansas PPO
P.O. Box 8200
Little Rock, AR 72221-8200
(501) 224-1235

CALIFORNIA

Kaiser Permanente Medical Center
441 N. Lakeview Ave.
Anaheim, CA 92807-3028
(714) 978-4000

Mullikin Medical Center
17821 South Pioneer Blvd.
Artesia, CA 90701-3968
(310) 860-6611

Wellpoint Pharmacy Management
27001 Agoura Rd., Ste. 325
Calabasas Hills, CA 91301-5334
(818) 878-2600

FHP, Inc.
18000 Studebaker Rd., Ste. 100
Cerritos, CA 90703-2674
(310) 809-5399

Community Health Group
740 Bay Blvd.
Chula Vista, CA 91910-5299
(619) 422-0422

Pacificare, Inc.
5995 Plaza Dr.
Cypress, CA 90630-5028
(714) 952-1121

RxNet
1931 North Fine Ave., Ste. 101
Fresno, CA 93727-1510
(209) 252-7142

Cigna Healthcare/Medical Group
505 N. Brand Blvd.
Glendale, CA 91203-1925
(818) 500-6262

United Health Plan
3405 W. Imperial Highway
Inglewood, CA 90303-2299
(310) 671-3465

Lakewood Health Plan
3300 E. South St., Ste. 200
Long Beach, CA 90805-4551
(310) 602-1563

Preferred Health Network
301 East Ocean Blvd., #900
Long Beach, CA 90802-4839
(310) 983-1616

Smart Care Health Plan/SCAN HP
3780 Kilroy Airport Way, Ste. 600
Long Beach, CA 90806-2460
(800) 762-7863

Kaiser Foundation Health Plan
1515 N. Vermont Ave.
Los Angeles, CA 90027-5328
(213) 667-4011

Managed Health Network, Inc.
5100 W. Goldleaf Cir., Ste. 300
Los Angeles, CA 90056-1293
(213) 299-0999

Maxicare
1149 S. Broadway
Los Angeles, CA 90015-2213
(213) 742-0900

Pacific Providers Medical Group
2080 Century Park E., Ste. 1703
Los Angeles, CA 90067-2020
(310) 553-2080

Watts Health Foundation
10300 South Compton Ave.
Los Angeles, CA 90002-3628
(213) 564-4331

Cost Care, Inc.
660 Newport Center Dr., Ste. 600
Newport Beach, CA 92660-6412
(714) 729-4500

Foundation Health Corporation
3500 E. Camino Ave., Ste. 110
Oxnard, CA 93030-8983
(805) 981-2800

Cigna Healthcare of Northern California
1999 Harrison St., Ste. 1000
Oakland, CA 94612-3517
(510) 237-8400

PruCare of Southern California
1100 Town & Country Rd., Ste.
  1600
Orange, CA 92868-4658
(714) 547-4088

Kaiser Permanente
393 E. Walnut
Pasadena, CA 91188-0001
(818) 405-3279

Intervalley Health Plan
P.O. Box 6002
Pomona, CA 91769-6002
(909) 623-6333

Integrated Pharmaceutical Services
3400 Data Dr.
Rancho Cordova, CA 95670-7956
(800) 867-6564

Omni Heathcare
2450 Venture Oaks, Ste. 300
Sacramento, CA 95833-3292
(209) 474-6664

Aetna Health Plans
1111 Bayhill Dr., Ste. 300
San Bruno, CA 94066-3035
(415) 952-2005

Cigna Healthcare of San Diego
9808 Scranton Rd., Ste. 400
San Diego, CA 92121-3706
(619) 457-5402

Foundation for Medical Care
P.O. Box 23545
San Diego, CA 92193-3545
(619) 268-7500

Premier
12730 Highbluff Dr., Ste. 300
San Diego, CA 92130-2078
(619) 481-2727

Blue Shield of California
P.O. Box 7168
San Francisco, CA 94120-7168
(415) 445-5000

Valley Health Plan
750 S. Bascom Ave.
San Jose, CA 95128-2603
(408) 885-4760

Monarch Health System
201 N. Salsipuedes, Ste. 206
Santa Barbara, CA 93103-3256
(805) 963-0566

Universal Care
1600 East Hill St.
Signal Hill, CA 90806-3682
(800) 635-6668

San Joaquin Foundation PPO
P.O. Box 210002
Stockton, CA 95210
(209) 951-4560

South Bay Independent Physicians
3480 Torrance Blvd., Ste. 220
Torrance, CA 90503-5813
(310) 543-8805

HealthNet
P.O. Box 9103
Van Nuys, CA 91409-9103
(818) 719-6800

CareAmerica Health Plans
6300 Canoga Ave.
Woodland Hills, CA 91367-2555
(818) 288-5050

Prudential Healthcare
5800 Canoga Ave.
Woodland Hills, CA 91367-6503
(818) 888-5861

COLORADO

Health Network—Colorado Springs
P.O. Box 828
Colorado Springs, CO 80901-0828
(719) 475-5025

Cigna Healthcare
3900 E. Mexico Ave., Ste. 1100
Denver, CO 80210-3946
(303) 782-9662

Colorado Access
501 S. Cherry, 7th floor
Denver, CO 80222-1325
(800) 211-5010

Community Health Plan Rockies
400 S. Colorado Blvd., Ste. 300
Denver, CO 80222-1238
(303) 355-3220

HMO Colorado
700 Broadway
Denver, CO 80203-3421
(303) 831-4114

Kaiser Permanente
10350 E. Dakota Ave.
Denver, CO 80231-1309
(303) 344-7200

Prudential Plus of Colorado
4643 S. Ulster St., Ste. 1000
Denver, CO 80234-2867
(303) 796-8788

Sloans Lake Managed Care
1355 S. Colorado Blvd., Ste. 902
Denver, CO 80222-3305
(303) 691-2200

FHP Health Care
6455 S. Yosemite St.
Englewood, CO 80111-5100
(303) 220-5800

Fort Collins IPA
1136 E. Stuart, Ste. 3220
Fort Collins, CO 80525-1196
(970) 484-3592

Rocky Mountain HMO
P.O. Box 10600
Grand Junction, CO 81502-5600
(970) 244-7760

Foundation Health
41 Montebello, Ste. 300
Pueblo, CO 81001-1366
(719) 583-7500

Preferred Choice, Inc.
1008 Minnequa Ave.
Pueblo, CO 81004-3733
(719) 560-5218

Qual-Med, Inc.
225 N. Main St.
Pueblo, CO 81003-3234
(800) 628-2287

CONNECTICUT

Connecticare, Inc.
30 Batterson Park Rd.
Farmington, CT 06032-2574
(860) 674-5700

Kaiser Foundation Health Plan
P.O. Box 4011
Farmington, CT 06034-4011
(860) 678-6000

Aetna Health Plan Southern New England
151 Farmington Ave.
Hartford, CT 06115
(860) 692-5000

Cigna Healthcare
900 Cottage Grove Rd.
Hartford, CT 06152-0001
(860) 726-6000

Aetna US Healthcare
1000 Middle St. MB66
Middletown, CT 06457-7527
(860) 636-8300

Blue Cross/Blue Shield of Connecticut
370 Bassett Rd.
North Haven, CT 06473-4201
(203) 239-4911

Constitution Health Care
P.O. Box 533 Blue Cross
North Haven, CT 06473-0533
(203) 234-2011

M D Health Plan
6 Devine St.
North Haven, CT 06473-2174
(203) 230-1000

Oxford Health Plans of New York
800 Connecticut Ave.
Norwalk, CT 06854-1631
(800) 889-7546

Physicians Health Service of Connecticut
120 Hawley Ln.
Trumbull, CT 06611-5347
(203) 381-6400

DELAWARE

Health Care Centers
200 Hygeia Dr.
P.O. Box 6008
Newark, DE 19714-6008
(302) 421-2466

Naticoke Memorial Health Plan
801 Middle Ford Rd.
Seaford, DE 19973-3636

AmeriHealth HMO, Inc.
919 N. Market St., Ste. 1200
Wilmington, DE 19801-3062
(610) 358-5650

Blue Cross/Blue Shield
P.O. Box 1991
Wilmington, DE 19899-1991
(302) 421-3056

Cigna Health Plan of New Jersey, Inc.
1 Beaver Valley Rd.
Wilmington, DE 19803-1115
(302) 477-3700

DISTRICT OF COLUMBIA

Capital Care, Inc.
550 12th St., S.W.
Washington, DC 20065-0001
(202) 479-8000

DC Chartered Health Plan, Inc.
820 First St. N.E., Ste. LL100
Washington, DC 2002-4243
(202) 408-4710

Humana Group Health Plan
4301 Connecticut Ave., N.W.
Washington, DC 20008-2304
(202) 364-2000

Providence Community Healthplan
1150 Varnum St., N.E.
Washington, DC 20017-2149
(202) 269-7022

U.S. Dept. of Veterans Affairs
810 Vermont Ave., N.W.
Mail Drop 111H
Washington, DC 20420-0001
(202) 273-5400

FLORIDA

Managed Care of America
999 Ponce De Leon Blvd., Ste. 940
Coral Gables, FL 33134-3047
(305) 529-1999

PacifiCare of Florida
1 Alhambra Plaza, Ste. 1000
Coral Gables, FL 33134-5217
(800) 887-6888

United Healthcare of Florida
75 Valencia Ave.
Coral Gables, FL 33134-6141
(305) 441-1140

Florida Health Choice Plan
5300 W. Atlantic Ave., Ste. 506
Delray Beach, FL 33484-8165
(561) 496-0505

Managed Care—Best Choice
1608 S.E. Third Ave., 3rd floor
Fort Lauderdale, FL 33316-2564
(954) 847-4534

Prudential Healthcare System
5900 N. Andrews Ave., #1000
Fort Lauderdale, FL 33309-2300
(954) 492-8244

Av-Med Health Plan
P.O. Box 749
Gainseville, FL 32602-0749
(352) 372-8400

Florida Health Care Plan
1340 Ridgewood Ave.
Holly Hill, FL 32117-2320
(904) 676-7193

HIP Network, Inc.
200 S. Park Rd., Ste. 410
Hollywood, FL 33021-8543
(800) 826-1013

American Life Insurance
1776 American Heritage Life Dr.
Jacksonville, FL 32224-6687
(904) 992-1776

Blue Cross/Blue Shield Florida
8900 Freedom Commerce Pkwy.
Jacksonville, FL 32256-8264
(800) 322-2808

Health Options, Inc.
8900 Freedom Commerce Pkwy.
Jacksonville, FL 32256-8264
(904) 791-6111

**Humana Health Plan of
Florida, Inc.**
P.O. Box 19080-F
Jacksonville, FL 32245-9080
(904) 296-7600

Humana Medical Plan
7825 Bay Meadows Way, Ste. 120B
Jacksonville, FL 32256-7557
(904) 281-8800

Prudential Health Care Systems
1200 Riverplace Blvd., Ste. 701
Jacksonville, FL 32207-1804
(904) 346-5800

**Lower Florida Keys Health
System**
P.O. Box 9107
Key West, FL 33041-9107
(305) 294-5531

Eckerd Health Services
8333 Bryan Dairy Rd.
Largo, FL 33777-1230
(813) 399-6022

Humana Health Plan
1060 Maitland Ctr. Comm., Ste. 300
Maitland, FL 32751-7246
(407) 661-6000

AvMed Health Plan Miami
P.O. Box 569004
Miami, FL 33256-9004
(305) 671-5437

**Blue Cross/Blue Shield/Health
Options**
3750 N.W. 87th Ave., Ste. 300
Miami, FL 33178-2430
(305) 591-9955

Family First
2901 N.W. 17th Ave.
Miami, FL 33142-6631
(305) 633-3015

Jackson Memorial Health Plans
1500 N.W. 12th Ave., Ste. 1001 W.
Miami, FL 33136-1051
(305) 585-7120

Mount Sinai
4300 Alton Rd.
Miami Beach, FL 33140-2800
(305) 674-2121

**Neighborhood Health
Partnership**
P.O. Box 02580
Miami, FL 33102
(305) 715-2200

Public Health Trust
1611 N.W. 12th Ave.
Miami, FL 33136-1005
(305) 585-1111

United Healthcare
8500 S.W. 117th Rd., Ste. 310
Miami, FL 33183-4841
(800) 752-7850

Humana Medical Plan
3400 Lakeside Dr.
Miramar, FL 33027-3238
(305) 621-4222

Blue Cross/Blue Shield Health
3191 Maguire Blvd., Ste. 125
Orlando, FL 32803-3723
(407) 894-3431

Medco Value Plus
7011 Grand National Dr.
Orlando, FL 32819-8329
(407) 345-9421

Kemper National Services PPO
1601 S.W. 80th Terrace
Plantation, FL 33324-4034
(954) 452-4000

Cigna Healthcare of Florida
5404 Cypress Center Dr.
Tampa, FL 33609-1044
(813) 281-1000

Capital Health Plan
2140 Centerville Pl.
Tallahassee, FL 32308-4300
(904) 386-3161

Healthplan Southeast
P.O. Box 13700
Tallahassee, FL 32317-3700
(904) 668-3000

Aetna Health Plans
4890 West Kennedy Blvd., Ste. 545
Tampa, FL 33609-1862
(813) 287-7250

AvMed Health Plan
2701 Rocky Point Dr., Ste. 1050
Tampa, FL 33607-5925
(813) 281-5650

Blue Cross/Blue Shield of Florida
4904 Eisenhower Blvd., Ste. 200
Tampa, FL 33634-6330
(813) 886-1663

Cigna Health Plan of Florida
3745 33rd St. N.
Saint Petersburg, FL 33713-1556
(813) 525-0006

Humana Health Care Plan
5401 W. Kennedy Blvd., Ste. 800
Tampa, FL 33609-2448
(813) 286-8829

Pharmacy Corporation of America
P.O. Box 30054
Tampa, FL 33630-3054
(813) 626-7788

Physicians Healthcare Plans
777 S. Harbor Island Blvd.
Tampa, FL 33602-5729
(813) 273-7474

Private Healthcare Systems, Inc.
1511 N. Westshore, #620
Tampa, FL 33607-4594
(813) 282-8200

Prucare of Tampa Bay
6200 Courtney Campbell Cwy., #200
Tampa, FL 33607-1400
(813) 288-0080

GEORGIA

Aetna US Healthcare
3500 Piedmont Rd. N.E., Ste. 300
Atlanta, GA 30305-1503
(404) 814-4300

Cigna Preferred Provider Organization
100 Peachtree St., Ste. 700
Atlanta, GA 30303
(404) 681-7000

Cost Care Physician Man Network
2727 Paces Ferry Rd., N.W. 2-600
Atlanta, GA 30339-4053
(770) 319-8101

Kaiser Permanente Medical Care
3495 Piedmont Rd., Bdg. 9
Atlanta, GA 30305
(404) 233-0555

PCA Health Plans of Georgia, Inc.
1349 West Peachtree St., Ste. 1000
Atlanta, GA 30309-2956
(404) 815-7160

Private Health Care Systems
1000 Abernathy Rd. N.E., Ste. 940
Atlanta, GA 30328-5650
(770) 394-1084

Prucare Plus Atlanta
2839 Paces Ferry Rd., Ste. 1000
Atlanta, GA 30339-5770
(770) 955-8010

Master Health Plan, Inc.
P.O. Box 16367
Augusta, GA 30919-2367
(706) 863-5955

Blue Cross/Blue Shield
2357 Warm Springs Rd.
Columbus, GA 31904-5668
(706) 571-5371

Circle of Care/Medical Center, Inc.
P.O. Box 790
Columbus, GA 31902-0790
(706) 660-6132

Physicians Group, Inc.
P.O. Box 5537
Columbus, GA 31906-0537
(706) 322-8872

Benescript Services
P.O. Box 921229
Norcross, GA 30092-7229
(770) 448-4344

United Healthcare
1854 Shackelford
Norcross, GA 30093-2924
(770) 935-3000

Healthsource Savannah, Inc.
7130 Hodgson Memorial Dr.,
 #4000
Savannah, GA 31406-2521
(912) 351-2410

Health Alliance
808 Gordon Ave.
Thomasville, GA 31792-6611
(912) 226-4122

HAWAII

Kaiser Foundation Health Hawaii
7111 Kapiolani Blvd.
Honolulu, HI 96813-5237
(808) 539-5500

ILLINOIS

Personalcare Health Management
510 Devonshire Dr.
Champaign, IL 61820-7306
(217) 366-1226

Aetna Health Plans of Midwest
100 N. Riverside Plaza
Chicago, IL 60606-1501
(312) 441-3000

Cigna Health Care of Illinois
525 W. Monroe St., Ste. 1800
Chicago, IL 60661-3629
(312) 648-2460

Community Healthplan
836 W. Wellington, Ste. 1707
Chicago, IL 60661-3629
(312) 648-2460

Healthstar
8745 W. Higgins Rd., Ste. 300
Chicago, IL 60657-5147
(312) 296-7827

Maxicare Illinois
111 East Wacker Dr., Ste. 1500
Chicago, IL 60601-3704
(312) 616-4700

Rush Prudential Health Plan
233 S. Wacker Dr., Ste. 3900
Chicago, IL 60606-6380
(312) 234-7000

United Healthcare of Illinois
1 S. Wacker Dr.
Chicago, IL 60606-4614
(312) 424-4460

University of Illinois
HMO, Inc.
2023 W. Ogden Ave., Ste. 205
Chicago, IL 60612-3713
(312) 996-3553

De Kalb Clinic Chapter
217 Franklin St.
De Kalb, IL 60115-3742
(815) 758-8671

Health Direct, Inc.
1011 East Touhy Ave., Ste. 500
Des Plaines, IL 60018-2808
(847) 391-9500

Trustmark
400 Field Dr.
Lake Forest, IL 60045-4809
(847) 615-1500

American Health Care Providers
142 Town Center Rd.
Matteson, IL 60443-2245
(708) 503-5000

John Deere Health Care
1515 5th Ave., Ste. 200
Moline, IL 61265-1367
(309) 765-1200

FHP of Illinois, Inc.
1 Lincoln Centre, Ste. 700
Oakbrook Terrace, IL 60181-4264
(630) 916-8400

John Deere Healthcare/Heritage
973 Featherstone, Ste. 300
Rockford, IL 61107-5908
(815) 227-1720

Health Alliance Medical Plans
P.O. Box 6003
Urbana, IL 61803-6003
(217) 337-8000

Medwest Business Medical Association
3201 Old Glenview Rd., Ste. 200
Wilmette, IL 60091-2964
(847) 853-6262

INDIANA

Sagamore Health Network
11555 N. Meridian St., Ste. 400
Carmel, IN 46032-6910
(317) 573-2900

Deaconess Health Partners
600 Mary St.
Evansville, IN 47747-0001
(812) 428-7625

Physicians Health Network
7100 Eagle Crest Blvd.
Evansville, IN 47715-8152
(812) 471-1100

Physicians Health Plan
8101 W. Jefferson Blvd.
Fort Wayne, IN 46804-4163
(219) 432-6690

Preferred Plan/FHP Preferred
7223 Engle Rd., Ste. 110
Fort Wayne, IN 46804-2228
(800) 535-8763

Anthem
120 Monument Circle
Indianapolis, IN 46204-4906
(317) 263-8000

**Healthsource Indiana Managed
Care**
225 S. East St., Ste. 240
Indianapolis, IN 46202-4059
(317) 685-8300

Healthstar, Inc.
8335 Allison Pointe Trail, Ste. 100
Indianapolis, IN 46250-1685
(800) 677-2552

Maxicare Indiana
9480 Priority Way W. Dr.
Indianapolis, IN 46206-1470
(317) 844-5775

M Plan
8802 N. Meridian, Ste. 100
Indianapolis, IN 46260-5318
(317) 571-5300

Prudential Healthcare
8425 Woodfield Crossing, Ste. 301
Indianapolis, IN 46240-2495
(317) 469-8000

Partners Health Plan
100 E. Wayne St., Ste. 502
South Bend, IN 46601-2354
(219) 233-4677

IOWA

Blue Cross & Blue Shield of Iowa
636 Grand Ave.
Des Moines, IA 50309-2502
(515) 245-4500

HMO Health Choices
P.O. Box 5002
Dubuque, IA 52004-5002
(319) 556-8070

Principal Healthcare of Iowa
4600 Westown Pkwy., #301 Reg 6
West Des Moines, IA 50266-1042
(515) 225-1234

KANSAS

**Cigna Health Care of Kansas/
Missouri**
7400 W. 110th St., Ste. 600
Overland Park, KS 66210-2346
(913) 339-4700

Kaiser Foundation Health Plan
10561 Barkley, Ste. 200
Overland Park, KS 66212-1839
(913) 722-2900

Blue Cross/Blue Shield Kansas
1133 SW Topeka Blvd.
Topeka, KS 66629-0001
(913) 291-7000

HMO Kansas, Inc.
P.O. Box 110
Topeka, KS 66601-0110
(913) 233-2751

Preferred Plus of Kansas
345 Riverview, Ste. 103
Wichita, KS 67203-4262
(316) 268-0390

KENTUCKY

HealthWise of Kentucky Ltd.
2409 Harrodsburg Rd.
Lexington, KY 40504-3329
(606) 296-6000

Anthem Blue Cross/Blue Shield
9901 Linn Station Rd.
Louisville, KY 40223-3808
(800) 880-2583

Humana Health Plan
500 W. Main St.
Louisville, KY 40202
(502) 580-1000

LOUISIANA

Gulf South Health Plans, Inc.
5615 Corporate Blvd., Ste. 3
Baton Rouge, LA 70808-2568
(504) 237-1700

MetraHealth
3900 N. Causeway Blvd., #860
Metairie, LA 70002-1746
(504) 832-7655

Willis Knighton Health Plan
2708 Greenwood Rd., 1st floor
Shreveport, LA 71109-4635
(318) 632-4590

MAINE

Martins Point Health Care Center
P.O. Box 9746
Portland, ME 04104-5040
(207) 774-5801

Medical Network, Inc.
P.O. Box 15253
Portland, ME 04112-5253
(207) 773-5116

Blue Cross/Blue Shield of Maine
2 Gannett Dr.
South Portland, ME 04106-6909
(207) 822-7000

MARYLAND

Capstone Pharmacy Services
2930 Washington Blvd.
Baltimore, MD 21230-1141
(410) 646-7373

Chesapeake Health Plan
814 Light St.
Baltimore, MD 21230-3963
(410) 539-8622

Prucare of Baltimore
2800 N. Charles St.
Baltimore, MD 21218-4026
(410) 554-7000

Total Health Care
2305 N. Charles St.
Baltimore, MD 21218-5128
(410) 383-8300

George Washington University HP
4550 Montgomery, Ste. 800
Bethesda, MD 20814-3304
(202) 416-0400

Cigna Health Care
9700 Patuxent Woods Dr.
Columbia, MD 21046-1526
(410) 720-5800

Columbia Medical Plan, Inc.
2 Knoll N. Dr.
Columbia, MD 21045-2298
(410) 997-8500

New York Life Healthplan
7601 Ora Glen Dr., Ste. 200
Greenbelt, MD 20770-3641
(301) 441-1600

Upper Chesapeake Health Systems
P.O. Box 777
Havre de Grace, MD 21078-0777
(410) 939-2566

Healthcare 2000
1407 York Rd., Ste. 302
Lutherville, MD 21093-6054
(410) 296-8326

Potomac Health
10455 Mill Run Circle
Owings Mills, MD 21117-4208
(800) 445-6036

Kaiser Permanente
2101 E. Jefferson
Rockville, MD 20852-4908
(301) 816-2424

Mid Atlantic Medical
4 Taft Ct.
Rockville, MD 20850-5310
(301) 294-5140

Optimum Choice, Inc.
4 Taft Court
Rockville, MD 20850-5310
(301) 738-7920

Principal Health Care, Inc.
1801 Rockville Pike
Rockville, MD 20852-1633
(301) 881-1033

MASSACHUSETTS

Kaiser Foundation Health Plan
170 University Dr.
Amherst, MA 01002-2247
(413) 256-0151

Blue Cross/Blue Shield
100 Summer St.
Boston, MA 02110-2190
(617) 832-5000

John Hancock Preferred Health
P.O. Box 111
Boston, MA 02117-0111
(617) 572-6000

Neighborhood Health Plan
253 Summer St.
Boston, MA 02210-1120
(617) 772-5500

HMO Blue at Goddard Medical Associates
1 Pearl St.
Brockton, MA 02401-2800
(508) 586-3600

Harvard Pilgrim Health Care
10 Brookline Pl. W.
Brookline, MA 02146-7226
(617) 431-1070

Lahey Clinic HMO
41 Mall Rd.
Burlington, MA 01805-0001
(617) 273-5100

Harvard University Group HP
75 Mount Auburn St.
Cambridge, MA 02138-4960
(617) 495-2074

MIT Health Plan
77 Massachusetts Ave., E23-308
Cambridge, MA 02139-4301
(617) 253-1322

Teamsters Union 25 Health
16 Sever St.
Sullivan Sq.
Charlestown, MA 02129-1304
(617) 241-9220

Cigna Healthplan of Massachusetts
20 Speen St., 3rd floor
Framingham, MA 01701-4680
(508) 935-2100

Pioneer Health Care PPO
P.O. Box 6600
Holyoke, MA 01041-6600
(413) 539-9900

CostCare
P.O. Box 1079
Lynnfield, MA 01940-3079
(617) 245-8500

Blue Cross/Blue Shield
20 Hamptson Ave., Ste. 150
Northampton, MA 01060-4403
(413) 586-9161

Massachusetts Mutual Pref Plus
1295 State St.
Springfield, MA 01111-0001
(413) 788-8411

Medical West Associates
360 Birnie St.
Springfield, MA 01107-1104
(413) 594-3111

Aetna Health Plans Boston
P.O. Box 357
Tewksbury, MA 01876-0357
(508) 640-6047

Private Healthcare System Boston
1100 Winter St.
Waltham, MA 02154-1227
(617) 895-7500

Tufts Associated Health Plan
333 Wyman St.
Waltham, MA 02154-1209
(617) 466-9400

United Healthcare
1 Research Dr.
Westborough, MA 01581-3922
(800) 410-3385

Fallon Community Health Plan
10 Chestnut St.
Worcester, MA 01608-2804
(508) 799-2100

Healthsource CMHC
100 Front St., Ste. 300
Worcester, MA 01608-1402
(508) 798-8667

MICHIGAN

M Care
2301 Commonwealth Blvd.
Ann Arbor, MI 48105-2945
(313) 747-8700

Mercy Health Plan
2000 Hogback Rd., Ste. 15
Ann Arbor, MI 48105-9735
(313) 971-7667

Choice One/Omni Care
1155 Brewery Park, Ste. 350
Detroit, MI 48207-2640
(800) 670-1172

Henry Ford Health System
1 Ford Pl.
Detroit, MI 48202-3450
(313) 876-8700

Health Alliance Plan of Michigan
2850 W. Grand Blvd.
Detroit, MI 48202-2643
(313) 872-8100

Total Health Care, Inc.
1600 Fisher Building
Detroit, MI 48202-3000
(313) 871-2000

Wellness Plan—Comp Health
2875 W. Grand Blvd.
Detroit, MI 48202-2623
(313) 875-4200

Health Plus
2050 S. Linden Rd.
Flint, MI 48532-4199
(810) 230-2000

Blue Care Network Great Lakes
611 Cascade W. Pkwy. S.E.
Grand Rapids, MI 49546-2107
(616) 957-5057

Grand Valley Health Plan
829 Forest Hill Ave. S.E.
Grand Rapids, MI 49546-2387
(616) 949-2410

Priority Health
1231 E. Beltline Ave. N.E.
Grand Rapids, MI 49505-4501
(616) 942-0954

Blue Care Network Health Central
1403 S. Creyts Rd.
Lansing, MI 48917-8507
(517) 322-8000

SVS Vision
140 macomb
Mount Clemens, MI 48043-5651
(810) 468-7612

Blue Care Network East Michigan
4200 Fashion Sq. Blvd.
Saginaw, MI 48603-1247
(517) 791-3200

Aetna Health Plans
26957 Northwestern Hwy.,
Ste. 140
Southfield, MI 48034-8456
(810) 468-7612

Blue Care Network of Southeastern Michigan
P.O. Box 5043
Southfield, MI 48086-5043
(810) 354-7450

Northmed/HMO, Inc.
109 E. Front St., Ste. 204
Traverse City, MI 49684-5705
(616) 935-0500

AmeriKinda Pharmacy Network
3100 West Big Beaver Rd., Ste. 235
Troy, MI 48084-3004
(800) 321-0103

MINNESOTA

Diversified Pharmaceutical Services
7760 France Ave. S., Ste. 310
Edina, MN 55435-5833
(612) 820-7000

Select Care/Allina Health Systems
P.O. Box 2042
Hopkins, MN 55343-3042
(612) 992-2500

Aetna Health Plans
901 Marquette Ave., 23rd floor
Minneapolis, MN 55402-3205
(612) 399-2550

Alliance Life Insurance
1750 Hennepin Ave.
Minneapolis, MN 55403-2115
(612) 347-6500

Hennepin County Medical Center
701 Park Ave.
Minneapolis, MN 55415-1623
(612) 347-2121

Metropolitan Health Plan
822 S. Third St., Ste. 140
Minneapolis, MN 55415-1200
(612) 347-8557

Bethesda Lutheran Care
559 Capital Blvd.
St. Paul, MN 55103-2101
(612) 232-2100

Blue Cross/Blue Shield of Minnesota
P.O. Box 64560
St. Paul, MN 55164-0560
(612) 456-8000

Pharmacy Gold
P.O. Box 64560
St. Paul, MN 55164-0560
(612) 456-5575

Ucare Minnesota
2550 University Ave. W., Ste. 201S
St. Paul, MN 55114-1904
(612) 627-4301

MISSISSIPPI

Magnolia Regional Health Center
611 Alcorn Dr.
Corinth, MS 38834-9368
(601) 293-1000

Blue Cross/Blue Shield
P.O. Box 1043
Jackson, MS 39215-1043
(601) 932-3704

North Mississippi Health Services
830 S. Gloster St.
Tupelo, MS 38801-4934
(601) 841-3000

MISSOURI

HealthLink HMO, Inc.
777 Craig Rd., Ste. 110
Creve Coeur, MO 63141-7138
(314) 569-7200

Healthnet
2300 Main St., Ste. 700
Kansas City, MO 64108-2458
(816) 221-8400

Medplan
10450 Holmes St., Ste. 100
Kansas City, MO 64131-3445
(816) 941-8003

Express Scripts
14000 Riverport Dr.
Maryland Heights, MO 63043-4827
(314) 770-1666

Blue Cross/Blue Shield
1831 Chestnut
St. Louis, MO 63103-2275
(314) 923-4444

Cigna Health Care
8182 Maryland Ave., Ste. 900
St. Louis, MO 63105-3786
(314) 726-7792

Group Health Plan
940 W. Port Plaza, Ste. 300
St. Louis, MO 63146-3116
(314) 453-1700

Managed Pharmacy Benefits
1100 N. Lindbergh Blvd.
St. Louis, MO 63132-2914
(314) 993-6000

United Healthcare of Midwest
77 W. Port Plaza, Ste. 500
St. Louis, MO 63146-3126
(314) 275-7000

NEBRASKA

Mutual of Omaha
Mutual of Omaha Plaza
Omaha, NE 68175-0001
(402) 351-2351

United Healthcare of Midlands
450 Regency Pkwy., Ste. 100
Omaha, NE 68114-3787
(402) 255-5600

NEVADA

FHP Health Care
700 E. Warm Springs
Las Vegas, NV 89119-4323
(702) 269-7500

Health Care, Inc.
2340 Paseo Del Prado, Bldg. D
#305
Las Vegas, NV 89102-4360
(702) 786-2600

Health Plan of Nevada
P.O. Box 15645
Las Vegas, NV 89114-5645
(702) 242-7000

Hometown Health Plan
400 S. Wells Ave.
Reno, NV 89502-1823
(702) 329-0101

St. Mary's Preferred Healthcare
5290 Neil Rd.
Reno, NV 89502-8526
(702) 829-3077

NEW HAMPSHIRE

Matthew Thornton Health Plan
43 Constitution Dr.
Bedford, NH 03110-6000
(800) 874-7122

Healthsource New Hampshire
P.O. Box 2041
Concord, NH 03302-2041
(603) 225-5077

NEW JERSEY

Oxford Health Plans
399 Thornall, 9th floor
Edison, NJ 08837-2238
(908) 632-9494

Aetna US Health Plans
55 Lane Rd.
Fairfield, NJ 07004-1011
(201) 334-2200

Preferred Health Strategies
401 Hackensack Ave.
Hackensack, NJ 07601-6411
(201) 487-6002

Quakerbridge Center
Mercerville, NJ 08619-1250
(609) 586-6700

Medco Containment
100 Summit Ave.
Montvale, NJ 07645-1712
(201) 794-7000

HMO Blue Cross
310 Plaza East
Newark, NJ 07105
(201) 466-4276

HIP Pro
825 Georges Rd.
North Brunswick, NJ 08902-3357
(908) 296-0820

HIP Rutgers Health Plan
1 HIP Plaza
North Brunswick, NJ 08902-3391
(908) 937-7600

Cigna Health Plan
100 Enterprise Dr., Ste. 610
Rockaway, NJ 07866-2120
(201) 361-3444

Prudential Health Care Plans
56 N. Livingston Ave.
Roseland, NJ 07068-1733
(201) 716-6000

Garden State Health Plan
CN 712
Trenton, NJ 08625
(609) 588-3526

HMO Blue
416 Bellvue
Trenton, NJ 08618-4513
(609) 396-4600

NEW MEXICO

FHP of New Mexico, Inc.
4300 San Mateo N.E. Blvd.
Albuquerque, NM 87110-1229
(505) 881-7900

Lovelace Health Plan
5301 Central Ave. N.E., Ste. 500
Albuquerque, NM 87018-1513
(505) 262-7075

Qual-Med Plans for Health
6100 Uptown Blvd. N.E., Ste. 400
Albuquerque, NM 87110-4143
(505) 889-8807

NEW YORK

Health Insurance Plan of Greater New York
7 W. 34th St.
New York, NY 10001-8190
(212) 630-5000

Multiplan
115 Fifth Ave.
New York, NY 10003-1004
(212) 780-2000

**National Health Plan
Corporation**
7 Penn Plaza, Ste. 910
New York, NY 1001-3900
(212) 279-3232

NYL Care
1 Liberty Plaza
New York, NY 10006-1404
(212) 437-1000

Ethix Southeast, Inc.
P.O. Box 222097
Charlotte, NC 28222-2097
(704) 529-0818

Maxicare North Carolina, Inc.
5550 77 Center Dr., Ste. 380
Charlotte, NC 28217-0700
(704) 525-0880

Prudential Healthcare Systems
2701 Coltsgate Rd., Ste. 300
Charlotte, NC 28211-3502
(704) 365-6070

**Blue Cross/Blue Shield of North
Carolina**
P.O. Box 2291
Durham, NC 27702-2291
(919) 489-7431

**Coastal Health Plan of North
Carolina**
P.O. Box 15309
Durham, NC 27704-0309
(919) 383-0367

Physicians Health Plan, Inc.
2307 W. Cone Blvd.
Greensboro, NC 27408-4032
(910) 282-0900

United Healthcare
P.O. Box 26722
Greensboro, NC 27417-6722
(800) 334-2400

**Cigna Healthcare of North
Carolina**
4011 W. Chase Blvd., #290
Raleigh, NC 27607-3954
(919) 839-7800

Healthsource North Carolina
701 Corporate Center Dr.
Raleigh, NC 27607-5071
(919) 460-1610

**Kaiser Foundation Health—
North Carolina**
3120 Highwoods Blvd.
Raleigh, NC 27604-1038
(919) 981-6000

**Pharmacy Network National
Corp.**
4000 Old Wake Forest Rd., Ste. 101
Raleigh, NC 27609
(919) 876-4642

MedCost, Inc.
P.O. Box 25347
Winston-Salem, NC 27114-5347
(910) 760-3090

Partners National Health Plans
P.O. Box 24907
Winston-Salem, NC 27114-4907
(910) 760-4822

Winston-Salem Health Care Plan
250 Charlois Blvd.
Winston-Salem, NC 27103-1508
(910) 768-4730

Blue Cross/Blue Shield
4510 13th Ave. S.W.
Fargo, ND 58121-0001
(701) 282-1100

Northern Plains Health Plan
1000 S. Columbia Rd.
Grand Forks, ND 58201-4032
(800) 675-2467

Heart of America HMO
802 S. Main Ave.
Rugby, ND 58368-2118
(701) 776-5848

Suma Health System
525 E. Market
Akron, OH 44304-1619
(330) 375-3000

Primary Health Services
P.O. Box 379
Aurora, OH 44202-0379
(216) 562-5711

Meridia South Pointe
4110 Warrensville Center Rd.
Beachwood, OH 44122-7024
(216) 491-6000

Aultman Hospital
2600 Sixth St. S.W.
Canton, OH 44710-1799
(330) 452-9911

Anthem Blue Cross Blue Shield
1351 William Howard Taft Rd.
Cincinnati, OH 45206-1721
(513) 872-8100

Blue Cross/Blue Shield of Ohio
2060 Reading Rd., Ste. 300
Cincinnati, OH 45202-1453
(513) 721-3388

Choicecare
655 Eden Park Dr.
Cincinnati, OH 45202-6000
(513) 784-5200

Cigna Preferred Provider Organization
600 Vine St., Ste. 602
Cincinnati, OH 45202-2427
(513) 629-2640

Cincinnati Health Plan
250 W. Court St., Ste. 100E
Cincinnati, OH 45202-1054
(513) 665-3580

Prudential Healthcare
312 Elm St., Ste. 1400
Cincinnati, OH 45202-2739
(513) 621-2620

United Healthcare
10560 Ashview Place, Ste. 205
Cincinnati, OH 45242-3738
(513) 554-1310

Continental Pharmacy Services
P.O. Box 94863
Cleveland, OH 44101-4863
(216) 459-2010

Emerald Health Network
1100 Superior Ave., 16th floor
Cleveland, OH 44114-2591
(216) 479-2030

Fairview Health System
18101 Lorain Ave.
Cleveland, OH 44111-5612
(216) 476-7217

Kaiser Permanente
1001 Lakeside Ave. E., #1200
Cleveland, OH 44114-1151
(216) 621-5600

Ohio Health Choice
1621 Euclid Ave., Ste. 1400
Cleveland, OH 44115-2107
(216) 436-4000

Qualchoice HMO
6000 Parkland Blvd.
Cleveland, OH 44124-4185
(216) 460-4040

Total Health Care Plan, Inc.
12800 Shaker Blvd.
Cleveland, OH 44120-2033
(216) 991-3000

United Healthcare
1 Cleveland Ctr.
1375 E. 9th, #700
Cleveland, OH 44114-1724
(216) 694-4080

Cigna Healthcare of Ohio
P.O. Box 182331
Columbus, OH 43218-2331
(614) 823-7500

Travelers of Columbus
Route OH 20-0175
P.O. Box 1138
Columbus, OH 43216-6676
(614) 433-2000

US Health Corporation
3555 Olentangy River Rd., #4000
Columbus, OH 43214-3912
(614) 566-5424

Trumbull Mahoning Medical Group
2600 Elm Rd.
Cortland, OH 44410-9393
(330) 399-9300

United Healthcare of Ohio
P.O. Box 751090
Dayton, OH 45475-1090
(937) 439-9355

Wright Health Associates
1222 South Patterson Blvd.
Dayton, OH 45402-2643
(937) 227-3800

EMH Regional Medical Center
630 E. River St.
Elyria, OH 44035-5902
(216) 329-7500

Holzer Health Plan
90 Jackson Pike
Gallipolis, OH 45631-1560
(614) 446-5187

Healthstar, Inc.
4807 Rockside Rd., Ste. 510
Independence, OH 44131-2192
(216) 642-3120

HealthFirst
P.O. Box 1820
Marion, OH 43301-1551
(614) 387-6355

Smith Clinic
1040 Delaware Ave.
Marion, OH 43302-6483
(614) 383-7900

Medina Area PPO
1000 E. Washington
Medina, OH 44256-2170
(330) 725-1000

Community Health Plan of Ohio
1915 Tamarak Rd.
Newark, OH 43055
(614) 348-4900

Kaiser Permanente
12301 Snow Rd.
Parma, OH 44130-1002
(216) 362-2000

Parma Preferred Providers Organization
7007 Powers Blvd.
Parma, OH 44129-5437
(216) 888-1800

Health Plan—Upper Ohio Valley
52160 National Rd. E.
St. Clairsville, OH 43950-9306
(614) 695-3585

Aetna Health Plans
1 Seagate, Ste. 690
Toledo, OH 43604-2614
(419) 249-2757

Blue Cross/Blue Shield
P.O. Box 943
Toledo, OH 43697-0943
(419) 473-7320

Blue Cross/Blue Shield
3737 Sylvania Ave.
Toledo, OH 43623-4482
(419) 473-7100

Family Health Plan
1001 Madison Ave.
Toledo, OH 43624-1535
(419) 241-6501

Paramount Health Care
P.O. Box 928
Toledo, OH 43697-0928
(419) 891-2500

MedE America
1933 Case Pkwy. N.
Twinsburg, OH 44087-2343
(216) 963-6721

US HealthPlan
300 E. Wilson Bridge Rd., Ste. 200
Worthington, OH 43085-2346
(614) 566-0123

OKLAHOMA

Cigna Health Care of Oklahoma
5100 N. Brookline Ave., 9th floor
Oklahoma City, OK 73112-3603
(405) 943-7711

PPO Oklahoma
P.O. Box 20040
Oklahoma City, OK 73156-0040
(405) 843-9551

Prudential Healthcare
4005 N.W. Expressway, Ste. 300
Oklahoma City, OK 73116-1679
(405) 879-1780

Bluelincs
P.O. Box 251128
Tulsa, OK 74121-1128
(918) 561-9900

Community Care HMO, Inc.
4720 South Harvard, Ste. 202
Tulsa, OK 74135-3071
(918) 749-1171

Pacificare/Secure Horizons
7666 East 61st
Tulsa, OK 74133-1143
(918) 459-1100

Prudential Health Care Plan
7912 E. 31st Court
Tulsa, OK 74145-1305
(918) 624-4664

OREGON

PACC Health Plans
12901 S.E. 97th Ave.
Clackamas, OR 97015-9748
(503) 659-4212

HMO of Oregon
P.O. Box 130
Medford, OR 97501-0204
(800) 828-0035

Blue Cross/Blue Shield of Oregon
P.O. Box 1271
Portland, OR 97207-1271
(800) 452-7390

Kaiser Permanente
500 N.E. Multnomah St., Ste. 100
Portland, OR 97232-2099
(503) 813-2800

Liberty Health Plan, Inc.
825 N.E. Multnomah St., Ste. 1600
Portland, OR 97232-2143
(503) 234-5345

Sisters of Providence Health Plan
1235 N.E. 47th Ave., Ste. 220
Portland, OR 97213-2100
(503) 215-7500

HMO Oregon
P.O. Box 12625
Salem, OR 97309-0625
(503) 225-5221

PENNSYLVANIA

Preferred Healthcare Systems
620 Howard Ave.
Altoona, PA 16601-4804
(814) 949-3099

Value Rx
3684 Marshall Ln., Exp 95 Ctr.
Bensalem, PA 19020-5914
(215) 638-7855

US Healthcare
980 Jolly Rd.
Blue Bell, PA 19422-1957
(215) 628-4800

Keystone Health Plan Central
P.O. Box 898812
Camp Hill, PA 17089-8812
(717) 763-3458

Pennsylvania Blue Shield
P.O. Box 890089
Camp Hill, PA 17089-0089
(717) 763-3151

Geisinger Health Plan
100 N. Academy Ave.
Danville, PA 17822-0001
(717) 271-8760

Alliance Health Network
1700 Peach St., Ste. 244
Erie, PA 16501-2118
(800) 866-1216

Capital Blue Cross
2500 Elmerton Ave.
Harrisburg, PA 17110-9764
(717) 255-0820

Healthamerica Pennsylvania, Inc.
2601 Market Pl.
Harrisburg, PA 17110-9363
(717) 540-6766

Health Central
2605 Interstate Dr., Ste. 140
Harrisburg, PA 17110-9364
(800) 968-7466

Prudential Healthcare
220 Gibralter Rd.
Horsham, PA 19044-2306
(215) 672-1944

Managed Care RX
20 Erford Rd.
Lemoyne, PA 17043-1163
(717) 730-9950

Central Susquehanna Insurance
1 Hospital Dr.
Lewisburg, PA 17837-9314
(717) 522-2748

Cigna Corporation
1 Liberty Pl., 1650 Market
Philadelphia, PA 19192-0001
(215) 761-1000

Health Partners of Philadelphia
4700 Wissahickon Ave.
Philadelphia, PA 19144-4248
(215) 849-9600

Healthpass
P.O. Box 41566
Philadelphia, PA 19101-1566
(800) 321-4462

Intracorp
1601 Chestnut St.
Philadelphia, PA 19192-0003
(215) 761-7100

Keystone Health Plan East
1901 Market St.
Philadelphia, PA 19103-1475
(215) 241-2001

Mercy Health Plan
200 Stevens Dr., Ste. 350
Philadelphia, PA 19113-1570
(215) 937-7300

Oxford Health Plans
601 Walnut St., #900
Independence Sq. W.
Philadelphia, PA 19106-3310
(215) 625-5631

Qual Med Plans for Help
1835 Market St.
Philadelphia, PA 19103-2968
(215) 209-6300

Travelers
3 Pkwy., Ste. 1310
Philadelphia, PA 19102-1321
(215) 557-6100

Advantage Health
121 Seventh St., Ste. 500
Pittsburgh, PA 15222-3408
(412) 391-9300

Healthamerica Pennsylvania, Inc.
5 Gateway Center
Pittsburgh, PA 15222-1209
(412) 553-5646

Pyramid Health
501 Holiday Dr., Bldg. 4
Pittsburgh, PA 15220-2749
(412) 937-1396

Sharon Regional Health System
740 E. State St.
Sharon, PA 16146-3328
(412) 983-3911

HIP Health Plan of Pennsylvania
6 Neshaminy Interplex, Ste. 600
Trevose, PA 19053-6942
(215) 633-7780

First Priority Health
70 N. Main St.
Wilkes-Barre, PA 18711-0300
(717) 829-7700

RHODE ISLAND

Blue Cross/Blue Shield
444 Westminster St.
Providence, RI 02903-3279
(401) 831-7300

Coordinated Health Partners
30 Chestnut St.
Providence, RI 02903-4138
(401) 459-5500

Harvard Pilgrim Health Plan
1 Hoppin St.
Providence, RI 02903-4120
(401) 331-3000

United Health Plans New England
475 Kilvert St., Metro Ctr.
Warwick, RI 02886-1360
(401) 737-6900

SOUTH CAROLINA

Blue Cross/Blue Shield of South Carolina
I-20 E. at Alpine Rd.
Columbia, SC 29219-0001
(803) 788-3860

Companion HealthCare
P.O. Box 6170
Columbia, SC 29260-6170
(803) 786-8466

Physicians Health Plan of South Carolina
110 Centerview Dr., Ste. 301
Columbia, SC 29210-8432
(803) 750-7400

Maxicare Southeast Health Plans
535 N. Pleasantburg Dr., Ste. 108
Greenville, SC 29607-2100
(864) 233-7437

Healthsource
146 Fairchild St.
Wando, SC 29492-7504
(803) 884-4063

TENNESSEE

Overlook Center, Inc.
280 Fort Sanders W. Blvd., Ste. 104
Knoxville, TN 37922-3352
(423) 531-5177

University of Tennessee HP
1111 Northshore Dr., Ste. N-400
Knoxville, TN 37919-4046
(423) 450-9000

Memphis Managed Care Corporation
P.O. Box 49
Memphis, TN 38101-0049
(901) 725-7100

Prudential Healthcare Systems
2620 Thousand Oaks Blvd., #4000
Memphis, TN 38118-2461
(901) 541-9400

Southern Health Plan
P.O. Box 97
Memphis, TN 38101-0049
(901) 725-7100

Aetna Health Plan of Tennessee
1801 W. End Ave., Ste. 500
Nashville, TN 37203-2509
(615) 322-1600

Cigna Healthcare of Tennessee
1801 W. End Ave., Ste. 800
Nashville, TN 37203-2526
(615) 340-3059

Cigna Medicare Service Organization
P.O. Box 1465
Nashville, TN 37202-1465
(615) 244-5600

Private Healthcare Systems
3319 W. End Ave., Ste. 400
Nashville, TN 37203-1075
(615) 386-9194

Prudential Healthcare Nashville
227 French Landing Dr., #300
Nashville, TN 37228-1605
(615) 248-7100

Tennessee Managed Care Network
210 Athens Way Metro Ctr.
Nashville, TN 37228-1308
(800) 269-3133

Tennessee Primary Care Network
205 Reidhurst Ave., Ste. N-104
Nashville, TN 37203-1618
(615) 329-2016

TEXAS

Harris Methodist Health Plan
611 Ryan Plaza Dr., Ste. 900
Arlington, TX 76011-4008
(817) 462-7000

FirstCare
12940 Research Blvd.
Austin, TX 78759
(512) 257-6215

Foundation Health Plan
9101 Burnet Rd., Ste. 104
Austin, TX 78758-5260
(512) 873-6100

HMO Blue
9020-11 Capital of Texas Highway North
Austin, TX 78759
(512) 345-0089

PCA Health Plans of Texas, Inc.
P.O. Box 9420
Austin, TX 78766-9420
(800) 234-7912

PCA Health Plans of Texas, Inc.
8303 North Mo-Pac Expressway, Ste. 450C
Austin, TX 78759-8369
(512) 454-6771

United Healthcare
9442 Capital of Texas Highway North, #600
Austin, TX 78759-7262
(800) 424-6480

Principal Healthcare of Texas
555 N. Carancahua St., Ste. 500
Corpus Christi, TX 78478-0301
(512) 887-0101

Aetna US Healthcare
2777 Stemmons Freeway
Dallas, TX 75207-2277
(214) 200-8000

Kaiser Foundation Health of Texas
12720 Hillcrest Rd., Ste. 600
Dallas, TX 75230-2043
(972) 458-5000

Prudential Healthcare System
4100 Alpha Rd., Ste. 400
Dallas, TX 75244-4327
(972) 991-0014

Prudential Health Care Plan, Inc.
100 N. Stanton, Ste. 1201
El Paso, TX 79901-1448
(915) 532-0700

Young Insurance/Advantage Care
P.O. Box 12609
El Paso, TX 79913-0609
(800) 854-2339

CorpHealth, Inc.
1300 Summit Ave., Ste. 600
Fort Worth, TX 76102-4420
(817) 332-2519

Aetna Health Plans
2900 N. Loop W., Ste. 300
Houston, TX 77092-8841
(713) 683-4500

Alliance Health Providers
9494 S.W. Freeway, Ste. 550
Houston, TX 70747-1420
(713) 683-2903

Cigna Health Care
2 Riverway St., Ste. 1200
Houston, TX 77056-1912
(713) 552-7600

MBC
24 Greenway Plaza, Ste. 725
Houston, TX 77046-2401
(713) 871-0821

National Association of Preferred Providers
15333 J F Kennedy Blvd., Ste. 505
Houston, TX 77032-2342
(713) 449-1313

Texas Children's Health Plan
P.O. Box 301011
Houston, TX 77230-1011
(713) 770-1000

United Healthcare of Texas
5 Post Oak Park, Ste. 550
Houston, TX 77027-3413
(713) 961-4300

Humana Health Care Plan
8431 Fredericksburg Rd., Ste. 360
San Antonio, TX 78229-3364
(210) 617-1000

Pacificare of Texas
8200 West IH 10, Ste. 1000
San Antonio, TX 78230-3878
(210) 524-9800

Prucare of Houston
1 Prudential Cir.
Sugar Land, TX 77478-3833
(713) 494-5000

UTAH

First Health
6975 Union Park Ctr., Ste. 600
Midvale, UT 84047-4183
(801) 568-5500

Union Pacific Railroad Health
3795 Kieesel Ave.
Ogden, UT 84405-1635
(801) 394-5741

FHP Administration
35 W. Broadway
Salt Lake City, UT 84101-2020
(801) 355-1234

Intermountain Health Care
36 South State St.
Salt Lake City, UT 84111-1453
(801) 442-2000

VERMONT

Blue Cross/Blue Shield of Vermont
P.O. Box 186
Montpelier, VT 05601-0186
(802) 223-6131

Community Health Plan Vermont
7 Park Ave.
Williston, VT 05495-9782
(802) 878-2334

VIRGINIA

Healthkeepers
3800 Concord Pkwy., Ste. 2000
Chantilly, VA 20151-1127
(800) 544-1901

Aetna Health Plans
7600 Leesburg Pike, Ste. A
Falls Church, VA 22043-2004
(703) 903-7100

Peninsula Health Care, Inc.
606 Denbigh Blvd., Ste. 500
Newport News, VA 23608-4439
(757) 875-5760

Aetna Health Plans
9030 Stony Point Pkwy.
Richmond, VA 23235-1936
(804) 330-8686

Cigna Health Plan of Virginia
P.O. Box 31353
Richmond, VA 23294-1353
(804) 273-1100

Prudential Health System
1000 Boulders Pkwy.
Richmond, VA 23225-5510
(804) 323-0900

Southern Health Services
P.O. Box 85603
Richmond, VA 23285-5603
(804) 747-3700

Virginia Health Network
7400 Beaufont Springs Dr., #505
Richmond, VA 23225-5519
(804) 320-3837

Cigna Healthcare of Virginia
200 Golden Oak Ct., Ste. 450
Virginia Beach, VA 23452-6756
(757) 463-8606

OPTIMA Health Plan
4417 Corporation Ln.
Virginia Beach, VA 23462-3147
(757) 552-7474

Priority Health Care
621 Lynnhaven Pkwy., Ste. 450
Virginia Beach, VA 23452-7300
(757) 463-4600

Sentara Health Plan
4417 Corporation Ln.
Virginia Beach, VA 23462-3114
(757) 552-7100

WASHINGTON D.C.

DC Chartered Health Plan, Inc.
820 First St. N.E., Ste. LL100
Washington, DC 2002-4243
(202) 408-4710

WASHINGTON

Group Health Northwest
3311 W. Clear Water, Ste. 1010
Kennewick, WA 99336-2776
(509) 783-3484

SelectCare
1338 Commerce St., Ste. 300
Longview, WA 98632-3732
(360) 577-4419

Group Health Cooperative Puget Sound
521 Wall St.
Seattle, WA 98121-1524
(206) 448-4137

Health First Partners
601 Union St., Ste. 700
Seattle, WA 98101-2327
(206) 667-8070

Sisters of Providence Health Plan
1501 Fourth Ave., Ste. 500
Seattle, WA 98101-1662
(206) 622-6111

Qual Med Washington Health Plan
P.O. Box 2470
Spokane, WA 99210-2470
(509) 459-6687

United PPO
1101 N. Agonne Rd., Ste. 107
Spokane, WA 99212-2699
(509) 928-2569

Pierce County Medical
1501 Market St.
Tacoma, WA 98402-3333
(206) 597-6520

WEST VIRGINIA

Charleston Area Health Plan, Inc.
P.O. Box 1711
Charleston, WV 25326-1711
(304) 348-2901

Mountain State Blue Cross
P.O. Box 1948
Parkersburg, WV 26102-1948
(304) 424-7700

Advantage Health
P.O. Box 470
Wheeling, WV 26003-0060
(304) 243-1489

WISCONSIN

Network Health Plan
P.O. Box 507
Appleton, WI 54912-0507
(414) 735-6440

United Health of Wisconsin
P.O. Box 507
Appletown, WI 54912-0507
(414) 735-6440

Group Health Cooperative
P.O. Box 3217
Eau Claire, WI 54702-3217
(715) 836-8552

Valley Health Plan
2270 Eastridge Ctr.
Eau Claire, WI 54701-3410
(715) 832-3235

ProVantage Prescription Management
408 Lombardi Ave.
Green Bay, WI 54304-3764
(414) 436-6162

Atrium Health Plan
2215 Vine St., Ste. E
Hudson, WI 54016-5802
(715) 386-6886

Greater La Crosse Health Plan
P.O. Box 38
La Crosse, WI 54602-0038
(608) 781-9692

Gundersen Clinic
1836 South Ave.
La Crosse, WI 54601-5494
(608) 782-7300

Dean Healthplan
P.O. Box 56099
Madison, WI 53705-9399
(608) 836-1400

Group Health Cooperative
P.O. Box 44971
Madison, WI 53744-4971
(608) 831-1766

Wisconsin Physicians Services
P.O. Box 8190
Madison, WI 53708-8190
(608) 221-4711

Security Health Plans
1000 N. Oak Ave.
Marshfield, WI 54449-5703
(715) 387-5621

Network Health Plan
P.O. Box 120
Menashe, WI 54952-0120
(414) 727-0100

Aetna Health Plans
2675 N. Mayfair Rd., Ste. 506
Milwaukee, WI 53226-1305
(414) 256-2294

Blue Mound Medical Center
P.O. Box 601
Milwaukee, WI 53201-0601
(414) 771-5600

**Compcare Health Services
Insurance Corp.**
401 W. Michigan St.
Milwaukee, WI 53203-2804
(414) 226-6171

Family Health Systems
11524 W. Theodore Trecker Way
Milwaukee, WI 53214-1142
(414) 256-0006

**Humana Wisconsin Health
Organization**
111 W. Pleasant St.
Milwaukee, WI 53212-3939
(414) 223-3300

**Managed Health Services
Insurance**
2040 W. Wisconsin Ave., Ste. 452
Milwaukee, WI 53233-2012
(414) 321-9001

**Maxicare Health Insurance of
Wisconsin**
733 N. Van Buren, Ste. 620
Milwaukee, WI 53202-4705
(414) 271-6371

Primecare Health Plan, Inc.
10701 W. Research Dr.
Milwaukee, WI 53226-3452
(414) 443-4000

Wausau Insurance Company
P.O. Box 8017
Wausau, WI 54402-8017
(715) 845-5211

WYOMING

Blue Cross/Blue Shield
P.O. Box 2266
Cheyenne, WY 82003-2266
(307) 634-1393

Bibliography

Abernathy DR, Andrawis NS, "Critical Drug Interactions: A Guide to Important Examples," *Drug Therapy*, Vol. Cot 15–27, 1993.

Aguglia E, Casacchi GB, et al, "Double Blinded Study of the Efficacy and Safety of Sertraline Versus Fluoxetine in Major Depression," *Int Clin Psychopharmacol*, Vol. 8, 1994, pp. 197–202.

Ahronheim J, "Practical Pharmacology for Older Patients: Avoiding Adverse Drug Effects," *Mt Sinai J Med*, Vol. 60(6), Nov 1993, pp. 497–501.

Akhtar M, Breithardt G, Camm AJ, Coumel P, Janse MJ, Lazzara R, Myerberg RJ, Schwartz PJ, Waldo AL, Wellens HJ, et al, "CAST and Beyond. Implications of the Cardiac Arrhythmia Suppression Trial. Task Force of the Working Group on Arrhythmias of the European Society of Cardiology [Review]," *Circulation*, Vol. 81(3), Mar 1990, pp. 1123–1127.

Alacon GS, Tracy IC, Stand GM, et al, "Survival and Drug Discontinuation Analyses in a Large Cohort of Methotrexate Treated Rheumatoid Arthritis Patients," *Ann Rheum Dis*, Vol. 54, 1995, pp. 708–712.

Albrich JM, "Geriatric Pharmacology" In: Schwartz GR, Bosker G, Grigsby JW, eds *Geriatric Emergencies*, Bowie, Md: Robert J. Brady Co., 1984.

Alderman J, "Drug Interactions: The Death Pen [Letter]," *JAMA*, Vol. 270(11), Sep 15, 1993, p. 1316.

Aloia JF, Vaswani A, Yeh JK, et al, "Calcium Supplementation With and Without Hormone Replacement Therapy to Prevent Postmenopausal Bone Loss," *Ann Intern Med*, Vol. 120, 1994, p. 97.

American College of Physicians, "Improving Medical Education in Therapeutics," *Ann Intern Med*, Vol. 108, 1988, pp. 145–147.

Ancill RJ, Carlyle WW, Liang RA, Holliday SG, "Agitation in the Demented Elderly: A Role for the Benzodiazepines?," *Int Clin Psychopharmacol*, Vol. 6(3), Winter, 1991, pp. 141–146.

Anderson IM, Tomenson BM, "Treatment Discontinuation With Selective Serotonin Reuptake Inhibitors Compared With Tricyclic Antidepressants: A Meta-analysis," *BMJ*, Vol. 310, 1995, pp. 1433–1438.

Anonymous, "Anti-anxiety Drug Usage in the United States," 1989 *Statistical Bulletin-Metropolitan Insurance Companies*, Vol. 72(1), Jan–Mar 1991, pp. 18–27.

Anonymous, "The Effects of Nonpharmacologic Interventions on Blood Pressure of Persons with High Normal Levels. Results of the Trails of Hypertension Prevention, Phase I [published erratum appears in JAMA 1992 May 6; 267(17):2330] [see comments]," *JAMA*, Vol. 267(9), Mar 4, 1992, pp. 1213–1220.

Anonymous, "Why Do GPs Overprescribe Antibiotics? [news]," *Br J Hosp Med,* Vol. 46(1), Jul 1991, p. 59.

Ballenger JC, Pecknold J, Rickles K, Sellers EM, "Medication Discontinuation in Panic Disorder [Review]," *J Clin Psychiatry,* Vol. 54 Suppl, Oct 1993, pp. 15–21; discussion 22–24.

Banks AT, Zimmerman HJ, Ishak KG, et al, "Diclofenac-associated Hepatotoxicity: Analysis of 180 Cases Reported to the Food and Drug Administration as Adverse Reactions," *Hepatology,* Vol. 22, 1995, pp. 820–827.

Barnett HJ, "Aspirin in Stroke Prevention. An Overview," *Stroke,* Vol. 21(12 Suppl), Dec 1990, p. IV40–3.

Bauer DC, for the Study of Osteoporotic Fractures Research Group, "Aspirin and NSAID Use in Older Women: Effect on Bone Mineral Density and Fracture Risk," *J Bone Miner Res,* Vol. 11, 1996, pp. 29–35.

Baxter JD, "Minimizing the Side Effects of Glucocorticoid Therapy [Review]," *Adv Intern Med,* Vol. 35, 1990, pp. 173–193.

Beers MH, Ouslander JG, Fingold SF, Morgenstern H, Reuben DB, Rogers W, Zeffren MJ, Beck JC, "Inappropriate Medication Prescribing in Skilled-Nursing Facilities," *Ann Intern Med,* Vol. 117(8), Oct 15, 1992, pp. 684–689.

Berger MS, "A Proposal for Using Generics," *Pa Med,* Vol. 96(5), May 1993, p. 10.

Blazer DG, et al, "The Risk of Anticholinergic Toxicity in the Elderly: A Study of Prescribing Practices in Two Populations," *J Gerontol,* Vol. 38(1), 1983, p. 31.

Bosker G, "Acute Otitis Media in Children; Overcoming Barriers to Clinical Cure," *Pediatric Emergency Medicine Reports,* Feb 1996, Atlanta, Georgia: American Health Consultants.

Bosker G, "Antibiotic Update," *Emergency Medicine Reports,* 1996, Atlanta, Georgia: American Health Consultants.

Bosker G, *Pharmatecture: Minimizing Medications to Maximize Results,* Facts and Comparisons, 1996, St. Louis.

Bosker G (Editor), *Geriatric Emergency Medicine,* 1993, St. Louis, Missouri: Mosby Yearbook Publishers.

Bosker G (Editor), *The Manual of Emergency Medicine Therapeutics,* 1996, St. Louis, Missouri: Mosby Yearbook Publishers.

Bosker G, Stander P (Editors) *The Quick Consult Manual of Primary Care Medicine,* 1997, Boston: Little, Brown and Company.

Bowler SD, Mitchell CA, Armstrong JG, "Corticosteroids in Acute Severe Asthma: Effectiveness of Low Doses [see comments]," *Thorax,* Vol. 74(8), Aug 1992, pp. 584–587.

Bradley C, Blenkinsopp A, "The Future for Self Medication," *BMJ,* Vol. 312, 1996, pp. 835–837.

Bradley CP, Bond C, "Increasing the Number of Drugs Available Over the Counter: Arguments For and Against," *Br J Gen Pract,* Vol. 45, 1995, pp. 553–556.

Bressler R, Katz MD, "Drug Therapy for Geriatric Depression [Review]," *Drugs Aging,* Vol. 3(3), May–Jun 1993, pp. 195–219.

Bridgen ML, "Oral Anticoagulant Thearapy. Newer Indications and an Improved Method of Monitoring [Review]," *Postgrad Med,* Vol. 91(2), Feb 1, 1992, pp. 285–288, 293–296.

Buchanan N, "Noncompliance with Medication Amongst Persons Attending a Tertiary Referral Epilepsy Clinic: Implications, Management and Outcome," *Seizure,* Vol. 2(1), Mar 1993, pp. 79–82.

Burris JF, "Hypertension Management in the Elderly [Review]," *Heart Disease Stroke,* Vol. 3(2), Mar–Apr 1994, pp. 77–83.

Burrows GD, Norman TR, Jud FK, Marriott PF, "Short-acting Versus Long-Acting Benzodiazepines: Discontinuation Effects in Panic Disorders [Review]," *J Psychiatr Res*, Vol. 24 Suppl 2, 1990, pp. 65–72.

Burrows GD, Norman TR, Judd FK, Marriott PF, "Short-acting Versus Long-acting Benzodiazepines: Discontinuation Effects in Panic Disorders," *J Psychiatr Res*, Vol. 24 Supp 2, 1990, pp. 65–72.

Busto UE, Sellers EM, "Anxiolytics and Sedative/hypnotics Dependence," *Br J Addict*, Vol. 86(12), Dec 1991, pp. 1647–1652.

Cadieux RJ, "Geriatric Psychopharmacology. A Primary Care Challenge [Review]," *Postgrad Med*, Vol. 93(4), Mar 1993, p. 281.

Canadian Medical Association, "Medication Use and the Elderly," *Can Med Assoc J*, Vol. 149(8), Oct 15, 1993, p. 1152A–D.

Cancellaro LA, "Appropriate Use of Neuroleptics and Antidepressants in the Geriatric Patient," *South Med J*, Vol. 84 (5 Suppl), May 1991, pp. S53–56.

Carvajal A, Prieto JR, Requejo AA, et al, "Aspirin or Acetominophen? A Comparison From Data Collected by the Spanish Drug Monitoring System," *J Clin Epidemiol*, Vol. 49, 1996, pp. 255–261.

Centers for Disease Control, "Immunization Practices Advisory Committee. General Recommendations on Immunization," *Ann Intern Med*, Vol. 111, 1989, p. 133.

Chapman KR, et al, "Effect of a Short Course of Prednisone in the Prevention of Early Relapse After the Emergency Room Treatment of Acute Asthma," *N Engl J Med*, Vol. 324, 1991, p. 788.

Ciraulo DA, Shader RI, "Fluoxetine Drug-drug Interactions II [Review]," *J Clin Psychopharmacol*, Vol. 10(3), June, 1990, pp. 213–217.

Closser MH, "Benzodiazepines and the Elderly. A Review of Potential Problems [Review]," *J Subst Abuse Treat*, Vol. 8(1-2), 1991, pp. 35–41.

Coleman TJ, "Non-redemption of Prescriptions. Linked to Poor Consultation," *BMJ*, Vol. 308(6921), Jan 8, 1994, p. 135.

Colley CA, Lucas LM, "Polypharmacy: The Cure Becomes the Disease [Review]," *J Gen Intern Med*, Vol. 8(5), May 1993, pp. 278–283.

Coons SJ, Kaplan RM, "Assessing Health-related Quality of Life: Applications to Drug Therapy," *Clin Ther*, Vol. 14(6), 1992, pp. 850–858; discussion 849.

Cooper JW, "Probable Adverse Drug Reactions in a Rural Geriatric Nursing Home Population: A Four-year Study," *J Am Geriatr Soc*, Vol. 44, 1996, pp. 194–197.

Cormack MA, Howelis E, "Factors Linked to the Prescribing of Benzodiazepines by General Practice Principals and Trainees," *Fam Pract*, Vol. 9(4), Dec 1992, pp. 466–471.

Crane JK, Shih HT, "Syncope and Cardiac Arrhythmia Due to an Interaction Between Itraconazole and Terfenadine," *Am J Med*, Vol. 95(4), Oct 1993, pp. 445–456.

Creutzfeldt W, "Risk-benefit Assessment of Omeprazole in the Treatment of Gastrointestinal Disorders [Review]," *Drug Saf*, Vol. 10(1), Jan 1994, pp. 66–82.

Danner SA, for the European-Australian Collaborative Ritonavir Study Group, "A Short-term Study of the Safety, Pharmacokinetics, and Efficacy of Ritonavir, an Inhibitor of HIV-1 Protease," *N Engl J Med*, Vol. 333, 1995, pp. 1528–1533.

Darnell JC, et al, "Medications Used by Ambulatory Elderly: An Inhome Survey," *J Am Geriatr Soc*, Vol. 34, 1986, p. 1.

Dartnell JGA, Anderson RP, Chohan V, et al, "Hospitalisation for Adverse Events Related to Drug Therapy: Incidence, Avoidability and Costs," *Med J Aust*, Vol. 164, 1996, pp. 659–662.

Dawson-Hughes B, Dallal GE, Krall EA, et al, "Effect of Vitamin D Supplementation on Wintertime and Overall Bone Loss in Healthy Postmenopausal Women," *Ann Intern Med*, Vol. 115, 1991, pp. 505–512.

De Geest S, Abraham I, Gemoets H, Evers G, "Development of the Long-term Medication Behavior Self-efficacy Scale: Qualitative Study for Item Development," *J Adv Nurs*, Vol. 19(2), Feb 1994, pp. 233–238.

Denke MA, Grundy SM, "Hypercholesterolemia in the Elderly: Resolving the Treatment Dilemma," *Ann Intern Med*, Vol. 112, 1990, pp. 780–792.

DeSantis G, Harvey KJ, Howard D, Mashford ML, Moulds RF, "Improving the Quality of Antibiotic Prescription Patterns in General Practice. The Role of Educational Intervention," *Med J Aust*, Vol. 160(8), Apr 18, 1994, pp. 502–505.

Devor M, Barrett-Connor E, et al, "Estrogen Replacement Therapy and Risk of Venous Thrombosis," *Am J Med*, Vol. 92, 1992, pp. 271–282.

Deyo RA, Inui TS, Sullivan B, "Noncompliance with Arthritis Drugs: Magnitude, Correlates, and Clinical Implications," *J Rheumatol*, Vol. 8, 1981, pp. 931–936.

Dichter MA, "Deciding to Discontinue Antiepileptic Medication," *Hosp Pract (Off Ed)*, Vol. 27(10A), Oct 30, 1992, pp. 16, 21–22.

DiMasi JA, "Success Rates for New Drugs Entering Clinical Testing in the United States," *Clin Pharmacol Ther*, Vol. 58, 1995, pp. 1–14.

Douglas RG, "Prophylaxis and Treatment of Influenza," *N Engl J Med*, Vol. 322, 1990, p. 443.

Doren M, Reuther G, Minne HW, et al, "Superior Compliance and Efficacy of Continuous Combined Oral Estrogen-Progestogen Replacement Therapy in Postmenopausal Women," *Am J Obstet Gynecol*, Vol. 173, 1995, pp. 1446–1451.

Dunner DL, "An Overview of Paroxetine in the elderly [Review]," *Gerontology*, Vol. 40(Supp), 1994, pp. 21–27.

Durnas C, Cusak BJ, "Salicylate Intoxication in the Elderly. Recognition and Recommendations on How to Prevent It [Review]," *Drugs Aging*, Vol. 2(1), Jan–Feb 1992, pp. 20–34.

Eagger SA, Levy R, Sahakian BJ, "Tacrine in Alzheimer's Disease [see comments]," *Lancet*, Vol. 337(8748), Apr 27, 1991, pp. 989–992.

Eisen SA, Miller DK, Woodward RS, Spitznagel E, Przybeck TR, "The Effect of Prescribed Daily Dose Frequency on Patient Medication Compliance," *Arch Intern Med*, Vol. 150(9), Sep 1990, pp. 1881–1884.

Ellmers SE, "Limiting the Drugs List. The Trouble with Generic Prescribing," *BMJ*, Vol. 306(6893), Jun 19, 1993, p. 1687.

Facchinetti F, for the Sumatriptan Menstrual Migraine Study Group, "The Efficacy and Safety of Subcutaneous Sumatriptan in the Acute Treatment of Menstrual Migraine," *Obstet Gynecol*, Vol. 86, 1995, pp. 911–616.

Falk GW, "Omeprazole: A New Drug for the Treatment of Acid-peptic Diseases [Review]," *Cleve Clin J Med*, Vol. 58(5), Sep–Oct 1991, pp. 418–427.

Falkeborn M, et al, "Hormone Replacement Therapy and the Risk of Stroke," *Arch Intern Med*, Vol. 153, 1993, pp. 1201–1209.

FDA Drug Experience Monthly Bulletin: Reports of Suspected Incidents of Adverse Reactions to Drugs, 1987, Rockville, Md: US Food and Drug Administration, Bureau of Medicine p. 87.

File SE, Andrews N, "Benzodiazipine Withdrawal: Behavioural Pharmacology and Neurochemical

Changes [Review]," *Biochem Soc Symp*, Vol. 59, 1993, pp. 97–106.

Flack JM, Wolley A, Esunge P, Grimm RH, "A Rational Approach to Hypertension Treatment in the Older Patient [Review]," *Geriatrics*, Vol. 47(11), Nov 1992, pp. 24–28, 33–38.

Fleming KC, Evans JM, "Pharmacologic Therapies in Dementia," *Mayo Clin Proc*, Vol. 70, 1995, pp. 1116–1123.

Fletcher A, Bulpitt C, "Quality of Life and Antihypertensive Drugs in the Elderly [Review]," *Aging (Milano)*, Vol. 4(2), Jun 1992, pp. 115–123.

Frank T, "Tapering Antihypertensives: Avoiding the Rebound," *Senior Patient*, June 16, 1990.

Freeman C, "Drug Treatment of Insomnia in the Elderly," *Conn Med*, Vol. 56(1), Jan 1992, pp. 35–37.

Frishman WH, "Beta-adrenergic Blocker Withdrawal," *Am J Cardiol*, Vol. 59, 1987, pp. 26F–32F.

Frishman WH, "Beta-adrenergic Blockers as Cardioprotective Agents," *Am J Cardiol*, Vol. 70(21), Dec 21, 1992, pp. 21–61.

Fuchs Z, Viskoper JR, Drexler I, Nitzan H, Lubin F, Berlin S, Almagor M, Zulty L, Chetrit A, Mishal J, et al, "Comprehensive Individualised Nonpharmacological Treatment Programme for Hypertension in Physician-nurse Clinics: Two Year Follow-up," *J Hum Hyptertens*, Vol. 7(6), Dec 1993, pp. 585–591.

Furberg C, for the PPP Project Investigators, "Design, Rationale, and Baseline Characteristics of the Prospective Pravastatin Pooling (PPP) Project—A Combined Analysis of Three Large-scale Randomized Trials: Long-term Intervention With Pravastatin in Ischemic Disease (LIPID), Cholesterol and Recurrent Events (CARE), and West of Scotland Coronary Prevention Study (WOSCOPS)," *American Journal of Cardiology*, Vol. 76, 1995, pp. 899–905.

Furguson RP, Wetle T, Dubitzky D, Winsemius D, "Relative Importance to Elderly Patients of Effectiveness, Adverse Effects, Convenience and Cost of Antihypertensive Medications. A Pilot Study," *Drugs Aging*, Vol. 4(1), Jan 1994, pp. 56–62.

Gabriel SE, Campion ME, O'Fallon WM, "A Cost-utility Analysis of Misoprostol Prophylaxis for Rheumatoid Arthritis Patients Receiving Nonsteroidal Anti-inflammatory Drugs," *Arthritis Rheum 1994*, Vol. 37(3), Mar 1994, pp. 333–341.

Garner EM, Kelly MW, Thompson DF, "Tricyclic Antidepressant Withdrawal Syndrome [Review]," *Ann Pharmacother*, Vol. 27(9), Sep 1993, pp. 1068–1072.

Garrad J, Makris L, Dunham T, Heston LL, Cooper S, Ratner ER, Zelterman D, Kane RL, "Evaluation of Neuroleptic Drug Use by Nursing Home Elderly Under Proposed Medicare and Medicaid Regulations [see comments]," *JAMA*, Vol. 265(4), Jan 23–30, 1991, pp. 463–467.

Gaspoz J-M, Kennedy JW, Orav EJ, et al, "Cost-effectiveness of Prescription Recommendations for Cholesterol-Lowering Drugs: A Survey of a Representative Sample of American Cardiologists," *J Am Coll Cardiol*, Vol. 27, 1996, pp. 1232–1237.

Gherpilli JK, Kok F, dal Forno S, Elkis LC, Lefevre BH, Diament AJ, "Discontinuing Medication in Epileptic Children: A Study of Risk Factors Related to Recurrence," *Epilepsia*, Vol. 33(4), Jul-Aug 1992, pp. 681–686.

Giovannucci E, Egan KM, Hunter DJ, et al, "Aspirin and the Risk of Colorectal Cancer in Women," *N Engl J Med*, Vol. 333, 1995, pp. 609–614.

Glassman AH, Roose SP, "Risks of Antidepressants in the Elderly: Tricyclic Antidepressants and Arrhythmia-revising Risks [Review]," *Gerontology*, Vol. 40 (Supp), 1994, pp. 15–20.

Goroll A (Editor), *Primary Care Medicine*, 1996, Philadelphia: Lippincott-Raven Publishers.

Gosney M, Tallis RL, "Prescription of Contraindicated and Interacting Drugs in Elderly Patients Admitted to Hospital," *Lancet*, Vol. 2, 1984, pp. 564–567.

Graham DY, White RH, Moreland LW, et al, "Duodenal and Gastric Ulcer Prevention with Misoprostol in Arthritis Patients Taking NSAIDs," *Ann Intern Med*, Vol. 119, 1993, p. 257.

Granek E, et al, "Medication and Diagnosis in Relation to Falls in a Long-term Care Facility," *J Am Geriatric Soc*, Vol. 35, 1987, p. 505.

Green LW, Purrell CO, Koop CE, et al, "Programs to Reduce Drug Errors in the Elderly: Direct and Indirect Evidence from Patient Education.," *Improving Medication Compliance*, 1985, Reston, Va: National Pharm Council.

Greenblatt DJ, Harmatz JS, et al, "Sensitivity to Triazolam in the Elderly," *N Engl J Med*, Vol. 324, 1991, pp. 1691–1698.

Greenblatt DJ, Miller LG, Shader RL, "Benxodiazepine Discontinuation Syndromes [Review]," *J Psychiatr Res*, Vol. 24 Suppl 2, 1990, pp. 73–79.

Greenblatt RM, Hollander H, McMaster JR, Henke CJ, "Polypharmacy Among Patients Attending an AIDS Clinic: Utilization of Prescribed, Unorthodox, and Investigational Treatments" *J Acquir Immune Defic Syndr*, Vol. 4(2), 1991, pp. 136–143.

Griffin MR, et al, "NSAID Use and Death From Peptic Ulceration in the Elderly," *Ann Intern Med*, Vol. 109, 1988, pp. 359–363.

Gross PA, Hermogenes AW, Sacks HS, et al, "The Efficacy of Influenza Vaccine in Elderly Persons: A Meta-analysis and Review of the Literature," *Ann Intern Med*, Vol. 123, 1995, pp. 518–527.

Gryfe CI, Gryfe BM, "Drug Therapy for the Aged: The Problems of Compliance and the Roles of Physicians and Pharmacists," *J Am Geriatr Soc*, Vol. 32(4), 1984, p. 301.

Gurwitz JH, Goldberg RJ, Chen Z, Gore JM, Alpert JS, "Beta-blocker Therapy in Acute Myocardial Infarction: Evidence for Underutilization in the Elderly," *Am J Med*, Vol. 93(6), Dec 1992, pp. 605–610.

Gurwitz JH, Noonan JP, Soumerai SB, "Reducing the Use of H2-Receptor Antagonists in the Long-term-care Setting [see comments]," *J Am Geriatr Soc*, Vol. 40(4), Apr 1992, pp. 359–364.

Hallas J, Harvald B, Worm J, Beck-Nielsen J, Gram LF, Grodum E, Damsbo N, Schou J, Kromann-Andersen H, Frolund F, "Drug Related Hospital Admissions. Results From an Intervention Program," *Eur J Clin Pharmacol*, Vol. 45(3), 1993, pp. 199–203.

Hallas J, Worm J, Beck-Nielsen J, Gram LF, Grodum E, Damsbo N, Brosen K, "Drug Related Events and Drug Utilization in Patients Admitted to a Geriatric Hospital Department," *Dan Med Bull*, Vol. 38(5), Oct 1991, pp. 417–420.

Hamilton RA, Gordon T, "Incidence and Cost of Hospital Admissions Secondary to Drug Interactions Involving Theophylline," *Ann Pharmacother*, Vol. 26(12), Dec 1992, pp. 1507–1511.

Haq IU, Jackson PR, Yeo WW, et al, "Sheffield Risk and Treatment Table for Cholesterol Lowering for Primary Prevention of Coronary Heart Disease," *Lancet*, Vol. 346, 1995, pp. 1467–1471.

Harris R, "Pharmacological and Nonpharmacological Approaches to the Treatment of Cardiovascular Disease in the Geriatric Patients," *Geriatr Med Today*, Vol. 1(3), 1982, p. 47.

Hartert TV, Windom HH, Peebles RS Jr, et al, "Inadequate Outpatient Medical Therapy for Patients With Asthma Admitted to Two Urban Hospitals," *Am J Med*, Vol. 100, 1996, pp. 386–394.

Harvey RP, Comer C, Sanders B, et al, "Model for Outcomes Assessment of Antihistamine Use for Seasonal Allergic Rhinitis," *J Allergy Clin Immunol*, Vol. 97, 1996, pp. 1233–1241.

Heimberger T, Chang H-G, Shaikh M, et al, "Knowledge and Attitudes of Healthcare Workers About Influenza: Why Are They Not Getting Vaccinated?," *Infect Control Hosp Epidemiol*, Vol. 16, 1995, pp. 412–414.

Held P, "Effects of Beta-blockers on Ventricular Dysfunction After Myocardial Infarction: Tolerability and Survival Effects," *Am J Cardiol*, Vol. 71(9), Mar 25, 1993, pp. 39C–44C.

Helling DK, Lemke LH, Semia TP, et al, "Medication Use Characteristics in the Elderly: The Iowa 65+ Rural Health Study," *J Am Geriatr Soc*, Vol. 35, 1987, pp. 4–12.

Hennekens CH, Jonas MA, Buring JE, "The Benefits of Aspirin in Acute Myocardial Infarction. Still a Well-kept Secret in the United States," *Arch Intern Med*, Vol. 154(1), Jan 10, 1994, pp. 37–39.

Henry D, Lim LL-Y, Rodriguez LAG, et al, "Variability in Risk of Gastrointestinal Complications With Individual Non-steroidal Anti-inflammatory Drugs: Results of a Collaborative Meta-analysis," *BMJ*, Vol. 312, 1996, pp. 1563–1566.

Heston LL, Garrard J, Makris L, Kane RL, Cooper S, Dunham T, Zelterman D, "Inadequate Treatment of Depressed Nursing Home Elderly," *J Am Geriatr Soc*, Vol. 40(11), Nov 1992, pp. 1117–1122.

Hetzel DJ, "Controlled Clinical Trials of Omeprazole in the Long-term Management of Reflux Disease [Review]," *Digestion*, Vol. 51 Suppl 1, 1992, pp. 35–42.

Hirsh J, Dalen JE, Foster V, Harker LB, Slazman EW, "Aspirin and Other Platelet-active Drugs. The Relationship Between Dose, Effectiveness, and Side Effects [Review]," *Chest*, Vol. 102 (4 Suppl), Oct 1992, pp. 327S–336S.

Hodsman GP, Johnston CL, "Angiotensin Converting Enzyme Inhibitors: Drug Interactions," *Hypertension*, Vol. 5, 1987, pp. 1–6.

Hoffman J, Barefield FA, Ramamurthy S, "A Survey of Physician Knowledge of Drug Costs," *J Pain Symptom Manage*, Vol. 10, 1995, pp. 432–435.

Holden MD, "Over-the-Counter Medications: Do You Know What Your Patients are Taking?," *Post-grad Med*, Vol. 91(8), Jun 1992, pp. 191–194, 199–200.

Hood JC, Murphy JE, "Patient Noncompliance Can Lead to Hospital Readmissions," *Hospitals*, Vol. 52, 1978, pp. 79–82, 84.

Hutchinson TA, et al, "Frequency, Severity, and Risk Factors for Adverse Drug Reactions in Adult Outpatients: Prospective Study," *J Chronic Diseases*, Vol. 39(7), 1986, p. 533.

Hux JE, Levinton CM, Naylor CD, "Prescribing Propensity: Influence of Life-expectancy Gains and Drug Costs," *J Gen Inter Med*, Vol. 9(4), April, 1994, pp. 195–201.

Imperiale TF, Speroff T, Cebul RD, et al, "A Cost Analysis of Alternative Treatments for Duodenal Ulcer," *Ann Intern Med*, Vol. 123, 1995, pp. 665–672.

Iserson KV, Hackney KU, "Anithistamines. In Haddad LM and Winchester JF," *Clinical Management of Poisoning and Drug Overdose*, 1983, Philadelphia: WB Saunders Co.

Jenck MA, Reynolds MS, "Anticonvulsant Drug Withdrawal in Seizure-free Patients [Review]," *Clin Pharm*, Vol. 9(10), Oct 1990, pp. 781–787.

Jerling M, "Dosing of Antidepressants: The Unknown Art," *J Clin Psychopharmacol*, Vol. 12, 1995, pp. 435–439.

Jones JK, "Assessing Potential Risk of Drugs: The Elusive Target," *Ann Intern Med*, Vol. 117(8), Oct 15, 1992, pp. 691–692.

Jordan LK 3d, Jordan LO, "Prudent Prescribing. Prescribing Suggestions for Physicians," *N C Med J*, Vol. 53(11), Nov 1992, pp. 585–588.

Jue SG, Vestal RE, "Adverse Drug Reactions in the Elderly: A Critical Review O'Malley K. Ed.," *Medicine in Old Age-Clinical Pharmacology and Drug Therapy*, 1985, London.

Kaplan NM, "Combination Therapy for Systemic Hypertension," *Am J Cardiol*, Vol. 76, 1995, pp. 595–597.

Kaplan NM, "How Bad are Diuretic-induced Hypokalemia and Hypercholesterolemia?," *Arch Intern Med*, Vol. 149, Dec 1989, p. 2649.

Kaplan NM, "The Potential Benefits of Nonpharmacological Therapy," *Am J Hypertens*, Vol. 3(5 Pt 1), May 1990, pp. 425–427.

Katon W, von Korff M, Lin E, Bush T, Ormel J, "Adequacy and Duration of Antidepressant Treatment in Primary Care," *Med Care*, Vol. 30(1), Jan 1992, pp. 67–76.

Katz IR, "Drug Treatment of Depression in the Frail Elderly: Discussion of the NIH Consensus Development Conference on the Diagnosis and Treatment of Depression in Late Life [Review]," *Psychopharmacol Bull*, Vol. 29(1), 1993, pp. 101–108.

Keen PJ, "What is the Best Dosage Schedule for Patients?," *J R Soc Med*, Vol. 84(11), Nov 1991, pp. 640–641.

Keller MB, et al, "Treatment Received by Depressed Patients," *JAMA*, Vol. 248(15), 1982, p. 1848.

Kernan WN, Castellsague J, Perlman GD, Ostfeld A, "Incidence of Hospitalization for Digitalis Toxicity Among Elderly Americans," *Am J Med*, Vol. 96(5), May 1994, p. 426.

Khosla S, Sornberg J, "Mild Heart Failure: Why the Switch to ACE Inhibitors?," *Geriatrics*, Vol. 48(11), Nov 1993, pp. 47–48, 51–54.

Kleerup EC, Tashkin DP, "Outpatient Treatment of Adult Asthma," *West J Med*, Vol. 163, 1995, pp. 49–63.

Knapp DA, et al, "Drug Prescribing for Ambulatory Patients 85 Years of Age and Older," *J Am Geriatr Soc*, Vol. 32(2), 1984, p. 138.

Knight JR, Campbell J, Williams SM, Clark DW, "Knowledgeable Noncompliance with Prescribed Drugs in Elderly Subjects: A Study with Particular Reference to Nonsteroidal Antiinflamatory and Antidepressant Drugs," *J Clin Pharm Ther*, Vol. 16(2), April, 1991, pp. 131–137.

Kranzelok EP, Anderson GM, Mirik M, "Massive Diphenhydramine Overdose Resulting in Death," *Ann Emerg Med*, Vol. 11(4), 1982, p. 212.

Kroenke K, Pinholt EM, "Reducing Polypharmacy in the Elderly. A Controlled Trial of Physician Feedback," *J Am Geriatr Soc*, Vol. 38(1), 1990, pp. 31–36.

Kushi LH, Folsom AR, Prineas RJ, et al "Dietary Antioxidant Vitamins and Death From Coronary Heart Disease in Postmenopausal Women," *N Engl J Med*, Vol. 334, 1996, pp. 1156–1162.

Laan RF, et al "Low-dose Prednisone Induces Rapid Reversible Axial Bone Loss in Patients with Rheumatoid Arthritis," *Ann Intern Med*, Vol. 119, 1993, pp. 963–968.

Lamy PP, "A Consideration of NSAID Use in the Elderly," *Geriatric Medicine Today*, Vol. 7(4), 1988, p. 30.

Lamy PP, "Drug Therapy in the Elderly," *Pharmacy International*, Vol. 7, 1986, p. 46.

Lamy PP, "Medication Management," *Clin Geriatr Med*, Vol. 4, 1984, pp. 623–638.

Lamy PP, "Renal Effects of Nonsteroidal Anti-inflammatory Drugs. Heightened Risk to the Elderly?," *J Am Geriatr Soc*, Vol. 34, 1986, pp. 361–367.

Larson EB, Kukull WA, Buchner D, et al, "Adverse Drug Reactions Associated with Global Cognitive Impairment in Elderly Persons," *Ann Intern Med*, Vol. 107, 1987, pp. 169–173.

Laucka PV, Hoffman NB, "Decreasing Medication Use in a Nursing-home Patient-care Unit," *Am J Hosp Pharm*, Vol. 49(1), Jan 1992, pp. 96–99.

Leape LL, for the ADE Prevention Study Group, "Systems Analysis of Adverse Drug Events," *JAMA*, Vol. 274, 1995, pp. 35–43.

LeMay P, "Quality of Life: Measuring Outcomes of Pharmaceutical Management. Summary of Workshop Proceeding," *Can J Public Health*, Vol. 83(3), May–June, 1992, pp. S5–16.

Levin GM, DeVane CL, "Prescribing Attitudes of Different Physician Groups Regarding Fluoxetine," *Ann Pharmacother*, Vol. 27(12), Dec 1993, pp. 1443–1447.

Limouzin-Lamothe MA, Mairon N, Joyce CR, Le Gal M, "Quality of Life After the Menopause; Influence of Hormonal Replacement Therapy," *Am J Obstet Gynecol*, Vol. 170(2), Feb 1994, pp. 618–624.

Lindley CM, Tully MP, Paramsothy V, Tallis RC, "Inappropriate Medication is a Major Cause of Adverse Drug Reactions in Elderly Patients," *Age Ageing*, Vol. 21(4), July, 1992, pp. 224–230.

Litchman HM, "Medication Noncompliance: A Significant Problem and Possible Strategies," *Rhode Island Medicine*, Vol. 76(12), Dec 1993, pp. 608–610.

Livingston J, Reeves RD, "Undocumented Potential Drug Interactions Found in Medical Records of Elderly Patients in a Long-term Care Facility," *J Am Diet Assoc*, Vol. 93(10), Oct 1993, pp. 1168–1170.

Magid D, Douglas JM Jr, Schwartz JS, "Doxycycline Compared With Azithromycin for Treating Women With Genital Chlamydia trachomatis Infections: An Incremental Cost-Effectiveness Analysis," *Ann Intern Med*, Vol. 124, 1996, pp. 389–399.

Marquardt D, "Antihistamines and the Heart," *West J Med*, Vol. 158(6), June 1993, pp. 613–614.

Maton PN, "Omeprazole [Review]," *N Engl J Med*, Vol. 324(14), Apr 4, 1991, pp. 965–975.

Mawhinney H, Spector SL, Heitjan D, Kinsman RA, Dirks JF, Pines I, "As-needed Medication Use in Asthma Usage Patterns and Patient Characteristics," *J Asthma*, Vol. 30(1), 1993, pp. 61–71.

May FE, Stewart RB, Cluff LE, "Drug Interactions and Multiple Drug Adminstration," *Clin Pharmacol Ther*, Vol. 22, 1977, pp. 322–328.

Mayer-Oakes SE, Kelman G, Beers MH, DeJong F, Matthias R, Atchison KA, Lubben JE, Schweitzer SO, "Benzodiazepine Use in Older, Community-dwelling Southern Californians: Prevalence and Clinical Correlates," *Ann Pharmacother*, Vol. 27(4), Apr 1993, pp. 416–421.

McCarthy DM, "Maintanance Therapy for Peptic Ulcer—Who Needs It? [Review]," *Gastroenterol Jpn*, Vol. 28, Suppl 5, May 1993, pp. 172–177.

McDonald CC, For the Scottish Cancer Trials Breast Group, "Cardiac and Vascular Morbidity in Women Receiving Adjuvant Tamoxifen for Breast Cancer in a Randomised Trial," *BMJ*, Vol. 311, 1995, pp. 977–980.

McNally DL, Wertheimer D, "Strategies to Reduce the High Cost of Patient Noncompliance," *Md Med J*, Vol. 41(3), Mar 1992, pp. 223–225.

McQuay H, Carroll D, Moore A, "Variation the Placebo Effect in Randomised Controlled Trials of Analgesics: All Is as Blind as It Seems," *Pain*, Vol. 64, 1995, pp. 331–335.

Meador KJ, Loring DW, Moore EE, et al, "Comparative Cognitive Effects of Phenobarbital, Phenytoin, and Valproate in Healthy Adults," *Neurology*, Vol. 45, 1995, pp. 1494–1499.

The Medical Letter on Drugs and Therapeutics, Vol. 36-39, 1994-1997, New Rochelle, New York: Medical Letter, Inc.

Messilia FS, "Fluoxetine: Adverse Effects and Drug-drug Interactions [Review]," *J Toxicol Clin Toxicol*, Vol. 31(4), 1993, pp. 603–630.

Monstad I, Krabbe A, Micieli G, et al, "Preemptive Oral Treatment With Sumatriptan During a Cluster Period," *Headache*, Vol. 35, 1995, pp. 607–613.

Montamat SC, Cusak B, "Overcoming Problems with Polypharmacy and Drug Misuse in the Elderly," *Clin Geriatr Med*, Vol. 8(1), Feb 1992, pp. 143–158.

Morganroth J, Bigger JT Jr, Anderson JL, "Treatment of Ventricular Arrhythmias by United States Cardiologists: A Survey Before the Cardiac Arrhythmia Suppression Trial Results Were Available," *Am J Cardiolog*, Vol. 23(2), Feb 1994, pp. 283–289.

Moriguchi Y, Consoni PR, Hekman PR, "Systemic Arterial Hypertension: Results of the Change From Pharmacological to Nonpharmacological Treatment," *J Cardiovasc Pharmacol*, Vol. 16, Suppl 8, 1990, pp. S72–74.

Morss SE, Lenert LA, Faustman WO, "The Side Effects of Antipsychotic Drugs and Patients' Quality of Life; Patient Education and Preference Assessment with Computers and Multimedia," *Proceedings – The Annual Symposium on Computer Applications in Medical Care*, Vol., 1993, pp. 17–21.

Nathan A, Sutters CA, "A Comparison of Community Pharmacists' and General Practitioners' Opinions on Rational Prescribing, Formularies and Other Prescribing-related Issues," *J R Soc Health*, Vol. 116(6), Dec 1993, pp. 302–307.

Nelson WL, Fraunfelder FT, et al, "Adverse Respiratory and Cardiovascular Events Attributed to Timolol Ophthalmic Solution, 1978-1985," *Am J Ophthalmol*, Vol. 102, 1986, pp. 606–611.

Nestico PF, Morganroth J, "Cardiac Arrhythmias in the Elderly: Antiarrhythmic Drug Treatment," *Cardiol Clin*, Vol. 4(2), 1986, pp. 285–303.

Newcomb PA, Storer BE, "Postmenopausal Hormone Use and Risk of Large-bowel Cancer," *J Natl Cancer Inst*, Vol. 87, 1995, pp. 1067–1071.

O'Connor HT, Richman RM, Steinbeck KS, et al, "Dexfenfluramine Treatment of Obesity: A Double Blind Trial With Post Trial Follow Up," *Int J Obes*, Vol. 19, 1995, pp. 181–189.

Ogren RA, Baldwin JL, Simon RA, "How Patients Determine When to Replace Their Metered-dose Inhalers," *Ann Allergy Asthma Immunol*, Vol. 75, 1995, pp. 485–489.

Olin B (Editor), *Drug Facts and Comparisons (1997 Edition)*, 1997, St. Louis, Missouri: Facts and Comparisons.

Opdycke RA, Ascione FJ, Shimp LA, Rosen RI, "A Systematic Approach to Educating Elderly Patients About Their Medications," *Pat Ed Coun*, Vol. 19(1), Feb 1992, pp. 43–60.

Oster G, Delea TE, Huse DM, et al, "The Benefits and Risks of Over-the-Counter Availability of Nicotine Polacrilex ('Nicotine Gum')," *Med Care*, Vol. 34, 1996, pp. 389–402.

Packer M, Gheorghiade M, Young JB, et al, "Withdrawal of Digoxin From Patients with Chronic Congestive Heart Failure Treated with Angiotensin-converting-enzyme Inhibitors," *N Engl J Med*, Vol. 329, 1993, pp. 1–7.

Palmer AJ, Fletcher AE, Rudge PJ, Andrews CD, Callaghan TS, Bulpitt CJ, "Quality of Life in Hypertensives Treated with Atenolol or Captopril: A Double-Blind Crossover Trial," *J Hyptertens*, Vol. 10(11), Nov 1992, pp. 1409–1416.

Pandey DK, Shekelle R, Selwyn BJ, et al, "Dietary Vitamin C and Beta-Carotene and Risk of Death in Middle-aged Men: The Western Electric Study," *Am J Epidemiol*, Vol. 142, 1995, pp. 1269–1278.

Park DC, Morrell RW, Frieske D, Kincaid D, "Medication Adherence Behaviors in Older Adults:

Effects of External Cognitive Supports," *Psychology & Aging,* Vol. 7(2), Jun 1992, pp. 252–256.

Parrish RH, "Understanding Physician Prescribing Behavior [letter]," *Am J Hosp Pharm,* Vol. 48(3), Mar 1991, p. 463.

Pearce LA, for the Stroke Prevention in Atrial Fibrillation Investigators, "Differential Effect of Aspirin Versus Warfarin on Clinical Stroke Types in Patients With Atrial Fibrillation," *Neurology,* Vol. 46, 1996, pp. 238–240.

Pecknold JC, "Discontinuation Reactions to Alprasolam in Panic Disorder," *J Psychiat Res,* Vol. 27 Suppl 1, 1993, pp. 155–170.

Pedersen TR, for the Scandinavian Simvastatin Survival Study Group, "Cholesterol Lowering and the Use of Healthcare Resources: Results of the Scandinavian Simvastatin Survival Study," *Circulation,* Vol. 93, 1996, pp. 1796–1802.

Peleg II, Lubin MF, Cotsonis GA, et al, "Long-Term Use of Nonsteroidal Antiinflammatory Drugs and Other Chemopreventors and Risk of Subsequent Colorectal Neoplasia," *Dig Dis Sci,* Vol. 41, 1996, pp. 1319–1326.

Petitti DB, Sidney S, Bernstein A, et al, "Stroke in Users of Low-dose Oral Contraceptives," *N Engl J Med,* Vol. 335, 1996, pp. 8–15.

Pfeffer M, "Angiotensin Coverting Enzyme Inhibition in Congestive Heart Failure: Benefit and Perspective," *Am Heart J,* Vol. 126 (3 Pt 2), Sep 1993, pp. 789–793.

The Physicians Desk Reference (1997 Edition), New Jersey: Medical Economics Company.

Pickering TG, "Predicting the Response to Nonpharmacologic Treatment in Mild Hypertension [editorial; comment]," *JAMA,* Vol. 267(9), Mar 4, 1992, pp. 1256–1257.

Piper JM, Ray WA, Daugherty JR, Griffin MR, "Corticosteroid Use and Peptic Ulcer Disease: Role of Nonsteroidal Anti-inflammatory Drugs," *Ann Intern Med,* Vol. 114(9), May 1, 1991, pp. 735–740.

Pollow RL, Stoller EP, Forster LE, Duniho TS, "Drug Combinations and Potential for Risk of Adverse Drug Reaction Among Community-dwelling Elderly," *Nurs Res,* Vol. 43(1), Jan-Feb 1994, pp. 44–49.

Prince RL, Smith M, Dick IM, et al, "Prevention of Postmenopausal Osteoporosis: A Comparative Study of Exercise, Calcium Supplementation, and Hormone Replacement Therapy," *N Engl J Med,* Vol. 325, 1991, pp. 1189–1195.

Psaty BM, Koepsell TD, et al, "The Relative Risk of Incident Coronary Heart Disease Associated with Recently Stopping the Use of B-blocker," *JAMA,* 1990, p. 263.

Raskind MA, "Geriatric Psychopharmacology. Management of Late-life Depression and the Noncognitive Behavioral Disturbances of Alzheimer's Disease [Review]," *Psychiatr Clin N Am,* Vol. 16(4), Dec 1993, pp. 815–827.

Reicher-Reiss H, for the Bezafibrate Infarction Prevention (BIP) Study Group, "Usefulness of Beta-blocker Therapy in Patients With Non-Insulin-dependent Diabetes Mellitus and Coronary Artery Disease," *Am J Cardiol,* Vol. 77, 1996, pp. 1273–1277.

Reveilleau S, Boissel JP, Alamercery Y, "Do Prescribers Know the Results of Key Clinical Trials? GEP (Groupe d'etude de la Prescription)," *Fundam Clin Pharmacol,* Vol. 5(4), 1991, pp. 265–273.

Rosenberg L, Palmer JR, Rao RS, Zauber AG, Strom BL, Warshauer ME, Harlap S, Shapiro S, "Case-Control Study of Oral Contraceptive Use and Risk of Breast Cancer," *Am J Epidmiol,* Vol. 143, 1996, pp. 25–37.

Rovner BW, Edelman BA, Cox MP, Shmuely Y, "The Impact of Antipsychotic Drug Regulations on

Psychotropic Prescribing Practices in Nursing Homes," *Am J Psychiatry*, Vol. 149(10), Oct 1992, pp. 1390–1392.

Rudd P, "Clinicians and Patients With Hypertension: Unsettled Issues About Compliance," *Am Heart J*, Vol. 130, 1995, pp. 572–579.

Rudd P, Marshall G, "Resolving Problems of Measuring Compliance with Medication Monitors," *J Compliance Health Care*, Vol. 2, 1987, pp. 23–25.

Sachs BA, "The Toxicity of Benadryl: Report of a Case and Review of the Literature," *Ann Intern Med*, Vol. 29, 1948, p. 135.

Sadler C, "A Pill For Every Ill?," *Nurs Times*, Vol. 87(9), Feb 27-Mar 1991, p. 21.

Sager DS, Bennett RM, "Individualizing the Risk/benefit Ratio of NSAIDs in Older Patients [Review]," *Geriatrics*, Vol. 47(8), Aug 1992, pp. 24–31.

Sagie A, Strasberg B, Kusnieck J, Selarovsky S, "Symptomatic Bradycardia Induced by the Combination of Oral Diltiazem and Beta Blockers [see comments]," *Clin Cardiol*, Vol. 14(4), Apr 1991, pp. 314–316.

Samuelsson K, Svensson J, "Aspirin: Optimal Dose in Stroke Prevention [letter; comment]," *Stroke*, Vol. 24(8), Aug 1993, pp. 1259–1261.

Schwartz JS, Abernethy DR, "Cardiac Drugs: Adjusting Their Use in Aging Patients," *Geriatrics*, Vol. 42(8), 1987, p. 31.

Sessler CN, "Theophylline Toxicity: Clinical Features of 116 Cases," *Am J Med*, Vol. 88, 1990, pp. 567–576.

Sessler CN, "Theophylline Toxicity: Clinical Features of 116 Cases," *Am J Med*, Vol. 88, 1990, pp. 567–576.

Seto TB, Taira DA, Davis RB, et al, "Effect of Physician Gender on the Prescription of Estrogen Replacement Therapy," *J Gen Intern Med*, Vol. 11, 1996, pp. 197–203.

Shaughnessy AF, Slawson DC, Bennett JH, "Teaching Information Mastery: Evaluating Information

Provided by Pharmaceutical Representatives," *Fam Med*, Vol. 27, 1995, pp. 581–585.

SHEP Cooperative Research Group, "Prevention of Stroke by Antihypertensive Drug Treatment in Older Persons with Isolated Systolic Hypertension," *JAMA*, Vol. 265, 1991, pp. 3255–3265.

Shinn AF, "Clinical Relevance of Cimetidine Drug Interactions [Review]," *Drug Saf*, Vol. 7(4), Jul–Aug 1992, pp. 245–267.

Shorr RI, Fought RL, Ray WA, "Changes in Antipsychotic Drug Use in Nursing Homes During Implementation of the OBRA-87 Regulations [see comments]," *JAMA*, Vol. 271(5), Feb 2, 1994, pp. 358–362.

Shorr RI, Ray WA, Daugherty JR, Griffin MR, "Concurrent Use of Nonsteroidal Antiinflammatory Drugs and Oral Anticoagulants Places Elderly Persons at High Risk for Hemorrhagic Peptic Ulcer Disease," *Arch Intern Med*, Vol. 153(14), July 26, 1993, pp. 1665–1670.

Shorr RI, Robin DW, "Rational Use of Benzodiazepine in the Elderly [Review]," *Drugs Aging*, Vol. 4(1), Jan 1994, pp. 9–20.

Shrimp LA, et al, "Potential Medication-related Problems in Noninstitutionalized Elderly," *Drug Intell Clin Pharm*, Vol. 19, 1985, p. 766.

Silverberg DS, Rotmensch HH, Iaina A, "Low-dose Thiazides in the Treatment of Hypertension: Benefits and Risks in Perspective," *J Hum Hypertens*, Vol. 9, 1995, pp. 869–873.

Simon GE, Lin EHB, Katon W, et al, "Outcomes of 'Inadequate' Antidepressant Treatment," *J Gen Intern Med*, Vol. 10, 1995, pp. 663–670.

Simons LA, Levis G, Simons J, "Apparent Discontinuation Rates in Patients Prescribed Lipid-lowering Drugs," *Med J Aust*, Vol. 164, 1996, pp. 208–211.

Singh RB, Niaz MA, Rastogi SS, et al, "Usefulness of Antioxidant Vitamins in Suspected Acute Myocardial Infarction (The Indian Experiment of Infarct Survival-3)," *Am J Cardiol,* Vol. 77, 1996, pp. 232–236.

Sloan RW, "Principles of Drug Therapy in Geriatric Patients [Review]," *Am Fam Phys,* Vol. 45(6), June, 1992, pp. 2709–2718.

So N, Gotman J, "Changes in Seizure Activity Following Anticonvulsant Drug Withdrawal," *Neurology,* Vol. 40(3 Pt 1), Mar 1990, pp. 407-413.

Soumerai SB, McLaughlin TJ, Avorn J, "Quality Assurance for Drug Prescribing [Review]," *Qual Assurance Health Care,* Vol. 2(1), 1990, pp. 37–58.

Stampfer MJ, et al, "Postmenopausal Estrogen Therapy and Cardiovascular Disease," *N Engl J Med,* Vol. 325, 1991, p. 11.

Stewart RB, "Advances in Pharmacotherapy: Depression in the Elderly—Issues and Advances in Treatment [Review]," *J Clin Pharm Ther,* Vol. 18(4), Aug 1993, pp. 243–253.

Stewart RM, Marks RG, Padgett PD, Hale WE, "Benzodiazepine Use in an Ambulatory Elderly Population: A 14-year Overview," *Clin Ther,* Vol. 16(1), Jan-Feb 1994, pp. 118–124.

"Stroke Prevention in Atrial Fibrillation Study Group. Preliminary Report of the Stroke Prevention in Atrial Fibrillation Study," *N Engl J Med,* Vol. 322, 1990, pp. 863–868.

Sullivan JT, Sellers EM, "Detoxification for Triazolam Physical Dependence," *J Clin Psychopharmacol,* Vol. 12(2), Apr 1992, pp. 124–127.

"Symposium: Managing Medication in an Aging Population: Physician, Pharmacist, and Patient Perspectives," *J Am Geriatr Soc,* Vol. Supp 30, 1985, p. 11.

Takami N, Okada A, "Triazolam and Nitrazepam Use in Elderly Outpatients," *Ann Pharmacother,* Vol. 27(4), Apr 1993, pp. 506–509.

Thapa PB, Meador KG, Gideon P, Fought RL, Ray WA, "Effects of Antipsychotic Withdrawal in Elderly Nursing Home Residents," *J Am Geriatr Soc,* Vol. 42(3), Mar 1994, pp. 280–286.

Thomas DR, "The Brown Bag and Other Approaches to Decreasing Polypharmacy in the Elderly," *N C Med J,* Vol. 52(11), Nov 1991, pp. 565–566.

Tilyard MW, et al, "Treatment of Postmenopausal Osteoporosis with Calcitriol or Calcium," *N Engl J Med,* Vol. 326(6), 1992, pp. 33357–33362.

Tjwa MKT, "Budesonide Inhaled via Turbuhaler: A More Effective Treatment for Asthma Than Beclomethasone Dipropionate via Rotahaler," *Ann Allergy Asthma Immunol,* Vol. 75, 1995, pp. 107–111.

Todd B, "Drugs and the Elderly: Identifying Drug Toxicity," *Geriatr Nurs,* Vol. 12, 1985, p. 213.

Tyring S, and the Collaborative Famciclovir Herpes Zoster Study Group, "Famciclovir for the Treatment of Acute Herpes Zoster: Effects on Acute Disease and Postherpetic Neuralgia: A Randomized, Double-blind, Placebo-controlled Trial," *Ann Intern Med,* Vol. 123, 1995, pp. 89–96.

U.S. Department of Health and Human Services, *Guidelines for the Study of Drugs Likely to be Used in the Elderly,* 1989, Rockville, Md: FDA, Center for Drug Evaluation and Research.

Udelman HD, Udelman DL, "Concurrent Use of Buspirone in Anxious Patients During Withdrawal from Alprazolam Therapy," *J Clin Psychiatry,* Vol. 51, Suppl, Sep 1990, pp. 46–50.

vanGijn J, "Aspirin: Dose and Indications in Modern Stroke Prevention," *Neurologic Clin,* Vol. 10(1), Feb 1992, pp. 193–207; discussion 208.

Vidt DG, Borazanian RA, "Calcium Channel Blockers in Geriatric Hypertension [Review]," *Geriatrics,* Vol. 46(1), Jan 1991, pp. 28–30, 33–34, 36–38.

Von Korff M, Galer BS, Stang P, "Chronic Use of Symptomatic Headache Medications," *Pain,* Vol. 62, 1995, pp. 179–186.

Walt RP, "Misoprostol for the Treatment of Peptic Ulcer and Antiinflammatory-drug-induced Gastroduodenal Ulceration," *N Engl J Med*, Vol. 327, 1992, p. 1575.

Ward RE, Gheorghiade M, Young JB, et al, "Economic Outcomes of Withdrawal of Digoxin Therapy in Adult Patients With Stable Congestive Heart Failure," *J Am Coll Cardiol*, Vol. 26, 1995, pp. 93–101.

Warram JH, Laffel LMB, et al, "Excess Mortality Associated with Diuretic Therapy in Diabetes Mellitus," *Arch Intern Med*, Vol. 151, 1991, pp. 1350–1356.

Wasserheil-Smoller S, Blaufox DM, et al, "Effect of Antihypertensives on Sexual Function and Quality of Life: The TAIM Study," *Ann Intern Med*, Vol. 114, 1991, pp. 613–620.

Weintrub M, "Compliance in the Elderly," *Clin Geriatr Med*, Vol. 6(2), May 1990, pp. 445–452.

West SL, Savitz DA, Koch G, et al, "Recall Accuracy for Prescription Medications: Self-report Compared With Database Information," *Am J Epidemiol*, Vol. 142, 1995, pp. 1103–1112.

Whelton A, et al, "Renal Effects of Ibuprofen, Piroxican, and Sulindac in Patients with Asymptomatic Renal Failure," *Ann Intern Med*, Vol. 112, 1990, pp. 568–576.

Wiklund I, Karlberg J, Mattsson LA, "Quality of Life of Postmenopausal Women on a Regimen of Transdermal Estradiol Therapy: A Double-Blind Placebo-controlled Study," *Am J Obstet Gynecol*, Vol. 168(3 Pt 1), Mar 1993, pp. 824–830.

Wilcox SM, Himmelstein DU, Woolhander S, "Inappropriate Drug Prescribing for the Community-dwelling Elderly," *JAMA*, Vol. 272(4), July 27, 1994, pp. 292–296.

Wood MJ, Kar R, Dworkin RH, et al, "Oral Acyclovir Therapy Accelerates Pain Resolution in Patients With Herpes Zoster: A Meta-analysis of Placebo-controlled Trials," *Clin Infect Dis*, Vol. 22, 1996, pp. 341–347.

World Health Organizations, "Health Care in the Elderly: Report of the Technical Group on the Uses of Medications in the Elderly," *Drugs*, Vol. 22, p. 279.

Wyngaarden JB, Severs MH, "The Toxic Effects of Antihistamine Drugs," *JAMA*, Vol. 145, 1951, p. 277.

Index

abortion, 313
Accolate (zafirlukast), 149, 152
Accupril (quinapril), 94, 95, 109
Accutane (isotretinoin), 135, 161, 166
acebutolol, 106–107
ACE inhibitors, 12, 16, 24, 47–48, 76–77, 94, 95, 104, 106, 109
acetaminophen (Tylenol), 176, 190, 212, 263, 264, 276, 279, 280
acetylsalicylic acid, *see* aspirin
aches and pains, 282–83
acid indigestion, medications for, 46, 193, 195–97
Aclovate, 169
acne medications, 161, 164–66
ACTH, 140, 176
Actifed (pseudoephedrine), 128, 134
Action Plan, *see* 12-Week Action Plan
Acutrim, 325
acyclovir (Zovirax), 141, 209, 226, 228, 260
Adalat, *see* nifedipine
Adderall, 74
addiction, 347
Adipex-P, 325
Advil, *see* ibuprofen
Aerobid (flunisolide), 148, 150

aidovudine (AZT), 253, 254, 255, 258
AIDS (acquired immunodeficiency syndrome), 253
Kaposi's sarcoma in, 246
see also HIV infection, medications for
airway openers (bronchodilators), 13, 46, 148, 149, 151, 152
Akineton, 135
albendazole, 214–15
albuterol (Proventil; Repetabs; Rotacaps; Ventolin; Volmax), 128, 140, 146, 148, 151, 152
alcohol, 127, 131, 354
Aldactazide, 17, 108
aldesleukin, 247
Aldomet (methyldopa), 111, 128, 136
Aleve, *see* naproxen
Alka-Seltzer, 196, 204
Allegra (fexofenadine), 154, 155, 157
Aller-Chlor, 158
allergic reactions:
to chemotherapy, 249
rashes, 162
allergy medications, 15–16, 34, 153–59
antihistamines, 135–36, 153–54, 155, 156–58
nasal sprays, 159

alpha reductase inhibitors, 290
alprazolam (Xanax), 119, 123, 127, 130, 141, 344
Altace (ramipril), 95, 109
Alteplase (tPA), 8
Alzheimer's disease, medications for, 6, 18, 46, 175–76, 360
for improving cognitive function, 178–80
for managing behavioral problems, 180–83
amantadine (Symmetrel), 185, 209–10
Ambien (zolpidem), 119, 120, 309–10
amiloride, 96
aminophylline, 145
Amipaque, 136
amitriptyline (Elavil; Endep), 12, 33, 114, 122, 127, 131, 138, 191
amlodipine (Norvasc), 16, 17, 33, 35, 77, 78, 96, 98, 104, 106
amlodipine/benazepril, 110
Amodopa (methyldopa), 111, 128, 136
amoxapine, 123
amoxicillin (Amoxil), 12, 31, 49–50, 64, 68–69, 218, 220, 230, 232
amoxicillin-clavulanate (Augmentin), 13, 67, 218, 220, 230, 232